HOME CARE

HOME CARE

Patient and Family Instructions

Second Edition

Deborah K. Zastocki, RN, MA, EdM

Christine Rovinski-Wagner, ARNP, MSN

W.B. SAUNDERS COMPANY
A Harcourt Health Sciences Company
Philadelphia   London   New York   St. Louis   Sydney   Toronto

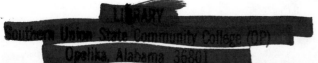

W.B. SAUNDERS COMPANY
A Harcourt Health Sciences Company

The Curtis Center
Independence Square West
Philadelphia, Pennsylvania 19106

Library of Congress Cataloging-in-Publication Data

Zastocki, Deborah K.

Home care: patient and family instructions / Deborah K. Zastocki, Christine Rovinski-Wagner.—2nd ed.

p.   cm.

Includes bibliographical references.

ISBN 0–7216–8442–4

1. Home nursing—Handbooks, manuals, etc.   I. Rovinski-Wagner, Christine.
   II. Title.
   [DNLM: 1. Home Nursing—Handbooks.   WY 49 Z38h 2000]

RT61.Z38 2000   362.1'4—dc21

DNLM/DLC   99–044465

Vice President, Nursing Editorial Director: Sally Schrefer
Acquisitions Editor: Terri Wood
Project Manager: Edna Dick
Production Manager: Natalie Ware
Illustration Specialist: Rita Martello
Book Designer: Marie Gardocky Clifton

HOME CARE: Patient and Family Instructions   ISBN 0–7216–8442–4

Printed in the United States of America.

Last digit is the print number: 9   8   7   6   5   4   3   2   1

To my husband Christopher J. Tighe

To my son Robert Rovinski

Contributors

Susan C. Becker, RN, BSN, CETN

Patient Care Clinician
Enterostomal Therapist/Coordinator Pain
  Management
Chilton Memorial Hospital
Pompton Plains, New Jersey

Elimination Alterations

Linda Cestaro, BS, RD

Clinical Dietitian
Chilton Memorial Hospital
Pompton Plains, New Jersey

Digestive Alterations

Judith Dedio, RN, BSN, CETN, CDE

Certified Enterostomal Therapy Nurse
Certified Diabetes Educator
Chilton Memorial Hospital
Pompton Plains, New Jersey

Endocrine Alterations

David Gourley, RRT, BS

President
Horizon Health Services
Riverdale, New Jersey
Home Care Surveyor
Joint Commission on Accreditation of
  Healthcare Organizations
Oakbrook Terrace, Illinois

Respiratory Alterations

Laura LaBarbera, RNC, BSN, MPA

Director of Patient Care Services
Family Wellness Administration
Chilton Memorial Hospital
Pompton Plains, New Jersey

Maternal Health

Elizabeth Lesnevich, MA, RD, CDE

Clinical Dietetics Manager
Chilton Memorial Hospital
Pompton Plains, New Jersey

Digestive Alterations

Michele Marchesa, BS, RD

Clinical Dietitian
Healthstart Nutritionist
Chilton Memorial Hospital
Pompton Plains, New Jersey

Digestive Alterations

Marylin Schulte, RN, IBCLC, FACCE

Private Practice
Hackettstown and Mt. Olive, New Jersey

Maternal Health

Leisa R. Venters, RN, CRNI

Nurse, Emergency Department
Jupiter Medical Center
Jupiter, Florida
Independent Intravenous Infusion Consultant
Jupiter, Florida

Infusion Therapy

Leilani C. Viney, MA, RD, CDE

Director of Dietetics
Chilton Memorial Hospital
Pompton Plains, New Jersey

Digestive Alterations

Preface

Home Care: Patient and Family Instructions, Second Edition, provides ready-to-use instructions for patient and family applications in the home setting. Much of the professional nurse's time spent in a patient's home involves teaching. With a ready-to-use tool, the preparation time needed for the teaching component of the home visit can be reduced. More importantly, teaching can be more effective and standardized within an agency.

ORGANIZATION

Section One of the book focuses on The Teaching-Learning Process. Reviewed in this section are principles of learning as well as crucial elements of effective documentation as they relate to patient teaching and to reimbursement

Section Two is divided into 15 units. Units 1 to 13 are classified systematically by health status alteration. Each instruction guide allocates space for tailoring the instruction to meet individualized patient and family needs, as well as space for an agency's identification and logo. Illustrations combined with the adjusted reading level enhance readability and patient/family comprehension. *Unit 14, Therapeutic Agents,* is categorized by major pharmacologic groups. The instructions are designed to offer general pharmacologic information for that drug category. The patient's specific drug information can be added to the basic instructions to promote compliance. *Unit 15, Maternal Health,* is new to this edition and addresses the unique needs of pre- and postpartum women.

The *Appendix* contains Equivalent Measures of Fluids and Illustrations of the body that provide a visual aid to assist with the teaching that involves anatomy. Near the back of the book is a Blank Monthly Calendar that can be photocopied and customized to fit the patient's routine.

USE

Home Care: Patient and Family Instructions, Second Edition, is a compilation of instruction guides in a format that allows for individualization to meet the needs of both the patient and family as well as the agency. The majority of instructions are in a format ready for photocopying. Also included with this edition is a CD-ROM containing the entire text of the book. This allows you the option of installing the patient instruction sheets on your computer to customize for your patients. Instructions for installing and printing from the CD-ROM are included.

This book can be utilized collaboratively by the home care nurse with acute care discharge planners to facilitate patient/family preparation for home care. Outstanding features include the following:

1. Instructions are provided for the most common learning needs of home care recipients.
2. Facilitation of documentation of patient and family teaching that is complete, consistent, and individualized for patient and family needs.
3. A format that is easy to use, photocopy, or customize and standardize within the agency.
4. Application of principles of the teaching-learning process to the home care setting.
5. Instructions that guide the development of the beginning home care nurse and supplement the knowledge base of the experienced practitioner.

Deborah K. Zastocki
Christine Rovinski-Wagner

Acknowledgments

We would like to acknowledge the following for their support, help, and encouragement: Christopher J. Tighe and Adam S. Wagner for their dedication and patience during the preparation of the manuscript; Charlene G. Taylor, M.L.S., for assistance in gathering resources; our editor, Terri Wood; friends and colleagues at Chilton Memorial Hospital, Pompton Plains, NJ; Valley Home and Community Care, Paramus, NJ; and our many colleagues who have provided professional expertise. A special acknowledgment goes to our families and friends for their unflagging confidence in this project and their understanding whenever the book came first.

About the Authors

Deborah K. Zastocki, RN, MA, EdM, received her B.S. in Nursing from the University of Rhode Island, Kingston, Rhode Island, and her M.A. in Nursing Education and Ed.M. in Community Health Nursing from Teachers College, Columbia University, New York. She has held a variety of clinical and academic positions including Director of Education, Training, and Research, which included community health education, and Director of Specialty Nursing, which included a skilled nursing, long-term ventilator unit; she has held academic appointments as adjunct faculty member at Kean College, Union, New Jersey, teaching the well family and community health; and adjunct faculty at Fairleigh Dickinson University. In addition, she has served in various capacities such as board member and professional advisory committee member for home health care agencies. She is a part-time faculty member at William Paterson University, Wayne, NJ. She is currently Senior Vice President of Clinical Services and Operations at Chilton Memorial Hospital, part of the Valley Health System which owns Valley Home Care and Community Care.

Christine Rovinski-Wagner, ARNP, MSN, received her B.S. in Nursing from Villanova University, Villanova, Pennsylvania, and her M.S. in Nursing from Seton Hall University, South Orange, New Jersey. She has worked in a variety of clinical and academic settings. Her home care experience includes administration, field nursing, clinical supervision, staff development, risk management, quality improvement, and finance. She is currently responsible for performance improvement at Tender Loving Care, Port St. Lucie, Florida.

Contents

SECTION 1

THE TEACHING-LEARNING PROCESS

OVERVIEW OF THE TEACHING-LEARNING PROCESS

Effective application of the teaching-learning process is one of the fundamental methods used by the home health care nurse to promote patient and family achievement of outcomes. The steps in the teaching-learning process can be organized into the familiar phases of assessment of the learner and the environment, planning of outcomes and teaching strategies, interventions in the teaching-learning session, and evaluation of learning. The teaching session must be well planned to be effective and to be accomplished within a very limited time frame. Since teaching is directed toward the achievement of behavior change and behavior change is a goal of nursing interventions, it is evident that the home health care nurse benefits by integrating the concepts of the teaching-learning process into his or her professional practice. Basically, the teaching-learning process requires determining what the learner needs to know, what the learner is capable of learning, how the learner can best be taught, and what the learner has learned. It is essential to integrate the teaching-learning process with culturally competent nursing care. This section is designed to offer an overview of the teaching-learning process and to sensitize the nurse to include cultural assessment into intervention strategies. It can serve as the basis for continued study by the novice as well as a refresher for the experienced practitioner.

LEARNING THEORY

Learning is considered a relatively permanent change in behavior, resulting from experience or training, whereas teaching is a system of actions designed to change behavior. Learning occurs in response to a felt need. With Maslow's hierarchy as an example, physiologic needs such as oxygen, food, and water represent basic levels of need, whereas safety, love and belonging, esteem, and self-actualization represent progressively higher levels of need. In Maslow's framework, basic "felt" needs must be satisfied before a person can be ready to satisfy needs on a higher level (Whitman, 1992). Understanding the learner's perceived felt needs and goals provides an opportunity for identifying learner readiness and motivational factors.

Contracting with the patient and family to meet their perceived needs, in addition to specific needs as identified by the home health care nurse, stimulates learner motivation and cooperation. Contracting establishes mutually agreed upon outcomes of care, which are described in measurable and observable terms (Falvo, 1994; Whitman et al., 1992). Although this "working agreement" can be renegotiated, it establishes priority setting and a mutual responsibility—a partnership relationship. To be most effective and to encourage compliance, the contract should focus on one behavior, involve another person, build on the learner's strengths, lead to a positive consequence, and clearly and specifically define responsibilities, expectations, time frame, and how the contract will be evaluated. Contracting needs to be individualized and may not be an effective strategy with all patients. The nurse should remain in contact with the patient during the duration of the contract. Success in achievement will likely reinforce the desired behavior and provide motivation for additional behavioral change. Providing a copy of the contract with supporting handout material helps the patient and family stay on track. Motivation is a key ingredient in learner outcome achievement and can be more important in successful learning than intelligence or formal education.

Learning is generally more effective when there is a planned educational experience with a focus on individualized instruction. Learning most readily progresses from simple to complex, from known to unknown. Organizing the content into distinct segments with subobjectives allows for incremental achievement (despite periodic plateaus in the learning process), timely positive feedback, interim evaluation of progress, and establishment of blocks of learning as a foundation to build on. Assisting the formation of connections to what the learner already knows helps him or her "experience" the information. As the learner begins processing the content, opportunities for discussion and interpretative exchanges occur. These exchanges during the teaching session allow the learner to develop a level of understanding that can be used to begin generalizing and applying the information and skills.

Using vocabulary that is easily understood, avoiding medical and technical jargon, and using short sentences enhance the learner's interest and minimize anxiety. Every learner has a saturation point; expectations of sessions lasting longer than 20 minutes may be unrealistic. Clues of learner saturation such as frequent position changes, restlessness, loss of eye contact, and initiation of unrelated side conversations indicate that the session should be brought to a close as soon as possible. These clues can also be a sign of lack of understanding or interest. It is best to pause when these signs are observed and to validate the observations with the patient and family to determine the source, if possible. A relationship built on trust and credibility between the patient and family and the home health care nurse is essential for effective learning. A dysfunctional relationship can be a source of patient noncompliance.

An environment that is conducive to learning is comfortable physically and psychologically. The area should be well lit, adequately ventilated, and of a comfortable temperature. Distractions should be controlled to the extent possible; a loud radio or television can be a major distraction. When engaging in adult education in a home with small children, plan for the children to participate in an age-appropriate activity, such as coloring or cutting out photographs from a magazine, that relate to the teaching focus. This tactic may successfully minimize the types of distractions children can provide. Controlling distractions enables learners to focus on the learning task at hand.

Promoting learner retention represents a challenge in the teaching-learning process. Verbally "giving" content without helping the patient and family reach a level of understanding results in limited short-term memory and retention. Retention rates are related to the amount of information given at one session, the patient's anxiety level, and the patient's amount of medical knowledge and intellectual level (Falvo, 1994). Teaching strategies, discussed later in the chapter, are designed to increase retention. Long-term memory is activated when the information is understood by the learner. Involving the learner's senses increases the amount of content that can be retained. Generally, people remember

- 10% of what they *read,*
- 20% of what they *hear,*
- 30% of what they *see,*
- 50% of what they *hear* and *see,*
- 70% of what they *say* or *write,*
- 90% of what they *say as they do a thing* (Wiman & Meierhenry, 1969).

The more senses involved in the learning process, the more likely the learner will be able to retain the information.

Age Group–Specific Needs

Learning theory refinements address the uniqueness of various age groups. Learning theory that focuses on how children learn differs somewhat from learning theory that focuses on how adults learn.

Children

Children have a short attention span. Teaching sessions should be short and allow for child participation. To fully appreciate learning theory as applied to children, review the way in which topics are presented on children's educational television programs. It is important to consider the stages of growth and development when approaching goal setting and when planning teaching strategies. Preschool-aged children, ages 3 to 6, learn largely through modeling; therefore assessing both the child and parents is important. School-aged children, ages 7 to 12, begin to demonstrate psychomotor, cognitive, and psychosocial skills, seeking a sense of mastery (Falvo, 1994; Whitman et al., 1992). Children benefit from play and active participation; they especially enjoy question periods in the session. Praise and support are significant factors with children. Parental involvement in the learning process can provide continuity and ongoing reinforcement. Including the child and the parents in goal setting is a successful strategy for effective teaching.

Adolescents

As the child reaches adolescence, ages 12 to 18, abstract thinking begins to develop. Important considerations for adolescents are peer influence, body image, and a developing sense of identity self-sufficiency (Falvo, 1994). With adolescents, parental presence during all teaching sessions may inhibit learning. Parental attendance at select sessions, however, can be part of the teaching plan. Adolescents want to be treated as individuals and to participate in goal setting. Despite the adolescent's projection of a rather cavalier attitude at times, particularly concerning knowledge of anatomy and physiology, a careful review of content is typically needed.

Adults

Although the outlook on life and the priorities of the young adult, ages 20 to 40, differ slightly from that of persons in the middle years, ages 40 to 65, the learning capacity remains similar (Whitman et al., 1992). Adults generally learn best when they see a need and an immediate use for what is to be learned. Learner motivation is stimulated by focusing on perceived "need to know" compared with "nice to know" information. Adults respond well when they are acknowledged and respected as people with worth and previous life experiences. Adults should be allowed to participate in setting goals and in sharing responsibility for the learning process.

Although this is true of all learning, the adult learning situation in particular should be nonthreatening and accompanied by a flexible approach to accommodate individual differences. Adults are a product of previous learning experiences and memories, both positive and negative. They have a great many life experiences to draw on. This wealth of life experiences can be advantageous for small group sharing and support, but the teaching-learning sessions must build on and draw analogies to these life experiences for them to be relevant. Although a problem-centered approach frequently works well, adults require a variety of methods to meet their individual needs. Adults also appreciate a comfortable environment and refreshment breaks.

Elderly

Those over 65 years old continue to have an ability and desire to learn. In reviewing the unique learning needs of the elderly, it is important to keep in mind the physiologic changes that occur with aging. Changes that occur to varying degrees are a decline in visual acuity, peripheral vision, and depth perception and difficulty discriminating detail and color perception, especially blue, green, and violet hues. Decreased auditory acuity includes difficulty discriminating high-frequency consonants such as "s," "f," and "k." Male voices are heard better than female voices. Sensitivity to touch, pressure, and temperature is diminished. Cerebral changes include a decreased sense of balance and fine movement. Cardiovascular and pulmonary changes can lead to fatigue and limited attention span, especially if the person is experiencing stress. Decreased muscle mass, tone, and strength can lead to diminished psychomotor reserve. Joint stiffness can also limit the ability to sit for long periods (Whitman et al., 1992). Teaching sessions need to be short, with intervals allotted for restroom activity and general movement to minimize joint stiffness. As with adult learning, plan to integrate the new into what is known; however, the rate of learning may be slower. The area should be well lit, with minimal glare and controlled extraneous noise. If visual aids are needed, use large, well-spaced letters in primary colors for best visual impact. Try to maintain the learner's usual routine as much as possible. Focus strategies on enhancing self-worth and independence. Use of community resources and social supports can improve compliance in the elderly (Falvo, 1994).

FUNDAMENTALS OF TEACHING

Assessment of the Learner and the Environment

As identified previously, the steps of the teaching-learning process are assessment of the learner and the environment, planning of outcomes and teaching strategies, interventions in the teaching-learning session, and evaluation of learning. During the assessment phase, individual learning styles and rates are a major focus. Each learner possesses a different "package" of life experiences, values, needs, goals, and beliefs. The learner's "world view" reflects his or her perceived relationship to nature, institutions, and people, including communication patterns. Communication variations encompass conversational style and pacing, personal space, eye contact, touch, and time orientation (Lipson et al., 1996). The assessment may also include the skills and willingness of family members to serve as interpreters. The person interpreting needs to be willing to communicate the content accurately without imposing personal perceptions or withholding information he or she may consider embarrassing. Nurses need to be aware of their own values and beliefs as well as their own communication patterns as they approach culturally diverse situations. Avoiding stereotypic assumptions is critical because of the individuality of each patient and family situation. Diversity includes the varying health beliefs and practices of racial, ethnic, socioeconomic status, sexual orientation, and disability groups (Falvo, 1994; Lipson et al., 1996). The assessment phase provides opportunities for promoting learner motivation and identifying barriers to learning. The goal is to eliminate or minimize value or cultural conflicts before the teaching session.

The Health Belief Model helps to explain readiness and motivational factors leading to health-related behavioral change (Becker, 1974). The model addresses the components of the person's:

- Perceived susceptibility to disease
- Perceived seriousness (severity) of disease
- Perceived benefits of preventive action
- Perceived barriers to preventive action.

Using this model, one can understand that in the absence of perceived susceptibility and seriousness, the perceived benefits of preventive health care, such as a yearly physical or dental check-up, may not be motivating enough to result in behavioral change. To take this thought one step further, it may be futile to explain to the learner that "doing this is good for you" if the learner's perceptions do not support the notion to the point of behavioral change. Addressing the patient's perceptions is the key to engaging the patient in self-care and to creating individualized teaching. Self-care requires the person's belief in his or her own ability (self-efficacy) to assume self-care (Damrosch, 1991). The home care nurse promotes self-care applying self-efficacy theory by

1. Persuading the patient that the plan will work
2. Teaching the patient
3. Helping the patient
4. Relating the patient's actions to the desired outcomes
5. Supporting the patient in valuing the outcomes sufficiently to maintain the behavior (Bohny, 1997).

Teaching the patient to make personal decisions increases the likelihood of compliance (agreement between the person's behavior and the expected goal). The home health care nurse must design strategies that realistically address perceived susceptibility and seriousness, promote the perceived benefits of action, and minimize the perceived barriers.

The parameters for completing the learner assessment are summarized for quick reference:

Biopsychosocial

　　Age, sex, developmental level

　　Medical diagnoses, nursing diagnoses

　　Ethnicity, race, culture, religion, language

　　Socioeconomic status, living arrangements

　　Support systems, marital relationship, roles of family members

　　Relationship with health care provider

Environmental

　　Occupation, job-related issues

　　Home and community resources

Functional abilities and limitations

　　Psychomotor areas

　　　　Sensory status

　　　　Mobility, dexterity

　　　　Comfort: psychological, physical and energy level

　　Cognitive areas

　　　　Ability to learn, identified best way to learn

　　　　Educational background, reading ability, functional illiteracy

　　　　Knowledge of disease and therapeutic plan

　　Affective (emotional) areas

　　　　Patient's and family's reactions and adjustment to patient's illness

　　　　Health beliefs and values

　　　　Compliance issues

　　　　Readiness and motivation for learning, prior learning experiences

　　　　Patient's self-image, personality

Readiness to learn and learning content also vary by health status. The health status categories of wellness, acute illness, and chronic illness suggest differing strategies for dealing with areas such as nutrition, activity, stress management, illness care, and health monitoring (Whitman et al., 1992). This approach also suggests that a person with an acute illness will attend to different content in different ways than a person dealing with an adjustment to chronic illness. The individual and dynamic nature of the teaching-learning process requires ongoing assessment as the patient experiences varying phases of health status.

During the assessment, sort the data into positive and negative findings. Plan to maximize the learner's strengths (positive findings) during the intervention phase. The negative findings form the basis for determining strategies during the planning phase. The definition of the learner's needs represents the individualized component to be factored into the learning plan. The negative findings, defined needs, are essential elements of documentation for successful third-party reimbursement.

Planning

After the learner assessment is completed, the teaching process continues with the planning phase. Establishing the expected outcomes in measurable terms is best accomplished through mutual goal setting with the patient and family. The most expedient approach to the challenge of establishing outcomes in a realistic and reimbursable manner is to focus on "survival skills." The survival skills are the core elements that reasonably predict whether the patient and family will be able to manage the therapeutic regimen safely within the defined parameters. It is not in the learner's best interest to have the teacher attempt to share as much knowledge as possible. Depositing knowledge on learners—the instructional dumping syndrome—is counterproductive. Not only do time and financial constraints make this unfeasible, but the learner may not want to know that much. Acknowledging that the patient's and family's mastery of core materials is a desirable outcome does not preclude providing supplemental resources or self-instructional materials for continued learning. National and local organizations, self-help groups, health care institutions, private medical practices, and equipment and pharmaceutical companies frequently offer free supplemental literature. Defining the learner's perceived needs and the survival skills in terms of desired outcomes is prerequisite to defining measurable objectives.

Developing Objectives

Developing meaningful objectives provides a prescription for action and serves as an evaluation tool. An objective is a written statement of the intended change in behavior. By identifying the behavior in precise, measurable terms, the teacher is able to focus and direct the teaching-learning process. Meaningful objectives convey a clear understanding of what content will be taught, the sequence of the content, how the content will be presented, what material is essential, the teaching methods and strategies that are most likely to be successful, and how the achievement of outcomes will be evaluated. The objective statement specifies:

- *Task*—terminal behavior that demonstrates learning has taken place; an action verb that prescribes action.
- *Criterion*—the standard against which the behavior will be measured; how well the learner must do.
- *Condition(s)*—the setting in which the behavior will be achieved; specifies the environment/situation, materials, equipment, and resources.

Objectives should be

- Measurable (quantitative),
- Specific, concise,
- Outcome focused (terminal behavior),
- Realistic and attainable,
- Time limited (when, how long, how often).

Teaching Strategies to Meet Learning Objectives

Educational objectives have been classified according to the type of behavioral change. Bloom has described these classifications as the cognitive, affective, and psychomotor domains of learning (Bloom, 1956; Krathwohl et al., 1964; Whitman et al., 1992). Organization of the objectives into the three classifications facilitates the development of effective teaching strategies (see table).

Teaching is a system of actions designed to bring about new and desired behavioral change. Teaching involves a series of planned, purposeful interventions that are designed to accomplish the expected outcomes in the most effective manner. Teaching strategies should target as many senses as possible without causing sensory overload. Teaching tools are devices that assist the instructor in the presentation of information. Written handouts, for example, should support and supplement your teaching; the material should not just be "read to" the learner. Handouts are most easily understood if written at the sixth- to eighth-grade level. To analyze the read-

Educational Objectives		
Category	**Examples**	**Teaching Strategies**
Cognitive objectives involve knowledge, comprehension, application, analysis, synthesis, and evaluation	Names, states, defines, lists, identifies, describes, understands, explains, evaluates, plans, selects, analyzes, applies, and recognizes	Written materials, audiovisual aids, lectures and presentations, discussions, and helping with problem solving
Affective objectives deal with attitudes and values that can be more difficult to define.	Appreciates, conforms, chooses, accepts, maintains, and uses psychomotor objectives related to physical performance	Talking with the learner, experience sharing, role playing, simulation, providing the learner with insight into feelings, and encouraging the learner to ventilate feelings
Affective objectives tend to require a greater time commitment for change to occur	Performs, demonstrates, exhibits, shows, and displays	Practice, participation, demonstration and return demonstration, use of models/ manikins, and coaching

ing grade level of written material, use one of the readability formulas currently available (Maynard, 1999; Murphy & Connally, 1997).

Other teaching tools include records, audiotapes, and videotapes. Visual aids can be inexpensively made by cutting photographs from magazines. For learners who are functionally illiterate, have language barriers, or have cognitive limitations, pictorial aids may prove most successful. Pictures can be used as medication compliance reminders: the sun, four glasses of water, or a line drawn through a salt shaker. The learner can be helpful in selecting pictures that best serve as memory aids. Games can make learning fun for all ages; they are commercially available from health and medical media firms or can be creatively self-designed. Models and manikins allow the learner to touch and "experience" the content. Mixing and matching teaching strategies and tools allows for highly individualized learning plans.

The use of computers in the teaching-learning process has many applications. Computer assisted learning with available software offers self-paced and diverse learning opportunities. Many Internet sites for health information are increasingly accessed by people through home, library, and community access centers such as schools. Although an exciting and helpful adjunct to learning, computers do not eliminate the need for one-on-one interactions with a health care educator for clarification, reinforcement, and discussion of misinformation.

Intervention

Teaching Behaviors

Completing the planning phase by defining the outcomes, objectives, and appropriate teaching strategies leads to the intervention phase. Developing and organizing the teaching session or lesson plan involve the following steps:

1. Introduction
   a. A brief opening statement to establish the direction and purpose of the session, as well as to establish a rapport with the learner
   b. A review of the mutually agreed on outcomes and objectives, with clarification of the learner's and teacher's expectations
2. Explanation of main points; be very specific yet brief
3. Summary of the main points (repetition).

The sequence is one of previewing the session, reviewing the content, promoting transfer of learning, and reaching closure by summarizing key points.

Teaching effectively requires a self-appraisal of one's current teaching style. Although talking is natural, the goal in teaching is to enhance the communication process. Using a tape recorder while presenting in front of a mirror is a relatively inexpensive way to begin a self-appraisal. A videotaped session, however, can be even more revealing. Consider the following:

- Are your hand movements distracting?
- Do you avoid eye contact?
- Do you look at the ceiling or the floor?
- Do you interject distracting words in your speech such as "ah," "um," or "you know"?
- Is your speech clear and spoken at a rate that is easy to follow?
- Do you vary your voice tone, or do you speak in a monotone?

Conveying a sense of confidence and self-esteem that is consistent with your voice, facial expression, and body language establishes a positive message. Maintaining eye contact and proper posture, using hand gestures only when appropriate, varying voice tones, and offering encouragement through nods and smiles support teaching effectiveness.

It goes without saying that thorough familiarity with the content and a clear picture of what you want the learner to understand are prerequisites for a successful teaching-learning session. It is important to convey expertise when establishing credibility, but one should not do so in a superior or critical manner. Try to make the session as interesting and enjoyable as possible; avoid overwhelming the learner with technicalities. Avoid IOBIIB thinking: "It's only beneficial if it's boring." Another useful teaching reminder is KISS: "Keep it simple and specific." Use words that are familiar to the learner, use analogies and illustrations to help clarify concepts, and stimulate learner participation through the use of open-ended questions. When asking questions, ask only one question at a time, and allow time for a response. Avoid rephrasing the question before the learner has had adequate time to formulate a response, since this tends to confuse the learner and to inhibit further responses.

Giving feedback effectively can greatly enhance the learning process. To be effective, feedback should be directed to behavior that the learner can do something about. Feedback should describe, not judgmentally evaluate, the behavior. For example, "you're good" is judgmental, compared with "you've changed the dressing exactly as you were instructed." Making the feedback specific increases the learner's ability to focus on behavioral change. Giving the feedback as soon as possible reinforces the desired behavioral change. When giving feedback, act as a facilitator; be supportive and nonthreatening.

The last steps of evaluation of learning and, most important, of documentation of the teaching-learning process flow logically if the preceding steps have been accomplished. To review, some of the key points in the teaching-learning process are listed:

1. Prepare yourself
   a. Know the learner
   b. Know the content
   c. Be aware of your teaching strengths and limitations
2. Clearly define and state the objectives in measurable terms
   a. Mutual goal setting and contracting are successful strategies
   b. Break learning sessions into manageable sections
3. Stimulate learner interest and motivation; set the tone
4. Sequence learning
   a. Arrange content from simple to complex
   b. Build on previous knowledge
5. Promote learner involvement and participation whenever possible
6. Evaluate progress and objective achievement
7. Document the progress or lack of progress toward outcomes

Evaluation

As stated previously, the evaluation phase should flow smoothly if the objectives have been defined in measurable terms. Evaluation is an integral ongoing part of the teaching-learning process. During the teaching-learning process, learning problems can occur. Using concepts of self-care and focusing on self-efficacy enhances compliance. Many patients do not experience maximum therapeutic benefit because of issues with compliance. Areas to evaluate for varying degrees of compliance include the following:

- The treatment plan
- Dietary and lifestyle changes
- Keeping up with appointments
- Medication plan

Some patients may need additional assistive interventions such as medication organizers to help with compliance.

Review the following questions to assist in diagnosing the learning problem:

1. What does the learner need to do differently?
2. Are there barriers to learning that were not initially assessed or addressed in the planning phase? Is the learner's world view or health belief system a barrier? Does the learner have a sensory impairment?
3. Were the goals mutually set with the learner? Was contracting used?
4. Were the objectives clearly defined in measurable terms? Were the objectives realistic?
5. Was the learner's individual learning style incorporated in the teaching plan?
6. Did the teaching strategies match the objectives?
7. Was the learner actively involved in the learning process?
8. Were there environmental distractions?
9. Was the learner's support system incorporated to promote compliance?

The diagnosis of learning problems should occur early in the learning process to allow for modifications in the plan.

DOCUMENTATION

Documentation is performed at each step of the teaching-learning process. The basis for successful third-party reimbursement is documentation in the clinical record of the patient's and family's needs and problems, the negative findings, as well as the outcomes and behaviorally defined objectives that are realistically achievable with short-term, intermittent skilled nursing intervention. Documentation needs to reflect clinical findings related to the current medical diagnoses and skilled nursing care. Teaching must focus on and support the need for skilled intervention. Is teaching necessary because the patient is newly diagnosed with insulin-dependent diabetes or because blood sugars are widely fluctuating in a previously stable individual? These findings and the use of terminology that support the need for skilled care are essential. *Instructed* or *taught* are acceptable terms, but words such as *reviewed*, *reinforced*, *stressed*, and *discussed* are not. Often the test of whether nursing instruction is reimbursable relates to the *skill* required to teach and not to the nature of what is being taught. A nurse is expected to teach at a higher level than a lay person. For example, "instructed about a 2-gram sodium diet" would indicate skill, whereas "instructed about a low-salt diet" typically does not. Skilled instruction includes, but is not limited to:

1. Teaching the self-administration of an injectable medication, a complex range of medications, or medical gases
2. Teaching self-catheterization
3. Teaching care for and maintenance of peripheral and central venous lines and administration of intravenous medications through such lines
4. Teaching bowel or bladder training when bowel or bladder dysfunction exists
5. Teaching proper body alignment and positioning and turning techniques of a bed-bound patient
6. Teaching the preparation and maintenance of a therapeutic diet
7. Teaching how to perform activities of daily living when the patient or care giver must use special techniques or adaptive devices due to loss of function

The written record should clearly communicate

the teaching plan and an evaluation of what was learned. It should reflect an evaluation of each session, with attention to progress or lack of progress toward outcomes and objectives. Documentation is focused on the material content covered and the teaching strategies and teaching tools that were used to meet the learner's learning style. The documentation of teaching strategies that were most successful in achieving the outcomes expedites future teaching and enhances the learning rate. The learner who has a language barrier or who is functionally illiterate may learn best with diagrams and photographs. With this information as part of the written record, involved professionals from all disciplines can approach the learner in the most effective manner. If care givers or family members have been incorporated to assist the patient with compliance, similar learning style information should be noted in the record. It is also helpful to identify the most competent learner in the home to facilitate the learning process. Names of reference materials left in the home should also be documented. Include documentation of self-study materials given to the learner and referrals to community resources that are used for health promotion needs as well as for learners who desire more information. Record any follow-up contacts with the learner in terms of learning retention.

Tools that assist with documentation include flow sheets and standardized patient instruction sheets. Flow sheets can include separate columns for instructions to the patient and family, supervision and return demonstration, and patient and family understanding. The Joint Commission on Accreditation of Healthcare Organizations (JCAHO, 1998) views documentation of patient and family understanding, as well as patient and family participation in goal setting, as one of the most important qualitative aspects of the written record. Standardized instruction sheets provide a framework from which individualized patient and family teaching can be designed. The standardized instruction sheets facilitate documentation, promote continuity and quality, provide a common base for communication with other members of the health care team (especially during case conferences), and increase productivity by requiring only writing supplemental instructions for an individualized plan.

The written record should reflect the entire teaching-learning process, including final outcomes. Clear, consistent documentation of all elements of the learning plan and process promotes favorable reimbursement decisions.

BIBLIOGRAPHY

American Nurses Association. (1998). ANA addressing cultural diversity in the profession. American Nurse, 30 (1), 25.

*American Nurses Association. (1996). Standards of community health nursing practice. Washington, D.C.: American Nurses Publishing.

*American Nurses Association. (1986). Standards of home health nursing practice. Washington, D.C.: American Nurses Publishing.

Arras, J. and Dubler, N. (1994). Bringing the hospital home: Ethical and social implications of high-tech home care. Hastings Center Report, 24 (5), 19–28.

*Becker, M. (ed.). (1974). The health belief model and personal health behavior. Thorofare, NJ: Charles B. Slack.

*Bloom, B.S. (ed.). (1956). Taxonomy of educational objectives: The classification of educational goals. Handbook I: Cognitive domain. New York: David McKay Co., Inc.

Bohny, B. (1997). A time for self-care: Role of the home health care nurse. Home Healthcare Nurse, 5 (4), 281–286.

Brent, N. (1997). Home healthcare fraud: Implications for the home healthcare agency and nurse. Home Healthcare Nurse, 15 (1), 38–40.

Capone, L. (1997). Home care: A family affair. Home Healthcare Nurse, 15 (1), 49–51.

Car, P. (1990). Needs to know, wants to know, ought to know. Home Healthcare Nurse, 8 (4), 34.

Damrosch, S. (1991). General strategies for motivating people to change their behavior. Nursing Clinics of North America, 26, 833–843.

Falvo, D. (1994). Effective patient education: A guide to increased compliance. Gaithersburg, MD: Aspen Publishers, Inc.

Foltz, A. and Sullivan, J. (1998). Get real: clinical testing of patients' reading abilities. Cancer Nursing, 21 (3), 162–166.

Friedman, M. (1997). The JCAHO clinical record review process. Home Healthcare Nurse, 15 (8), 541–548.

Harris, M.D. and Dugan, M. (1996). Evaluating the quality of homecare services using patient outcome data. Home Healthcare Nurse, 14 (6), 463–468.

Hellwig, K. (1990). Health teaching: The crux of home care nursing. Home Healthcare Nurse 8 (4), 35–37.

Jette, A., Smith, K., and McDermott, S. (1996). Quality of Medicare-reimbursed home health care. The Gerontologist, 36 (4), 492–501.

Joint Commission on Accreditation of Healthcare Organizations—1999–2000. (1998). Oakbrook Terrace, IL: JCAHO.

Jones, E. (1997). Telemedicine fosters homecare. Health Measures, 2 (1), 20–25, 37.

Krathwohl, D.R., Bloom, B.S., and Masia, B.B. (1964). Taxonomy of educational objectives: The classification of educational goals. Handbook I1: Affective domain. New York: David McKay Co., Inc.

Lipson, J., Dibble, S., and Minarik, P., (eds.). (1996). Culture and nursing care: A pocket guide. San Francisco, CA: UCSF Nursing Press.

Maynard, A.P. (1999). Preparing readable patient education handouts. Journal for Nurses in Staff Development, 15 (1), 11–18.

Medicare Home Health Agency Manual (HIM II). (1998). Washington, D.C.: HCFA.

Meleis, A., Isenberg, M., Koerner, J., and Stern, P. (1995). Diversity, marginalization, and culturally competent healthcare: Issues in knowledge development. Washington, D.C.: American Academy of Nursing.

Murphy, P. and Connally, T. (1997). When low literacy blocks compliance. RN, October, 58–63.

*Asterisk indicates a classic or definitive work on this subject.

Pennington, J. (1994). Bowes & Church's food values of portions commonly used, 16th ed. Philadelphia: J.B. Lippincott Co.

Price, J. and Cordell, B. (1984). Cultural diversity and patient teaching. Journal of Continuing Education in Nursing, 25 (4), 163–166.

Radu, V. (1997). Making the connection: Understanding and documenting the major medical diagnoses and related psychosocial indicators. Chattanooga, TN: Medical Social Work Solutions.

Rovinski, C. (1996). Psychiatric homecare chart review. Dimensions in Home Health, 1 (8), 8–9.

U.S. Department of Health & Human Services. (1990). Health information resources. Washington, D.C.: U.S. Government Printing Office.

Whitman, N. and Graham, BA. (1992). Teaching in nursing practice: A professional model, 2nd ed. Gleit, C. and Boyd, M.D. (eds): Norwalk, CT: Appleton & Lange.

Wilson, F. (1996). Patient education materials nurses use in community health. Western Journal of Nursing Research, 18 (2), 195–205.

*Wiman, R.V. and Meierhenry, W.C. (eds.). (1969). Educational media: Theory into practice. Columbus, OH: Charles Merrill.

Winter, A. and Winter, R. (1993). Consumer's guide to free medical information. Englewood Cliffs, NJ: Prentice-Hall.

---

*Asterisk indicates a classic or definitive work on this subject.

SECTION 2

PATIENT AND FAMILY INSTRUCTIONS

General Resources

Child Safety in the Home

GENERAL INFORMATION

Accidental injury is one of the major threats to the safety of a child. Many of the injuries can be prevented by following safety guidelines.

BURNS

1. Preventing burns
   a. Reduce the temperature of your hot water to 120°F.
   b. Always test the temperature of bath water before placing the child in the water. Use your elbow, it is more sensitive to heat. **Never leave your child alone in the tub.** Do not let your child play with the faucet.
   c. Never leave hot liquids or foods near your child. Do not carry your child and hot foods at the same time.
   d. Do not allow your child to crawl or play near a hot stove, hot appliance, fireplaces, wood burning stoves, or heaters. It is best to place your child in a playpen or highchair or to play safely away from the "hot" areas.
   e. Do not allow appliance cords or tablecloths to dangle within a child's reach. Turn handles of pots and pans toward the back of the stove.
   f. Lock up all chemicals and keep them out of reach.
   g. Use safety outlet covers.
   h. Keep lighters and matches out of the reach of children.
   i. Check the temperature of the car seat and seat belt before putting your child in the seat. Cover the seat with cloth.
2. Treating burns
   a. Put cold water on the burned area immediately.
   b. Loosely cover the area with a clean bandage or cloth.
   c. Call your doctor or emergency service number for serious burns.
   d. Call the Poison Control Center for chemical burns.
   e. Call the Fire Department for fire.

POISONINGS

1. Preventing poisonings
   a. Keep all household products, chemicals, and medicines completely out of children's reach and out of sight. Use safety locks for cabinets.
   b. Remember children like to put things such as medicines, chemicals, plants, toys, and perfumes in their mouths. Inside the house check the bathroom, bedroom, kitchen, garage, and basement. Outside the house check for poisonous plants, mushrooms, and pesticides.
   c. Remove sources of lead poisoning.
      - Check for chipped paint on walls, window sills, and doors. Also check cribs for chipped paint.
      - Lead crystal and some types of ceramic and pottery contain lead.
      - Old pipes, solder, and fixtures can contain lead and contaminate the drinking water.
   d. Watch your child when you are visiting or when guests are visiting you. An unattended purse may contain medications.
2. Treating poisonings. If you think your child has swallowed or come in contact with a poison:
   a. **Act immediately**—do not wait to see if your child becomes ill.
   b. Call the Poison Control Center for advice. Have the container with you when you call.
   c. Keep ipecac syrup in the house. **Do not use it unless directed by your doctor or the Poison Control Center.** Sometimes vomiting can cause more harm.

FALLS

1. Preventing falls
   a. Never leave a baby alone on a changing table.
   b. Use gates on stairways and doors. Use guards on windows. Be sure the bars are no more than 2⅜ inches apart so that your baby's head doesn't get stuck.
   c. Cover or remove sharp edged furniture where the child plays.
   d. Remove chairs or stools away from tables or counters to prevent your child from climbing to high places.
   e. Lock the doors to dangerous areas.
2. Treating falls.
   a. If your child has a serious fall, call your doctor or the emergency services number.
   b. If your child has a minor bruise or scrape,
      - For a bruise, apply ice wrapped in a clean cloth for no more than 15 minutes.

- Clean a minor scrape with warm soap and water or an antiseptic, then apply a Band-aid.
c. Call your nurse or doctor if minor bruises or scrapes do not heal.

EMERGENCY NUMBERS

POISON CENTER　　　　　　＿＿＿＿＿＿＿＿＿＿＿＿＿＿＿＿

EMERGENCY SERVICES　　　＿＿＿＿＿＿＿＿＿＿＿＿＿＿＿＿

DOCTOR　　　　　　　　　＿＿＿＿＿＿＿＿＿＿＿＿＿＿＿＿

FIRE DEPARTMENT　　　　　＿＿＿＿＿＿＿＿＿＿＿＿＿＿＿＿

OTHER INSTRUCTIONS

Intramuscular Injections

STEPS

1. Gather your equipment. You need
   - A sterile _____-milliliter syringe with an attached _____-gauge needle
   - Prescribed medication
   - Alcohol wipes
2. Wash your hands. Hand washing is the single most important factor in the prevention of infection.
3. Prepare the medication.
   a. *Vial.* If you are using the vial, follow these instructions:
      - Remove the metal cap. Open an alcohol wipe. Use it to clean the rubber top of the vial.
      - Uncap the needle and draw _____ milliliters of air into the syringe. (If you accidentally contaminate the needle, get a fresh one and begin the procedure again.)
      - Insert the needle into the rubber top of the vial and inject the air. Do not remove the needle and syringe from the vial.
      - Turn the vial, needle, and syringe upside down. Withdraw _____ milliliters of medication. Remove the needle and syringe from the vial.
      - If air bubbles are in the syringe, hold the syringe with the needle pointed up. Draw the plunger back slightly.
      Tap the barrel gently until the bubbles rise to the top. Push the plunger in slightly to get the air out of the syringe. Recap the needle.
   b. *Prefilled Syringe.* If you are using a prefilled syringe, follow these instructions: Check the syringe label for the correct name and amount of medication. If you have been instructed to remove some of the medication, gently push on the syringe plunger until you reach the correct amount.

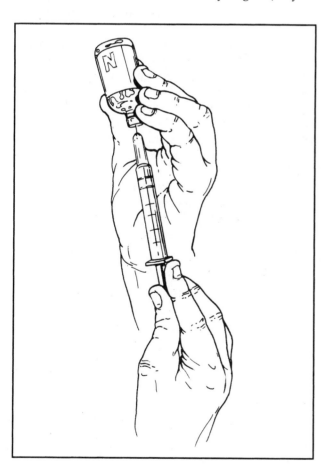

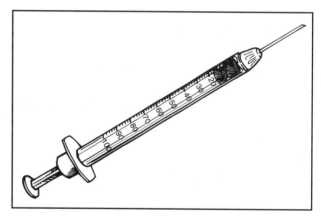

4. Select the injection site. Look for a site that is not reddened, hard, sore, bruised, scarred, or swollen. Use the picture for acceptable sites for intramuscular injections.

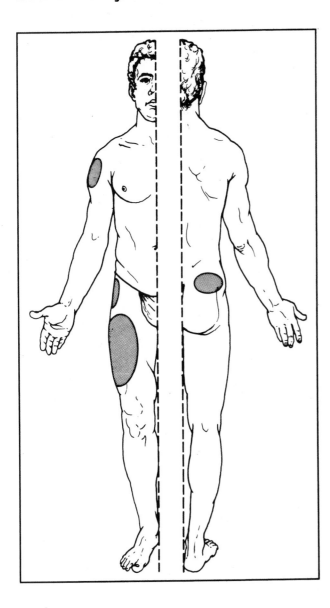

5. Open an alcohol wipe and use it to clean the selected site. Start at the center of the site and wipe in a circular motion, widening the circle to a 2-inch area.

6. Uncap the needle.

7. Spread the skin at the injection site tightly between your thumb and index finger. (If the muscle mass is small at the selected site, grasp the muscle firmly between your thumb and index finger.)

8. Hold the syringe like a pencil and insert the needle quickly into the injection site at a 90-degree angle.

9. Release the skin after the needle is inserted.

10. Hold the syringe in place and pull back gently on the plunger. Be careful not to pull the needle out of the skin. If blood appears in the syringe, withdraw the needle and put pressure on the injection site. Prepare a new needle and syringe and select another site for injection.

11. If no blood appears in the syringe, push the plunger in slowly until all the medication has been injected.

12. Withdraw the needle quickly from the injection site.

13. Gently rub the site with a fresh alcohol wipe. This helps the body absorb the medication.

14. Put used needles/syringes into a sharps container or a metal or hard plastic container such as a coffee can or laundry detergent bottle with a tight lid. Keep out of reach of children.

15. Dispose of full receptacle according to your town's requirements.

16. Keep a record of
    - The date and time you gave the injection,
    - How much medication you gave,
    - The site of the injection,
    - The effect of the medication on the patient.

INTRAMUSCULAR INJECTIONS RECORD

(Name of Prescribed Medication)

Date	Time	Amount	Site	Effect

OTHER INSTRUCTIONS

Making the Home Environment Safe

Completing the following checklist provides you with a safety assessment of your home. The nurse can help you determine which questions are applicable to your home and situation. Safety hazards in a home can usually be remedied very easily. If you answer "no" to any applicable question, the nurse can teach you what you have to do to answer "yes" and increase your home's safety.

SAFETY QUESTIONS

	YES	NO
1. Bathroom		
a. Are there handgrips by the tub/shower?	____	____
b. Are there handgrips by the toilet?	____	____
c. Is there a nonskid mat in the tub/shower?	____	____
d. Is there a seat in the tub/shower?	____	____
e. Is there a seat by the sink?	____	____
f. Does the toilet have a high-rise seat?	____	____
2. Electric Outlets and Devices		
a. Are unused outlets covered?	____	____
b. Are appliances disconnected when not in use?	____	____
c. Are all electric cords free from fraying or cracking?	____	____
d. Do all electric plugs fit snugly into their sockets?	____	____
e. Do electric cords run along walls?	____	____
f. Are all electric devices protected from and not exposed to moisture?	____	____
3. Fire		
a. Is there a home fire safety/drill plan?	____	____
b. Are exits available from all locations in the house?	____	____
c. Do the following areas have smoke alarms?		
• Hallways	____	____
• Kitchen	____	____
• Bedrooms	____	____
• Attic	____	____
• Basement	____	____
d. Does the fireplace have a smoke screen?	____	____
e. Is maintenance for the fireplace/woodstove scheduled and completed on a regular basis?	____	____
f. Are curtains and other flammable items kept away from the stove and other open flame areas?	____	____
g. Are there an adequate number of glass or ceramic ashtrays?	____	____
4. Floors		
a. Is nonskid wax used on the floors?	____	____
b. Are scatter rugs secured by nonskid backing?	____	____
c. Are large rugs anchored at the edges?	____	____
d. Are pathways and hallways cleared of toys, excess furniture, etc.?	____	____
5. Heating System		
a. Are examinations/cleanings done on a regular basis by a utility expert?	____	____
6. Lighting		
a. Is lighting adequate throughout the house?	____	____
b. Are burned-out light bulbs replaced?	____	____
c. Are nightlights used along routes/areas traveled after dark?	____	____

			YES	NO
7.	Stairwells			
	a.	Are there nonskid treads on steps?	————	————
	b.	Are different colors used to mark changes in levels?	————	————
	c.	Are handrails present and securely fastened?	————	————
8.	Miscellaneous			
	a.	Are the following items in secured areas out of the reach of children and confused individuals?		
		• Medications	————	————
		• Sharp objects (knives, axes, etc.)	————	————
		• Dangerous tools	————	————
		• Cleaning substances	————	————
		• Poisons (bug killer, weed killer, etc.)	————	————
	b.	Is snow and ice removal adequate and efficient?	————	————
	c.	Are sidewalks, curbs, and outside stairs maintained?	————	————
	d.	Is the water heater temperature kept under 120°F?	————	————
	e.	Is wheeled furniture secured by caster plates?	————	————

OTHER INSTRUCTIONS

Medication Compliance

GUIDELINES

These guidelines will help you take your medications. Taking your medications properly can make the difference in your health. The table lists some problems that might tempt you to stop taking your medications and some solutions to help you stay on track.

TO TAKE MEDICATIONS PROPERLY

1. Be sure you understand
   a. Each medication's name
   b. Why you are taking the medication
   c. How much medication you should take
   d. How to take the medication:
      - With meals or on an empty stomach
      - The same time each day
      - The number of hours between dosages
   e. The side effects
   f. The side effects (symptoms) you should report to your nurse or doctor
2. Always ask your nurse or doctor about any questions you have.
3. Take your medications exactly as instructed.
   a. Do not take anyone else's medications.
   b. Do not take medications you can buy without prescription (over the counter) unless they are approved by your nurse or doctor.
   c. Do not use alternative medicine or herbal or vitamin supplements unless they are approved by your nurse or doctor.
   d. Follow any special safety precautions, such as
      - Avoid taking aspirin with certain medications
      - Keep your medications separate from other family members' medications.
4. Let your family and friends help you.
5. Ask your nurse or doctor about community groups that may be able to help you.
6. Your nurse can help you with
   a. Fitting your medication into your daily routine. Try to keep your routine as simple as possible.
   b. Tips to help you remember to take your medication, such as
      - Using a calendar, grease board, or checklist with the medication times marked,
      - Using an egg carton to arrange medications for the day,
      - Scheduling your medications around usual routines such as meals,
      - Using pictures or colored dots on bottles. For example red dots or a picture of a sun will tell you to take the medication in the morning.
      - Using an index card with a picture of the medication by your toothbrush could remind you to take the medication in the morning and at bedtime
      - Using a medication organizer on the next page, for example
   You or your family can fill the organizer for the week.

Problems Encountered with Taking Medications

Problem	Solution
1. You think you do not need the medication because a. You are feeling better; you do not feel ill.	1a. Do not stop taking your medication unless instructed to do so by your nurse or doctor.
b. You do not understand the reason for taking the medication.	1b. Ask your nurse or doctor why the medication has been prescribed for you.
2. You experience side effects from the medication.	2. Tell your nurse or doctor about the symptoms of any side effects you experience.
3. The child-proof bottles are too hard to open.	3. Get a different bottle from your pharmacy.
4. You are tired of taking the medications; your illness has lasted a long time.	4. Talk to your nurse or doctor about how you feel.

5. You do not understand how to take the medication, especially when
   a. You must take three or more medications at different times of the day.
   b. There have been new changes in the medications.
   c. You must adjust the dosage.
	5. Ask your nurse or doctor about ways to remember when to take your medications. Ask your nurse or doctor any questions you have.

Medication Compliance

SUN	MON	TUE	WED	THU	FRI	SAT
Morn	Morn	Morn	Morn	Morn	Morn	Morn
Noon	Noon	Noon	Noon	Noon	Noon	Noon
Eve	Eve	Eve	Eve	Eve	Eve	Eve
Bed	Bed	Bed	Bed	Bed	Bed	Bed

7. When traveling,
   a. Carry your medications on your person. Do not put them in your luggage.
   b. Carry your doctor's name and phone number. Your doctor may give you a prescription to take with you.
   c. Carry a list of your medications with you.

Drug Name	Use	Color/shape	Directions: When and how to take

OTHER INSTRUCTIONS

Reading a Thermometer and Taking a Temperature

GENERAL INFORMATION

Thermometers come in different types. Glass oral mercury thermometers may have a longer, thinner bulb; have a blue or clear bulb; or be marked "oral." Glass rectal mercury thermometers may have a shorter, rounder bulb; have a red bulb; or be marked "rectal." Chemical dot and electronic thermometers may come in different shapes and brands; follow the directions on your brand.

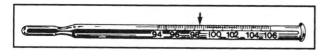

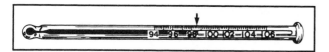

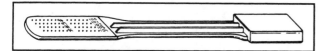

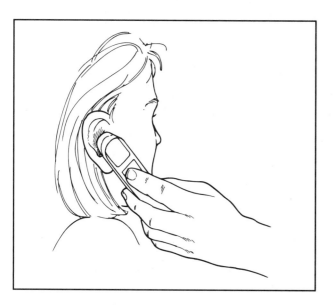

EQUIPMENT

- Thermometer
- Watch or clock with a sweep hand
- Lubricant (if taking a rectal temperature)

READING A GLASS THERMOMETER

Thermometers come with Fahrenheit (F) or with Celsius (C) markings. Each large line is one degree. Each degree is divided into parts. Each part is 2 tenths of a degree (0.2).

1. Hold the tip of the thermometer (end opposite the bulb) at eye level.
2. Turn the thermometer slowly until you can see the mercury column (silver in color) and the numbers.
3. The temperature reading on the top thermometer is 98.6°F.

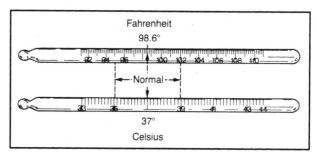

Fahrenheit
98.6°

←--Normal--→

37°
Celsius

TAKING A TEMPERATURE WITH A GLASS THERMOMETER

Special Notes

1. Glass thermometers can break easily if not used properly.
2. If a thermometer breaks inside the body, call the emergency room immediately.
3. Always check the thermometer for any breaks or cracks before you use it.
4. Glass thermometers can lose their accuracy with age.

Steps

1. Take the thermometer out of the package. Rinse it completely in cool water.
2. Hold the tip end of the thermometer firmly between your thumb and first finger. Shake the

thermometer until the mercury line is below the number 95°F (35°C).

Choose *oral*, *rectal*, or *axillary* for the next step.

Oral

1. Place the oral thermometer under the tongue. Keep the lips closed—do not bite down.

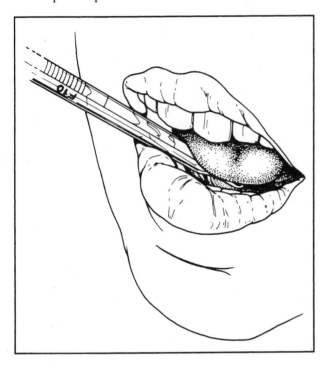

2. Keep the thermometer under the tongue for 5 to 8 minutes. Take an oral temperature on a cooperative child older than 4 or 5 years of age.
3. When the timing is up, hold the thermometer at eye level. Read the number exactly where the fluid stops.

Special Notes

1. The normal reading is between 96.4°F and 99.1°F (35.8°C and 37.8°C).
2. Do not take the oral temperatures of
   a. Infants,
   b. Persons who can breathe only through their mouths,
   c. Persons who are unconscious,
   d. Persons who may bite the thermometer.
3. Wait at least 30 minutes after a person has eaten or drunk before taking the temperature.

Rectal

1. Have a tissue and lubricating jelly on hand.
2. Have the person lie comfortably on his or her side, stomach, or back.

3. Put a small amount of lubricating jelly on the bulb end of the rectal thermometer.
4. Separate the skin of the buttocks to have a clear view of the rectum.
5. Insert the thermometer into the rectum about one inch in an adult or about one half inch in an infant or child. Hold the infant still with one hand. An axillary temperature may be better for an uncooperative child or a child less than 4 years old. Hold the thermometer in place for 3 minutes.

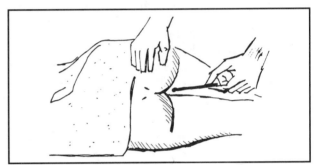

From Rambo BJ and Wood LA: Nursing Skills for Clinical Practice, 3rd ed. Philadelphia, WB Saunders, 1982.

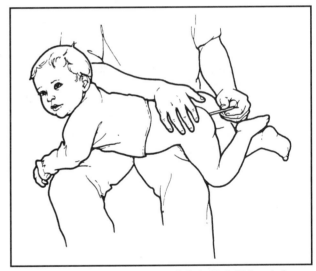

From Wong D and Hess C: Wong and Whaley's Clinical Manual of Pediatric Nursing, 5th ed. Copyright 2000 by the CV Mosby Co., St. Louis.

6. When the time is up, remove and wipe off the thermometer with a tissue. Hold it at eye level and read the number exactly where the fluid stops.

Special Notes

1. The normal reading is between 97.2°F and 100°F (36.2°C and 37.8°C).
2. Check with the nurse or doctor before taking the

rectal temperature of someone who has had rectal surgery or who has heart disease.

3. Use only a rectal thermometer. An oral thermometer with a long bulb could injure the rectum.

Axillary

1. With the person lying or sitting, put the bulb of the oral thermometer in the center of the armpit. Taking an axillary temperature is better for an uncooperative child of any age or for a child less than 4 years old.

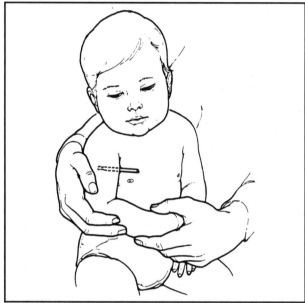

From Wong D and Hess C: Wong and Whaley's Clinical Manual of Pediatric Nursing, 5th ed. Copyright 2000 by the CV Mosby Co., St. Louis.

2. Make sure the armpit is dry. There should be no clothing between the arm and the chest.
3. Keep the thermometer in place for 10 minutes. Keep the arm at the person's side.
4. When the time is up, hold the thermometer at eye level and read the number.

Special Notes

1. The normal reading is between 96.6°F and 98°F (35.9°C and 36.7°C).
2. Use the underarm only if the oral or rectal areas cannot be used.
3. Wait at least 15 minutes after a person has bathed before taking the temperature. Make sure the area is completely dry.

General Notes

1. Write down the time, the place on the body used to take the temperature (oral, rectal, or axillary), and the temperature reading. Body temperatures can vary with age, the time of day, and the part of the body used.
2. Call your nurse or doctor:
   a. If the temperature is _____ .
   b. If there are signs of infection or fever.
3. After using a glass thermometer, wash it with warm (not hot) soapy water. Rinse it with cool water and dry it.
4. Store the glass thermometer in a container to prevent breakage.
5. If using an electronic oral or ear thermometer, follow the instructions in the package. Pay careful attention to the beeping tones, which tell you when to remove the thermometer.

OTHER INSTRUCTIONS

Subcutaneous Injections

STEPS

1. Gather your equipment. You need
   - A sterile _____-milliliter syringe with an attached _____-gauge needle
   - Prescribed medication
   - Alcohol wipes
2. Wash your hands. Hand washing is the single most important factor in the prevention of infection.
3. Prepare the medication.
   a. *Vial.* If you are using the vial, follow these instructions:
      - Remove the metal cap. Open an alcohol wipe. Use it to clean the rubber top of the vial.
      - Uncap the needle and draw _____ milliliters of air into the syringe. (If you

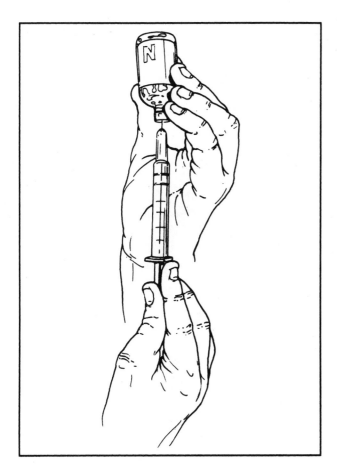

accidentally contaminate the needle, get a fresh one and begin the procedure again.)
      - Insert the needle into the rubber top of the vial and inject the air. Do not remove the needle and syringe from the vial.
      - Turn the vial, needle, and syringe upside down. Withdraw _____ milliliters of medication. Remove the needle and syringe from the vial.
      - If air bubbles are in the syringe, hold the syringe with the needle pointed up. Draw the plunger back slightly. Tap the barrel gently until the bubbles rise to the top. Push the plunger in slightly to get the air out of the syringe. Recap the needle.
   b. *Prefilled Syringe.* If you are using a prefilled syringe, follow these instructions:
      - Check the syringe label for the correct name and amount of medication.
      - If you have been instructed to remove some of the medication, gently push on the syringe plunger until you reach the correct amount.

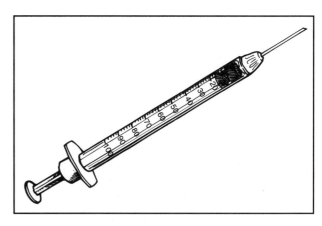

4. Select the injection site. Look for a site that is not reddened, hard, sore, bruised, scarred, or swollen. Use the picture for acceptable sites for subcutaneous injections.

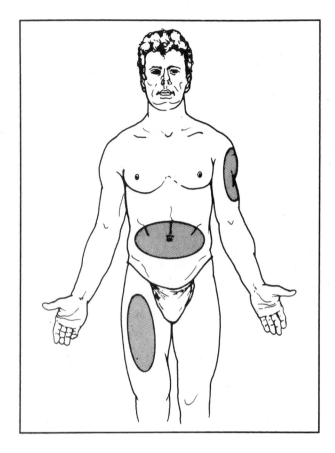

6. Uncap the needle.
7. Pinch the skin at the injection site.
8. Insert the needle quickly into the injection site at a 45-degree angle. (For obese people, use a 90-degree angle; for very thin people, use a 15- to 30-degree angle.)
9. Release the skin after the needle is inserted.
10. Hold the syringe in place and pull back gently on the plunger. Be careful not to pull the needle out of the skin. If blood appears in the syringe, withdraw the needle and put pressure on the injection site. Prepare a new needle and syringe and select another site for injection.
11. If no blood appears in the syringe, push the plunger in slowly until all the medication has been injected.
12. Withdraw the needle quickly from the injection site.
13. Gently rub the site with a fresh alcohol wipe. This helps the body absorb the medication.
14. Put used needles/syringes into a sharps container or a metal or hard plastic container such as a coffee can or laundry detergent bottle with a tight lid. Keep out of reach of children.
15. Dispose of full receptacle according to your town's requirements.
16. Keep a record of
    • The date and time you gave the injection
    • How much medication you gave
    • The site of the injection
    • The effect of the medication on the patient.

5. Open an alcohol wipe and use it to clean the selected site. Start at the center of the site and wipe in a circular motion, widening the circle to a 2-inch area.

SUBCUTANEOUS INJECTIONS RECORD

(Name of Prescribed Medication)

Date	Time	Amount	Site	Effect

OTHER INSTRUCTIONS

Cardiovascular Alterations

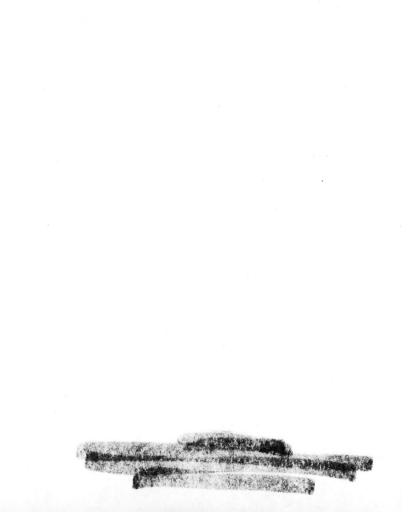

After Your Heart Attack

GENERAL INFORMATION

A heart attack is death of part of the heart muscle. That part of the heart muscle turns into a scar. It takes about 6 weeks for the scar to be strong.

Guidelines

These guidelines can help your recovery. Your nurse or doctor will give you instructions that are important for you to follow.

1. To help you have fewer problems with your heart, you should follow healthy heart steps. Ask your nurse or doctor for a copy of *Healthy Heart* instructions.
2. Follow your diet. It should be
   a. Low in cholesterol and saturated fat, which helps to reduce heart disease risk,
   b. Low in sodium (salt), which helps to reduce fluid retention,
   c. High in fiber and bulk, which helps with bowel movements.
   d. Your nurse or doctor will give you a copy of your diet.
3. Keep your weight under control.
   a. Extra weight causes your heart to work harder.
   b. If you are overweight, your nurse or doctor can help you with a weight loss plan.
4. Regular exercise is an important part of your recovery.
   a. Until your first visit to the doctor, 5 minutes of slow walking once or twice a day may be all that is allowed. Your doctor will tell you about your activity plan.
   b. Always begin exercise with a warm-up: 5 minutes of slow walking and stretching.
   c. Exercise at your target heart rate. Your target heart rate is how fast your heart should beat during exercise.
      • Count your pulse during the exercise.
      • Your nurse or doctor will tell you what your heart rate should be.
      • Your activity will increase as you recover.
   d. After exercise, cool down by slow walking for at least 5 minutes. End with stretching.
   e. Stop and rest for 15 to 30 minutes if you feel tired.
   f. Avoid activity in very hot or very cold temperatures.
   g. Stop if you experience chest pressure, tightness, pain in the chest, shortness of breath, or dizziness.
5. Plan for rest and relaxation.
   a. Try to sleep 6 to 8 hours every night.
   b. Rest or take naps during the day.
   c. Space your activities. Do not push yourself.
   d. Make time for fun and recreation.
   e. Learn to feel relaxed. Worry and stress increase your heart rate and blood pressure.
   f. Your nurse or doctor can help with ways to relax.
6. Sex after a heart attack.
   a. Sexual relations usually are allowed by your doctor about 3 to 4 weeks after the heart attack.
   b. You can show affection and caring by touching, holding, and caressing. These activities use little energy, so you can use them as soon as you are home.
   c. Avoid sexual relations when you
      • Are tired and feeling stressed,
      • Have just eaten a large meal (wait about 2 hours),
      • Are in a very hot or very cold area.
   d. If you feel your medication is making you feel ill, notify your doctor before stopping it.
7. Take your medications as instructed.
   a. Do not skip or stop taking any medication without first checking with your doctor.
   b. Keep a list of the name, the dose, how you should take it, the reason you are taking it, and the side effects for each medication.
   c. If you have diabetes, be sure to monitor blood glucose levels as part of your exercise plan. Always plan to carry a source of sugar (such as hard candy) when exercising.
8. Do not smoke.
   a. Smoking makes the heart beat faster and raises the blood pressure.
   b. Many groups have classes to help stop smoking. Your nurse or doctor can give you more information.
   c. Ask your doctor about medications to help you stop smoking.
9. Avoid straining and holding your breath while doing activities.
   a. Do not strain during bowel movements. If you have trouble with constipation, call your nurse or doctor.

b. Do not lift heavy objects, especially above your head or when bending at the waist.

c. Refrain from vacuuming or carrying heavy objects for the first 4 to 6 weeks.

10. Life after a heart attack

a. Set goals you can reach at home and at work.

b. Talk out your feelings with your family.

c. Tell your nurse or doctor about your home and work demands.

d. Call the American Heart Association for the name of the self-help group that meets in your area. This is a group of people who have recovered from a heart attack. They help others recovering from heart attacks.

e. Have regular check-ups with your doctor.

f. Your nurse or doctor can discuss your personal risk factors for heart disease and how to change them.

11. Know the signs of a heart attack:

a. Pressure, fullness, tightness, or pain in the center of the chest for more than 2 minutes

b. Pain that spreads to the neck, jaw, shoulders, or arms

c. Shortness of breath

d. Nausea or vomiting

e. Fainting, dizziness, or weakness

f. Sweating

g. Your signs may be mild. They may go away and then return. If you have diabetes, you may not experience chest pain because of nerve changes.

12. If you have these signs, act *immediately.*

a. Call the emergency service number.

b. Never drive yourself to the hospital.
   • Call an ambulance.
   • If the ambulance cannot come immediately, you may need to have someone drive you.

c. Talk to your nurse or doctor about your emergency plan.

OTHER INSTRUCTIONS

Angina

GENERAL INFORMATION

Angina is the name used to describe the discomfort caused when the heart muscle temporarily does not get enough oxygen and blood. This is your body's warning to stop and rest until the heart muscle's demand for oxygen and blood can be supplied. Angina attacks usually last only a few minutes and go away if you rest and take nitroglycerin.

There are different types of angina. Your nurse or doctor can teach you about your type of angina. An angina attack is not the same as a heart attack. Each person may have different symptoms. It is important for you to get to know your symptoms and what causes you to have symptoms. Your angina will usually feel about the same each time. Angina usually lasts a few minutes.

COMMON SYMPTOMS

The most common symptoms are

1. Pain, tightness, aching, or numbness in the chest, arm, neck, shoulder, jaw, or throat,
2. Shortness of breath,
3. Sweating,
4. Dizziness,
5. Extreme fatigue.

WHAT TO DO WHEN YOU HAVE SYMPTOMS

1. Stop what you are doing at the first sign of symptoms.
2. Sit and, if possible, look at the time.
3. If nitroglycerin pills are prescribed for you,
   a. Take one pill at the first sign of symptoms.
      • Put the pill under your tongue.
      • Do not swallow your saliva until the pill is gone.
   b. If the symptoms are not gone after 5 minutes,
      • Take another nitroglycerin pill.
      • Look at the time.
      • Wait 5 minutes.
   c. If the symptoms still are not gone after taking two pills and waiting a total of 10 minutes:
      • Take one more nitroglycerin pill.
      • Look at the time.
      • Wait 5 minutes more.
   d. If the symptoms are not gone after 15 to 20 minutes from the time when the pain began:
      • Call your doctor or the emergency services number.
      • Keep these telephone numbers by the phone.
      • Do not drive yourself to the emergency room.
4. When the symptoms are gone, you can begin some activity.

SYMPTOMS TO REPORT TO YOUR DOCTOR OR TO YOUR EMERGENCY ROOM

1. Symptoms that
   a. Last 20 minutes and are not relieved by medication,
   b. Become worse (last longer, hurt more, hurt in other parts of your body than usual),
   c. Happen more often,
   d. Occur while you are at rest,
   e. Are different from those you have had before,
   f. Happen with less activity than usual.
2. Shortness of breath.
3. Fainting spells.
4. Irregular pulse (heart beat) or a heart beat below 60 or over 100 beats per minute.
5. If you think you may be having a heart attack, call an ambulance immediately.
   a. Heart attack symptoms usually feel "different" than your angina symptoms.
   b. Heart attack symptoms last longer than 2 minutes.
6. For safety, carry some form of medical identification with you at all times.

GENERAL TIPS FOR HEALTHFUL LIVING

1. Learn to take your pulse, which tells you
   a. Your number of heart beats per minute,
   b. How regular your heart is beating.
2. Plan a daily program of exercise and activity that does not lead to symptoms.
   a. Before starting an exercise or activity program, check with your doctor.
   b. Pace yourself.
      • Angina can be caused by hard, fast-paced activity.

- It is better to exercise more slowly for a longer time.
c. Take your pulse before and after the activity.
   - Check for the regularity of rhythm.
   - If your heart rate does not return to normal 10 minutes after the activity, call your physician before doing that activity again.
d. Include a warm-up and a cool-down period in your program:
   - Warm-up—walk slowly for 5 minutes, then stretch,
   - Exercise as directed,
   - Cool-down—walk slowly for 5 minutes. End with stretching.
e. Avoid physical activity
   - For 1 to 2 hours after eating,
   - If you are not feeling well,
   - After drinking alcohol.
f. Rest before and after sexual activity.
g. If your doctor prescribes nitroglycerin pills, you may be told to take one pill before the activity. This may prevent angina symptoms.

3. Avoid situations or activities that put too much strain on the heart or cause you to have angina symptoms, such as
   a. Sudden bursts of activity like walking up stairs or hills or lifting heavy objects (children, grocery bags),
   b. Walking against a strong wind,
   c. Very hot or very cold temperatures
      - Avoid very hot or very cold water/bathing.
      - Avoid physical activities out of doors during very hot or very cold weather. In the winter, cover your nose and mouth with a scarf.
   d. Higher altitudes than you are used to,
   e. Emotionally stressful situations (anger or excitement),
   f. Anal stimulation (rectal temperatures), because this leads to a slow heart rate.
4. Eating for a healthy heart:
   a. Limit intake of caffeine (coffee, tea, colas, chocolate).
   b. Drink alcohol only if permitted by your doctor.
   c. Avoid overeating and large meals; it is better to eat smaller, more frequent meals.
   d. Eat foods high in fiber (if your doctor recommends) such as bran, raw fruits and vegetables, and whole grains.
   e. Consume foods low in fat and cholesterol, such as chicken, fish, and skim milk.
5. Plan to take all of your medications in the way you have been told.

a. Do not take any medication (especially diet pills, herbal or alternative medications, or nasal decongestants) without talking to your doctor first.
b. Do not stop taking medications without talking to your doctor first.
c. Your nurse or doctor can teach you about your medication
   - Its name,
   - What it does,
   - When and how often you should take it,
   - Any side effects,
   - Any effects you should report to your physician.
6. If your doctor has prescribed nitroglycerin, you should know that it
   a. Can help bring more blood to the heart,
   b. Comes in different forms (pills, patches, and ointment).
7. Nitroglycerin pills
   a. Relieve the symptoms within 2 minutes —you should always carry some with you if prescribed for you,
   b. Burn or sting slightly when placed under the tongue,
   c. Should be stored carefully in a dark, closed, glass container and protected from heat, wetness, air, and light. Keep your nitroglycerin pills in a separate container.
   d. Lose strength—buy only a 6-month supply,
   e. May cause mild side effects that should go away quickly.
      - If you feel dizzy or faint, sit down, lower your head between your legs, and breathe deeply.
      - A mild headache or flushing of the face and neck is common.
8. Follow your health plan as prescribed by your doctor.
   a. Keep your blood pressure under control.
   b. Stop smoking.
   c. Control stress.
      - List those things in life that are stressful for you.
      - List ways to handle the stress.
   d. Keep your follow-up appointments.
9. Ask your nurse or doctor about community resources that can help you, such as
   a. The American Heart Association
   b. Programs to stop smoking
   c. Weight control programs
   d. Stress management programs
   e. Cardiac rehabilitation
   f. Support groups for angina patients and their families.

ANGINA RECORDS

Doctor's telephone number _____   Emergency services telephone number _____

Medication Name and Dose   **Special Instructions**

_____

_____

_____

_____

Guidelines for Describing an Angina Attack

Date:

Time:

What were you doing?

How did it feel?

How long did it last?

How many nitroglycerin pills did you take?

Time #1 _____ Result _____

Time #2 _____ Result _____

Time #3 _____ Result _____

OTHER INSTRUCTIONS

Healthy Heart

GENERAL INFORMATION

Your heart is a muscle that pumps blood through your body. The heart muscle gets its blood supply from arteries (the coronary arteries). Atherosclerosis ("hardening of the arteries") is a disease that narrows the arteries so that less blood flows through. Atherosclerosis can be slowed down by following healthy heart steps.

HEALTHY HEART STEPS

1. Do not smoke cigarettes.
   a. It is not too late to stop.
   b. Smoking makes the heart beat faster and narrows the arteries.
   c. Your nurse or doctor can give you information to help you stop smoking. The American Lung Association also has information.
2. Control high blood pressure.
   a. High blood pressure is called a "silent killer." Untreated, high blood pressure can lead to heart attack, stroke, and kidney failure.
   b. Have your blood pressure checked regularly.
   c. High blood pressure cannot be cured. It can be controlled by treatment.
   d. Treatment may include reducing weight if you are overweight, limiting salt (sodium) intake, and taking medication.
      • Omit salt by avoiding pickled foods, lunch meats, salty snacks, monosodium glutamate, and use of added salt. Read all labels: frozen, canned, and packaged foods often contain a lot of sodium.
      • If you have a prescription, take your medication as your nurse or doctor has instructed.
3. Reduce saturated fat and cholesterol in the diet.
   a. Saturated fats and cholesterol lead to atherosclerosis ("hardening of the arteries").
   b. A diet should be balanced with plenty of water and the right amount of calories for weight control.
   c. What you eat has an important effect on how you feel and how your body works.
   d. Limit fatty meats, lard, butter, and whole-milk dairy products, which are high in saturated fats.
   e. Limit egg yolks and organ meats, which are high in cholesterol.
   f. Have meals of fish and poultry. For meat, use lean cuts and trim off the fat.
   g. Use skim milk and skim milk products. Cook with polyunsaturated oils and margarine.
   h. Your nurse or doctor can help you with diet. The American Heart Association also has information.
4. Control your weight.
   a. Being overweight can raise your blood pressure and blood fat levels. It makes your heart work harder and can lead to diabetes.
   b. Check with your nurse or doctor before starting a weight loss diet. You can harm your health by cutting out important foods.
   c. Plan to weigh yourself once a week at the same time of day.
   d. Plan to lose ½ to 1½ pounds a week, no more.
   e. To lose one pound a week, you should eat about 500 calories less a day.
   f. Eat foods high in fiber and bulk; they
      • Are lower in calories and help you feel full,
      • Help to keep bowel movements regular.
   g. Plan to eat three to four times a day.
   h. Spread calories throughout the day:

      _____ calories breakfast,

      _____ calories lunch,

      _____ calories snack,

      _____ calories dinner.
   i. Avoid large meals and overeating.
5. Exercise regularly.
   a. Exercise helps blood circulate and helps relieve tension.
   b. Check with your nurse or doctor before starting an exercise program.
   c. Pick an exercise that you like and that can be done year-round.
      • Some exercises are walking, hiking, bicycling, and swimming.
      • Many people walk in shopping malls when the weather is bad.
      • Avoid exercise in very hot or very cold temperatures.
   d. Weightlifting may build muscle, but it does not help the heart.
   e. Always start exercise with a warm-up of 5 minutes of slow walking and stretching.

f. Exercise at your target heart rate. Your target heart rate is how fast your heart should beat during exercise.
- Take your pulse during exercise.
- Your nurse or doctor will tell you what your heart rate should be.
- Exercise in the target heart rate zone for 20 to 30 minutes.
- Exercise at least three times a week.
- Wait 2 hours after eating to exercise.

g. After exercise, cool down by slow walking for at least 5 minutes. End with stretching.

h. Stop and rest for 15 to 30 minutes if you feel tired.

i. If you have signs of a heart attack, get help immediately.
- Pressure, fullness, tightness, or pain in the center of the chest for more than 2 minutes.
- Pain spreading to the neck, jaw, shoulders, or arms,
- Shortness of breath,
- Nausea or vomiting,
- Fainting, dizziness, or weakness.

6. Your nurse or doctor may tell you to use a perceived exertion rating scale. You will be asked to use a number or words to describe how the exercise feels.
- For example, the range can be from rest (6) to fairly light (11–12) to hard (15–16) to exhaustion (20).
- Using the scale helps to better describe how you feel when you are exercising.

7. Plan for regular rest and relaxation.
   a. Stress can make your heart beat faster and can raise your blood pressure.
   b. If you feel stressed, take two or three deep breaths and think about something relaxing.
   c. Relaxation can be doing a hobby, exercising, or watching a movie. Do what you enjoy.
   d. Limit caffeine intake. Caffeine is a stimulant that increases your heart rate.

8. Have regular medical check-ups.
   a. A check-up will show if you have diabetes, high blood pressure, or other problems that can lead to a heart attack.
   b. If you have heart disease, check-ups are an important part of your treatment.

9. The American Heart Association has information about heart disease and ways to keep healthy.

OTHER INSTRUCTIONS

Pacemaker

GENERAL INFORMATION

A pacemaker is used to keep the heart beating as it should. A pacemaker uses batteries to send signals to the heart muscle to make your heart pump. People of all ages have pacemakers and are able to have normal lives. There are different types of pacemakers. Your nurse or doctor can teach you about yours. Yours is a _____ pacemaker.

GUIDELINES

These guidelines can help you with your pacemaker:

1. Carry your pacemaker identification card at all times.
   a. The card should have information about
      • The name of the company (model and serial number) that made the pacemaker battery and wire,
      • The type of pacemaker you have and the date and site of insertion.
      • The magnet rate at which the pacemaker is set. Your rate should be _____ per minute,
      • The names and phone numbers of your doctor and nurse,
      • The name of the hospital where it was put in,
      • Any extra equipment you have, such as a magnet or special transmitter.
   b. When you travel, visit another doctor or nurse, or enter the hospital, you may need to show your pacemaker information.
   c. You also may want to wear a medical chain or bracelet identification tag.
2. Follow your nurse's or doctor's instructions for keeping your pacemaker incision clean and dry until it is healed.
   a. Follow the activity and bathing instructions given to you.
   b. Check your incision site every day for signs of infection during the first month.
3. Call your nurse or doctor right away if you have any of these signs of infection at the incision:
   a. Swelling,
   b. Redness,
   c. Pain,
   d. Fever,
   e. Opening in the skin or drainage at the pacemaker insertion site.
4. See your doctor or nurse for check-ups.
   a. Be sure to have your pacemaker sutures or staples removed on time. Your sutures should be removed on _____ .
   b. Your nurse or doctor can tell you about
      • Proper diet,
      • Activity and rest plan,
      • Any limits on travel, bathing, sex, heavy lifting, running or contact sports. It takes about 8 weeks for the pacemaker to settle in place. Be careful not to hit or rub the insertion site during this time.
   c. Tell your doctor or nurse your new address if you move.
   d. Be sure to have your pacemaker checked as scheduled.
   e. Your nurse or doctor will give you instructions about which ways are best for you to check your pacemaker. These are some of the ways to check a pacemaker:
      • In person at the nurse's or doctor's office or clinic,
      • By checking your pulse.
      • By phone, using a special transmitter, electrodes (wrist, finger tip, or chest) and possibly a special magnet.

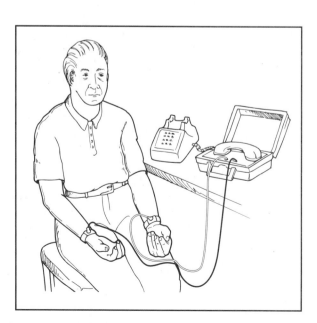

5. Learn the most common symptoms of pacemaker problems:
   a. Dizziness,
   b. Fainting spells or light-headedness,
   c. Shortness of breath,
   d. Blurred vision,
   e. Confusion,
   f. Irregular heart beat (change from your regular heart rhythm and rate),
   g. Pulse rate that is 4 to 5 beats slower than the rate set on the pacemaker,
   h. Long-lasting hiccups,
   i. Chest pain,
   j. Sudden drop of heart beat to 40 or 50 beats per minute.
   k. Heart beat that is rapid and irregular, above 100 beats per minute,
   l. Weight gain and swelling of legs or ankles.

6. Know what to do when you have symptoms that your pacemaker is not working right:
   a. Turn the equipment off immediately or move at least 5 feet away from any electrical equipment.
   b. Take your pulse.
   c. If you feel better after you have moved, do not use the equipment again until you talk to your doctor or nurse.
   d. If you do not feel better after you have moved, call your nurse, doctor, or emergency service number immediately.

7. Show anyone who treats you your pacemaker card:
   a. A dentist, physical therapist, chiropractor, or any new doctor or nurse.
   b. Technicians who perform any treatments or tests using electric equipment, such as radiation or diathermy.

8. Do not "fiddle" or play with your pacemaker. It could become damaged.

9. Most electric equipment in the home will not bother your pacemaker.
   a. Keep electrical equipment in good repair.
   b. Computers, microwaves, vacuum cleaners, power tools, and the like are okay to use.

10. Stay away from areas marked with high-voltage signs because your pacemaker may not work well around:
    a. Electrical power plants,
    b. Radar stations or high-voltage wires,
    c. Industry using heavy-duty equipment such as electric arc welders,
    d. Radio and television transmitters,
    e. High-powered amplifiers for ham and CB radios (ordinary CB radios should be fine),
    f. Very strong magnets such as an MRI (medical test).

11. Do not work on large running motors like those of cars or boats. The motor creates an electrical field.

12. If in doubt about the effect an electric appliance or a piece of equipment may have on your pacemaker, have someone with you (who knows you have a pacemaker) the first time you use it.
    a. If you become dizzy or lightheaded, turn off the equipment or move 5 feet away from it.
    b. You should feel better as soon as you are out of range.

13. When passing through security devices (airport and libraries), your pacemaker may cause the screening device to alarm.
    a. The screening device will not harm your pacemaker.
    b. Have your pacemaker identification card ready to show the security staff.

14. You can wear any clothes you like.
    a. Your doctor or nurse may tell you to wear loose tops until the pacemaker incision heals.
    b. Avoid tight straps over the pacemaker area.

15. Your nurse or doctor can tell you how to get more information about pacemakers:
    a. American Heart Association,
    b. Your pacemaker company.

16. Take your pulse as often as the doctor or nurse advises.
    a. Count it for 1 full minute.
    b. Write down the number of beats, the date, and the time.
    c. If your pulse is less than _____ or more than _____ per minute, call your nurse or doctor.

OTHER INSTRUCTIONS

Taking a Pulse

GENERAL INFORMATION

You can count your own heartbeat. This is called taking your pulse. When you take a pulse the right way, you can feel your artery give a little jump each time your heart beats. The number of times you feel the pulse in a minute is your pulse rate. Your pulse rate is the same as your heart rate.

WHEN TO TAKE YOUR PULSE

Your nurse or doctor will tell you when to count your pulse. Some people take their pulse rates

- Before getting out of bed every day,
- Before taking certain medications,
- Before and after exercise/activity.

EQUIPMENT

Use a watch or clock with a sweep second hand or a digital watch that shows seconds.

STEPS FOR TAKING A RADIAL PULSE

1. Put the watch or clock where it can be seen.
2. Find the radial artery.
3. Use the pads of your middle three fingers. Do not use your thumb.
4. Press lightly until you feel the pulse. If you press too hard, you may stop the flow of blood; then you would not be able to feel the pulse.
5. If using a sweep second hand, begin counting when the sweep hand reaches the "12." Count each pulse until the sweep hand reaches the "6." Any number can be used to start counting the 30 seconds.
6. If using a digital watch, count the pulse for 30 seconds.
7. After counting the pulse for 30 seconds, double the number. For example, 35 pulses felt during 30 seconds equals 70 heartbeats per minute.

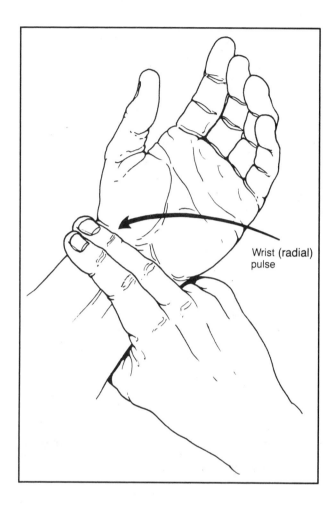

Wrist (radial) pulse

8. If you prefer, take your pulse for 10 seconds and use the pulse rate chart.

STEPS FOR TAKING A CAROTID PULSE

1. Put the watch or clock where it can be seen.
2. Find the carotid artery. First look at the neck for skin movement with each heartbeat. Look just to the side of the windpipe and in front of the neck muscles.

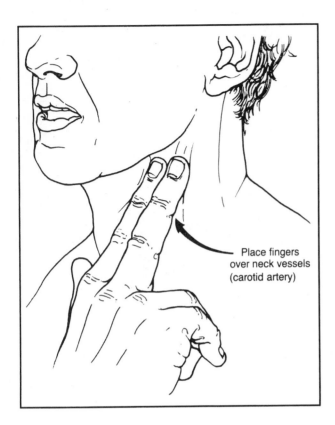

Place fingers over neck vessels (carotid artery)

3. Use the tips of the index and middle fingers. Do not use your thumb.
4. Place the two fingers lightly on either side of the windpipe.
   a. Slide the fingers gently to the groove between the windpipe and the neck muscle on the middle of the neck.
   b. Press lightly until you feel the pulse.

c. If you cannot feel a pulse on one side of the neck, try the other side of the neck.
d. Do not press on both sides of the neck at the same time. Do not press hard or massage this area while finding your pulse.
5. If using a sweep second hand, begin counting when the sweep hand reaches the "12." Count each pulse until the sweep hand reaches the "6." Any number can be used to start counting the 30 seconds.
6. If using a digital watch, count the pulse for 30 seconds.
7. After counting the pulse for 30 seconds, double the number. For example, 35 pulses felt during 30 seconds equals 70 heartbeats per minute.
8. If you prefer, take your pulse for 10 seconds and use the pulse rate chart.

10 SECOND COUNT PULSE RATE CHART (BPM = BEATS PER MINUTE)

8 = 48 BPM	18 = 108 BPM
9 = 54 BPM	19 = 114 BPM
10 = 60 BPM	20 = 120 BPM
11 = 66 BPM	21 = 126 BPM
12 = 72 BPM	22 = 132 BPM
13 = 78 BPM	23 = 138 BPM
14 = 84 BPM	24 = 144 BPM
15 = 90 BPM	25 = 150 BPM
16 = 96 BPM	26 = 156 BPM
17 = 102 BPM	27 = 162 BPM

RECORDS

Use this log for keeping track of your pulse rate.

PULSE RATE LOG

Date	Time	Pulse Rate	Comments

OTHER INSTRUCTIONS

Respiratory Alterations

Apnea Monitoring

GENERAL INFORMATION

Apnea is a pause in breathing. The pause in breathing can cause the heart to beat more slowly (bradycardia) or cause your baby to turn pale or bluish (cyanotic). There are many reasons why a baby has periods of apnea. In some babies it is unclear why there are pauses in breathing.

GUIDELINES

Use the following guidelines to help you remember how to take care of the Apnea Monitor and your baby and how to respond to the monitor's alarms.

The Monitor

1. Keep the monitor on a hard surface at the baby's bedside. Do not put the monitor on a mattress or padding, as this can muffle the sounds of the alarm.
2. Keep the Apnea Monitor alarm log and pencil with the monitor. Keep the telephone nearby, too, if possible.
3. Do not place the monitor on electric equipment.
4. Make sure the monitor has at least 8 inches of ventilation above and behind it.
5. Keep the monitor out of the reach of children.
6. Do not reset the monitor controls.
7. Use a grounded outlet or a grounding adapter. Do not plug the monitor into a circuit that carries other heavy-use equipment like a heater, hairdryer, etc.
8. Do not use an extension cord with the monitor.
9. Unplug the power cord from the wall when it is unplugged from the monitor.

10. Keep enough extra supplies on hand. A battery pack, two sets of lead wires, and four sets of disposable patches are recommended.
11. Keep the manufacturer's manual near the monitor.

The Baby

1. If there is any adhesive on the skin, remove all the adhesive by soaking a cotton ball or swab in baby oil or vegetable oil and gently rubbing the skin.
2. Always remove the monitor leads from the baby before washing the baby.
3. Wash the baby with mild soap and warm water only. Do not use baby bath products, lotions, and oils. Rinse away all soap and dry the baby well.
4. Check the baby's skin every day for redness or dry patches. Avoid placing electrodes on these areas.
4. Thread the leads out the lower ends of the baby's clothes.
5. Remove the leads from the baby unless they are attached to the monitor.
6. Remove, replace, and reposition the electrodes and belt every 2 days or if the electrode attachment becomes loose. Wash the belt by hand when it becomes dirty.
7. Place the electrodes symmetrically on the sides of the baby's chest.
8. Do not use an electrode belt on babies less than 9 pounds unless directed to do so by your doctor or nurse.

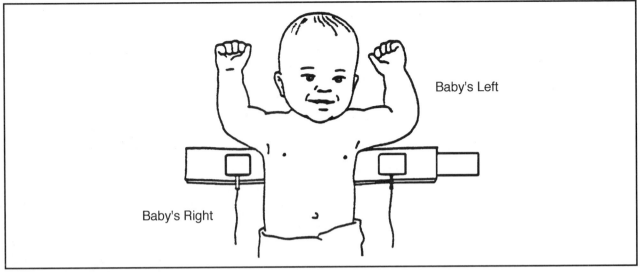

Courtesy of Respironics, Inc.

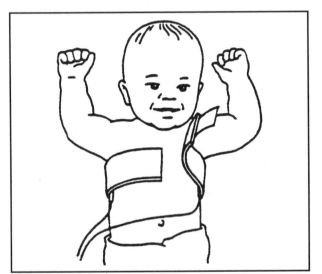

Courtesy of Respironics, Inc.

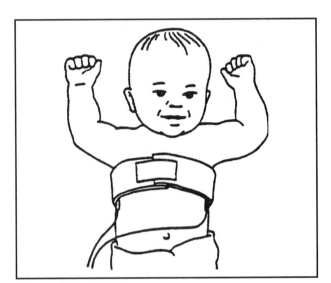

Courtesy of Respironics, Inc.

9. To feed the baby, put him or her in an infant seat that is inclined 35 to 45 degrees, or hold the baby in your arms, with his or her shoulders 30 degrees higher than the feet. Keep the baby in this position for 45 to 60 minutes after the baby finishes eating. Remove the belt and wires for 2 to 3 hours every day at a time when you can closely watch the baby.

10. Watch the baby carefully when he or she is not attached to the monitor. This is very important if you have a baby who falls asleep easily.

11. Be aware of the baby's skin color and how it changes when the baby is feeding, sleeping, and passing a stool and when the room temperature changes.

The Alarm

Responding to Alarms

The monitor can alarm for several reasons: apnea, bradycardia, loose-lead, low battery, or accidental shut off.

1. Respond to all alarms. You should reach the baby *before* 10 beeps (seconds).

2. Look at the baby.

3. If the baby's

   a. Color has changed (baby's color is gray, pale, or blue), gently touch the baby.

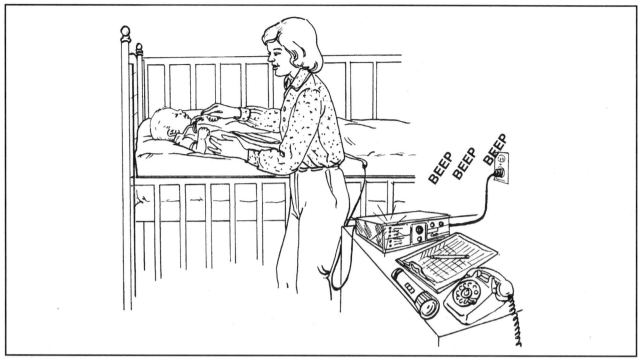

From Ross Laboratories: Apnea: Monitoring Your Baby at Home. 1993.

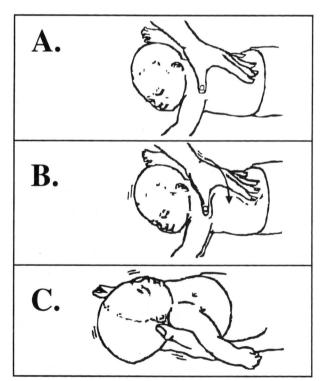

Courtesy of Respironics, Inc.

   b. Breathing has changed or stopped, wait until 10th beep *without touching* the baby.
   c. Check the pulse after the 10th beep.
4. For real apnea or low heart rate
   a. Gently touch the baby.
   b. Gently rub the baby's back.
   c. If your baby still does not respond, pick up your baby carefully, support the head, and turn the baby onto his back. **Never shake your baby**—you can cause injury.
   d. If the baby makes no response, start CPR. Ask a family member to call the Emergency Medical Services number.
5. For false alarms (the baby is breathing and pink)
   a. Check all connections and wires,
   b. Check the chest and the leads,
   c. If a battery is used, make sure the battery is charged,
   d. Reapply the belt securely,
   e. Change the wires,
   f. Check the manufacturer's manual; the response to the alarm may vary from monitor to monitor.

6. It is important to be able to hear the alarm. Do not shower, vacuum, use a hairdryer, or do anything else that would drown out the noise of the alarm, unless more than one person is at home with the baby.

7. Keep a written record of
   a. All alarms, how often they sound, and how long they last,
   b. The status of the baby during the alarms,
   c. The baby's symptoms before the alarms,
   d. How much stimulation the baby needed to be aroused after the alarms,
   e. All nonalarm periods of apnea and bradycardia, how often they occur, and how long they last.

8. Call the nurse or doctor if
   a. there is an increase in the number of "real" alarms,
   b. your baby's lips or skin turns pale, gray and/or blue,
   c. your baby needs stimulation to make the alarms stop,
   d. short episodes of apnea or bradycardia that do not set off the alarms occur frequently or persistently.

9. If your monitor does not have battery power when traveling in a car
   a. you must be able to keep your eyes on the baby at all times,
   b. you should have another person in the car when driving.

OTHER INSTRUCTIONS

CRITERIA FOR CONCERN
(to be filled in by the nurse)

When any of the following occur, call the nurse.

1. _____

2. _____

3. _____

When any of the following occur, call the doctor.

1. _____

2. _____

3. _____

When any of the following occur, call the emergency services.

1. _____

2. _____

3. _____

APNEA MONITOR ALARM LOG

SETTINGS: **Slow Heart Rate** _____   **Fast Heart Rate** _____   **Apnea Delay** _____

Event				
Date _____				
Time—AM or PM _____				
Number of Beeps Counted _____				
Baby				
Awake _____				
Asleep _____				
Breathing _____				
NOT BREATHING _____				
Color				
Normal Color _____				
Pale _____				
Blue _____				
Monitor				
Apnea Alarm _____				
Heart Rate Alarm _____				
Equipment Alarm _____				
Action				
Real Alarm _____				
Baby corrected _____				
Gentle touch _____				
Turn baby over _____				
CPR _____				
Other _____				

COMMENTS:

Bronchopulmonary Health

GUIDELINES

Your bronchopulmonary (respiratory) system, like any other part of your body, needs to be taken care of. The following are suggestions to guide you in helping your respiratory system work the best way it can.

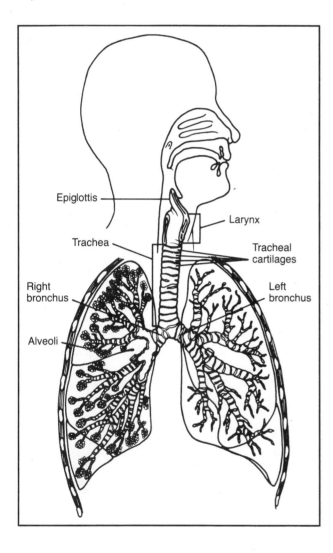

Epiglottis
Larynx
Trachea
Tracheal cartilages
Right bronchus
Left bronchus
Alveoli

Reduce Irritation to Your Respiratory System

1. Check air pollution levels and pollen counts every day. Avoid outdoor activity when the levels are high.
2. Keep the temperature in your home at about 70°F during the day and about 65°F during the night.
3. Use radiant heat and air conditioning.
4. Change or clean the air filters in forced air-conditioning systems at least monthly.
5. Do not use fireplaces and coal- or wood-burning stoves.
6. Use an exhaust fan in the kitchen and bathroom.
7. Avoid having heavy drapes and carpets in your home.
8. Cover mattress, box springs, and pillows with zippered covers (plastic or others approved by your doctor).
9. Wash bedding once a week. Wash and dry pillows once per month.
10. Wear a face scarf in cold weather.
11. Avoid people with colds and other respiratory infections.
12. Avoid cigarette smoke. Do not smoke. The benefits of not smoking include
    a. Coughing less,
    b. Renewed sensitivity to taste and smell,
    c. Increased resistance to respiratory infections,
    d. Reduced sputum (thick mucus) production.
13. Having a pet can be irritating to your airways. If you have a pet you may need to
    a. Bathe your pet regularly (weekly or monthly),
    b. Vacuum frequently,
    c. Use a HEPA air filter.
14. If you use a humidifier or vaporizer, thoroughly clean it regularly to remove mold.
15. Take your medications as directed.
16. Learn to avoid substances that trigger respiratory symptoms, especially if you have asthma. Examples are
    a. Strong odors such as perfumes / colognes, cleaning solutions, certain flowers, or pollen,
    b. Dust, pet hair, or feather pillows, especially where you sleep.
17. Drink warm fluids to minimize coughing spasms. Drink at least eight to ten 8-oz glasses of water every day.
18. Cough up lung secretions as much as possible. Call your doctor or emergency services immediately if you or your child
    a. Has difficulty breathing,
    b. Has severe wheezing,
    c. Needs to take medications, like an inhaler, more often than every 4 hours,
    d. Coughs up blood,
    e. Has a fever for more than 2 to 3 days.

OTHER INSTRUCTIONS

Oral Suctioning

GENERAL INFORMATION

The purpose of oral suctioning is to remove secretions (mucus, thick saliva, excess saliva) from the patient's mouth and upper airway. Suctioning is needed when the patient is unable to cough up the secretions, when he or she is drooling and is restless.

GUIDELINES

1. Wash your hands. Handwashing is the single most important factor in controlling the spread of infection.
2. Gather your equipment. You need
   - A suction machine,
   - A connecting tube,
   - A suction catheter with a control device,
   - Two nonsterile gloves,
   - A clean basin filled with tap water,
   - Two clean towels,
   - A clean 4×4 gauze pad,
   - A rubber band.
3. Help the patient into a comfortable sitting position, with the head and neck well supported. Turn the patient's head toward you. If the patient is unconscious, place him or her in a side-lying position, facing you.
4. Put a clean towel under the patient's chin.
5. Attach the connecting tube to the suction machine.
6. Turn on the suction machine.
7. Put on the gloves.
8. Attach the suction catheter to the connecting tube.
9. Put the tip of the suction catheter into the tap water and apply suction. This wets the suction catheter and lets you make sure the suction is working.
10. Take the suction catheter out of the water and release the suction.
11. Put the suction catheter into the patient's mouth, advancing it gently along one side to the back of the mouth. Do not apply suction while inserting the catheter.
12. The patient may cough while the catheter is being inserted. This is normal. Continue to insert the catheter to the back of the patient's mouth.
13. Apply suction and gently roll the catheter between your fingers as you withdraw it.
14. Suction for no more than 15 seconds. If the patient begins to make a crowing sound, stop suctioning, give the patient oxygen, and call the ambulance right away.
15. Put the catheter tip into the water and apply suction. This flushes the catheter.
16. Take the suction catheter out of the water and release the suction.
17. Repeat steps 11 to 16 until the patient's mouth is free of excess secretions or the patient is coughing out the excess secretions.
18. Put fresh tap water into the basin. Thoroughly flush the suction catheter and the connecting tube.
19. Turn off the suction machine.
20. Detach the suction catheter from the connecting tube. Cover the end of the connecting tube with a clean gauze pad, secure it with a rubber band, and hang it on the suction machine, with the tip pointing up.
21. Rinse the suction catheter with running tap water.
22. Dry the catheter and store it in a clean towel until its next use.
23. Wash the basin with warm water and soap. Dry it and put it away.
24. Remove your gloves and throw them away.
25. Help the patient into a comfortable position.
26. Wash your hands.

CARE OF SUCTIONING EQUIPMENT

1. Keep enough supplies on hand and ready for use.
2. Throw away collection canisters, connecting tubes, and suction catheters that are hard or cracked.
3. Attach a clean connecting tube to the suction machine as needed.
4. Empty the collection canister once a day.
5. Disinfect reusable equipment (collection canister, connecting tubes, suction catheters, basins) at least once a week.
   a. Thoroughly wash the equipment in warm soapy water. Rinse completely.
   b. Boil the equipment in tap water for 15 minutes.
   c. Let the equipment cool.
   d. Dry the equipment with clean towels.
   e. Store the equipment in clean plastic bags, fresh jars, or freshly laundered towels.

CALL THE NURSE

If any of the following happen, call the nurse or doctor:

1. The patient has a fever over 101°F.

2. The color of the secretions changes.
3. The secretions smell bad.
4. The patient has an increase in the amount of secretions, or the suctioning does not seem to be removing enough of the secretions.

OTHER INSTRUCTIONS

Oxygen Therapy

GUIDELINES

Oxygen can be dangerous if it is not used carefully and correctly. Follow the guidelines below to help you remember how to use oxygen safely at home.

1. Oxygen is a medication. Do not change the flow rate or pattern of oxygen use from that prescribed by your doctor. Your oxygen flow rate is _____ .
2. You may be asked to use a pulse oximeter to measure the amount of oxygen in your blood. When your baby needs oxygen, use the pulse oximeter at all times. The pulse oximeter range should be _____ .
3. Oxygen can be very drying to the nose. A bottle of water may be attached to the tubing for humidity.
4. Do not smoke near the oxygen. Oxygen makes smoldering fires, like cigarettes, burst into flame. Put easily seen "No Smoking" signs in the rooms where the oxygen is used or kept.
5. Do not use or store the oxygen near stoves, space heaters, or other heat sources. Oxygen under pressure explodes if it gets too hot.
6. Keep the oxygen at least 5 feet away from electric outlets and appliances. Do not use electric blankets or heating pads near the oxygen. Oxygen supports combustion.
7. Use all-cotton bed linens and clothing to prevent static electricity. Do not use polyester or nylon bed linens and clothing.
8. Do not use skin care products that contain oil or alcohol while using oxygen and for up to 6 hours after use. Do not use grease, oil, or petroleum-based products with oxygen. They are flammable, and oxygen remains in your clothing for as long as 6 hours after it is shut off.
9. Do not run oxygen tubing under clothes, bed linens, furniture, rugs, and similar objects. You should be able to see the oxygen tubing clearly at all times.
10. Keep the oxygen container in an upright position.
11. Turn off the oxygen when it is not being used.

This prevents oxygen leaks and lessens the chance of unexpected combustion.
12. Alert the electric company, the local fire department, and the local ambulance about the use and storage of oxygen in your home. Put their numbers and the number of your oxygen supplier next to the telephone.

SPECIAL REMINDERS FOR SPECIFIED OXYGEN DELIVERY SYSTEMS

Oxygen Concentrator

1. Do not use with extension cords.
2. Clean the filter at least twice each week.
3. If a power failure occurs, turn off the concentrator and use a back-up oxygen tank until power is restored.
4. Turn off the concentrator, use a back-up oxygen tank, and call your oxygen supplier if any of the following happen:
   a. The alert buzzer does not come on when the power switch is pushed.
   b. The power light goes out, and the alert buzzer goes on during use.
   c. The alert buzzer sounds.

Liquid Oxygen

1. Always keep the unit upright in a well-ventilated area.
2. Avoid touching the unit's metal parts with your bare hands, since frostbite may occur.

Compressed Oxygen

1. Keep the oxygen tank away from congested areas in your home.
2. Check your oxygen supply every morning. Always keep at least a 1 to 2 day supply of oxygen at your home.
3. Open the windows and call your oxygen supplier if
   a. The oxygen tank empties too quickly,
   b. The oxygen tank makes a hissing sound.
4. Keep in a well-ventilated area.

OTHER INSTRUCTIONS

Percussion and Postural Drainage

PERCUSSION

Percussion helps mucus move in the lungs. It is also called "cupping" or "clapping."

Infant

To percuss an infant, tent two or three fingers together. Use a brisk, but gentle, up and down wrist motion so that a hollow sound, like removing a suction cup, is produced. The sound should not be a slapping sound.

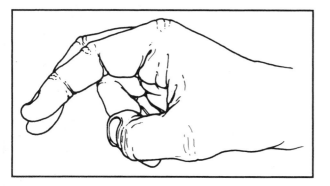

Child and Adult

To percuss an older child or an adult, cup your whole hand tightly together. Be careful not to use only your fingers or only the heel of your palm. Use a brisk, but gentle, up and down wrist motion so that a hollow sound, like removing a suction cup, is produced. The sound should not be a slapping sound. Use both hands in an alternating, rhythmic pattern. Percussion is done for 1 to 3 minutes in each prescribed position of postural drainage.

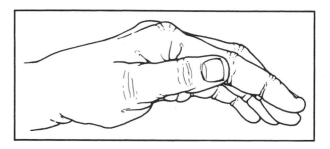

POSTURAL DRAINAGE

The patient can be put in a series of positions known as postural drainage positions so that gravity helps secretions move out of the lungs. The positions recommended for the patient differ according to which parts of the patient's lungs are most affected by the mucus. An infant or young child can be positioned on a pillow in bed or on your lap. Older children and adults can be positioned on an inverted chair, pillows, a stack of newspapers covered by a blanket, or a padded board. The following pictures show the various postural drainage positions.

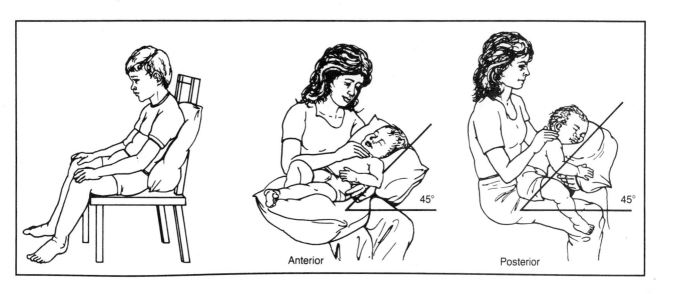

Anterior   Posterior

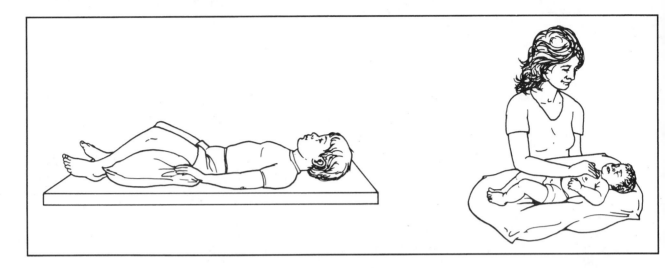

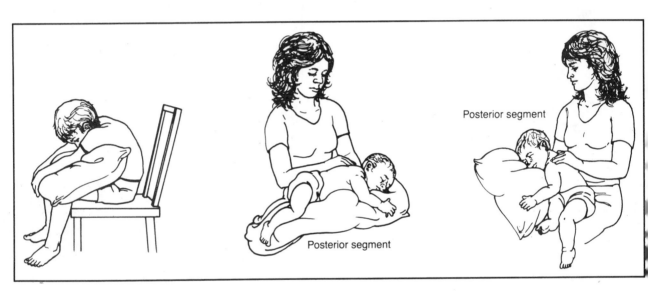

Posterior segment

Posterior segment

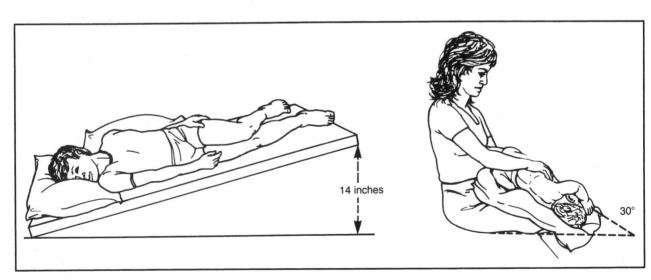

14 inches

30°

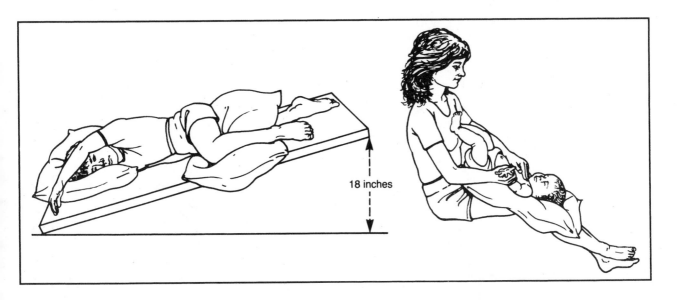

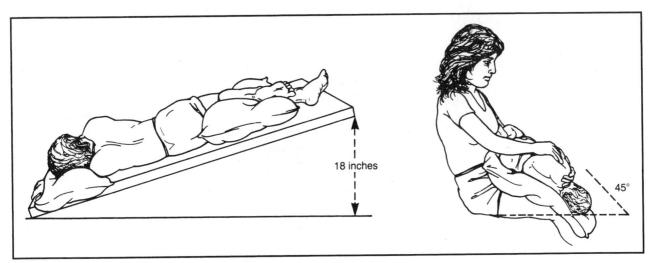

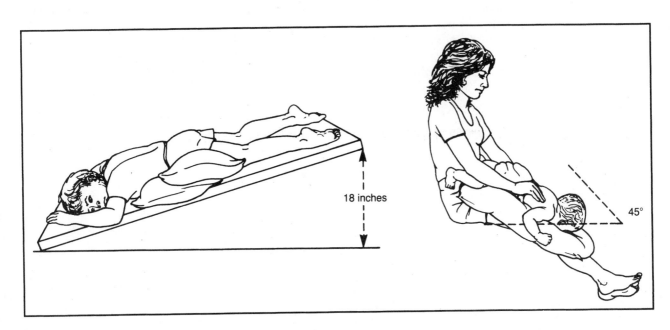

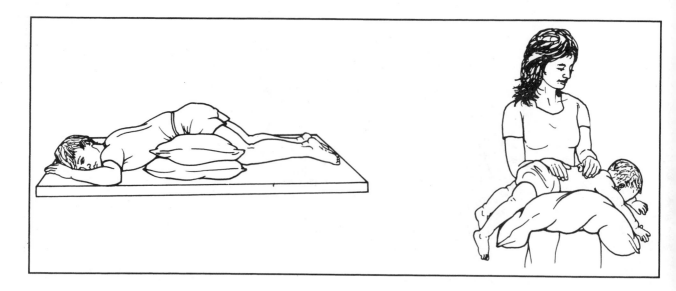

PERCUSSION AND POSTURAL DRAINAGE

General Guidelines

1. Percussion and postural drainage should be done at least twice a day: on arising in the morning and at bedtime. Percussion and postural drainage should be done more often when the patient has a cold or has a lot of secretions he or she is unable to cough up.

2. Percussion and postural drainage should be done long enough before meals so that the patient has enough time to rest before eating.

3. Nebulization therapy is done either before or after postural drainage, depending on the doctor's order. Your doctor has ordered nebulization BEFORE / AFTER postural drainage.

4. Protect the patient's skin from irritation during postural drainage. Have the patient wear a lightweight cotton shirt. Place a thin towel over the area to be percussed. You should not wear rings, bracelets, or low-hanging necklaces while percussing the patient.

5. If the patient has high blood pressure, dizziness, or arthritis, do not put the patient in a head-hanging-down position for percussion and postural drainage.

6. Do not percuss or do postural drainage when the patient is coughing up blood or having asthmatic episodes.

7. Limit the number of positions for postural drainage used in any one session. Four to six different positions are usually all a child can tolerate in one session.

8. Do not percuss over the patient's breast bone, spine, and kidneys. Do not percuss over any body areas that are tender.

9. Percuss and drain the areas of greatest involvement first.

10. The patient should cough two to three times after each position used during postural drainage. It is important to remind the patient not to suppress any cough.

OTHER INSTRUCTIONS

Tracheostomy Care

GUIDELINES

Use the following guide as a reminder of how to suction a tracheostomy, change a tracheostomy tube, and do routine tracheostomy care.

Tracheostomy Suctioning

The purpose of tracheostomy suctioning is to remove thick mucus and secretions from the patient's trachea and lower airway. Suctioning is needed when tracheostomy care is done or when the patient is restless, has blue-tinged lips, is wheezing, or is unable to cough up the secretions.

1. Gather your equipment. You need
   - A suction machine,
   - A connecting tube,
   - A sterile or disinfected suction catheter with a suction device,
   - A manual resuscitator attached to a source of oxygen,
   - Two nonsterile gloves,
   - A clean basin filled with normal saline or boiled tap water that is cooled to room temperature,
   - A clean 4×4 gauze pad,
   - A rubber band.
2. Help the patient into a comfortable sitting position with his or her head and neck well supported.
3. Wash your hands. Handwashing is the single most important factor in controlling the spread of infection.
4. Adjust the flow meter on the source of oxygen to 12 to 14 liters per minute.
5. Attach the connecting tube to the suction machine.
6. Turn on the suction machine. (Suction machine pressure for older children and adults is 100–120 mm mercury and 50–100 mm mercury for younger children.)
7. Put on the gloves.
8. Attach the suction catheter to the connecting tube.
9. Put the tip of the suction catheter into the filled basin and apply suction. This wets the suction catheter and lets you make sure it is working.
10. Take the catheter tip out of the basin and release the suction.
11. Tell the patient to turn his or her head to the left. This makes it easier to suction the left bronchus or airway.

12. Put the suction catheter into the tracheostomy. Gently advance the catheter until resistance is met. Pull the catheter back slightly. Do not apply suction while inserting the catheter.
13. The patient may cough while the catheter is being inserted. This is normal. Continue to insert the catheter.
14. Apply suction and gently roll the catheter between your fingers as you withdraw it. Steps 12 to 14 are called a pass of the suction catheter.
15. Suction for no more than 15 seconds.
16. Put the catheter tip into the basin and apply suction. This flushes the catheter.
17. Take the catheter tip out of the basin and release the suction.
18. Give the patient three hyperinflations from the manual resuscitator between each pass of the suction catheter. If the patient has a lot of thick secretions, increase the liter flow on the patient's regular oxygen delivery system and use it instead.
19. Tell the patient to turn his or her head to the right. This makes it easier to suction the right bronchus or airway. Repeat steps 12 to 18.
20. Repeat steps 11 to 19 until the patient's tracheostomy is cleared of secretions.
21. Put fresh saline or water in the basin. Thoroughly flush the suction catheter and connecting tube.
22. Turn off the suction machine.
23. Detach the suction catheter from the connecting tube.
24. Cover the end of the connecting tube with a clean gauze pad. Secure the gauze with a rubber band.
25. Hang the connecting tube on the suction machine, with the tip pointing up.
26. Rinse the suction catheter and store it with the other equipment that needs to be disinfected.
27. Wash the basin with soap and warm water. Dry it and put it away.
28. Remove and discard your gloves.
29. Help the patient into a comfortable position.
30. Wash your hands.

Changing a Tracheostomy Tube

The tracheostomy tube should be changed at least every 30 days. Change the tube before a feeding or wait at least 2 hours after a feeding.

1. Gather your equipment. You need

- A sterile or disinfected tracheostomy tube with an obturator,
- Clean tracheostomy ties (twill or bias tape) or tube holder,
- Clean 4×4 gauze pads,
- Water-soluble lubricant,
- Clean scissors.

2. Wash your hands.
3. Help the patient into a comfortable sitting position.

When Using Tracheostomy Ties

1. Measure and cut two pieces of twill or bias tape that are long enough to fold in half and fit around the patient's neck.

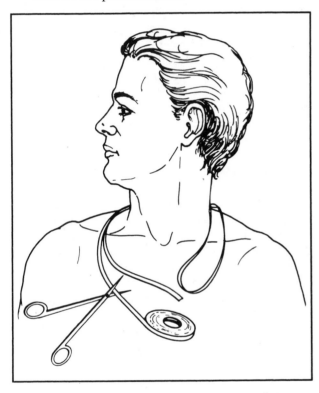

2. Fold one piece of string in half and bring it up through one hole of the tracheostomy faceplate.

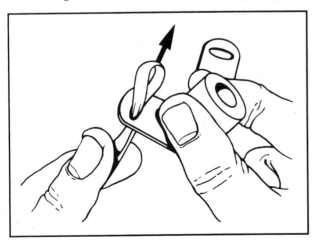

3. Bring the loose ends of the tape through the loop created by the folded end.

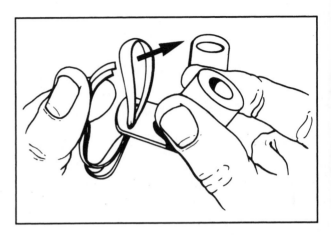

4. Pull the loose ends of the tape to tighten the knot on the faceplate.

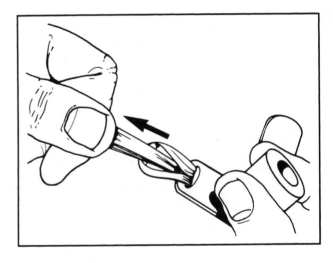

5. Remove the inner cannula of the disinfected tracheostomy tube and insert the obturator.
6. Lubricate the outer cannula and obturator tip with the water-soluble lubricant.
7. Cut the dirty tracheostomy ties that are around the patient's neck.
8. Remove the tracheostomy tube from the patient's neck by pulling it steadily downward and outward. The patient may begin coughing while the tracheostomy tube is being withdrawn. Wait until the patient stops coughing before continuing to pull out the tube.
9. Remove the dirty gauze dressing.
10. Tell the patient to take a deep breath as you insert the lubricated tracheostomy tube and obturator. If the patient begins to cough, hold the tube in place until the coughing stops.
    NOTE: If you are unable to insert the new tra-

cheostomy tube, reposition the patient's head and try again. If still unsuccessful, try to insert the tube you removed. If unable to do this, insert a suction catheter into the tracheostomy stoma (hole) and cut the catheter off about 6 inches above the stoma. *DO NOT LET GO OF THE CATHETER.* Take the patient to the emergency room. Do not leave the patient alone.

11. Remove the obturator.
12. Tie the tracheostomy ties. Pull the tape snugly and tie a square knot to one side of the patient's neck. There should be enough space for one finger between the tape and the patient's neck.
13. Insert the inner cannula and lock it in place.
14. Apply a fresh gauze dressing under the tracheostomy ties and faceplate by folding it as shown below.

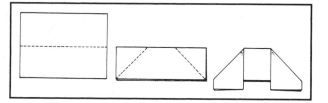

15. Discard the old tracheostomy ties and gauze dressing.

When Using a Tube Holder

1. Thread the long narrow fastener strips through the openings on the sides of the tracheostomy faceplate.

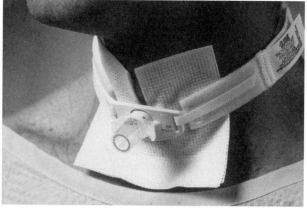

Courtesy of Dale Medical Products, Plainville, MA. Product No. 240: Tracheostomy Tube Holder.

2. Bring the strips over the flange on the faceplate and secure the rough side of the strip to the soft material on the band. Thread the long narrow fastener strips through the openings on the

sides of the strip to the soft material on the band. Allow a longer loop on the fastener tabs to keep the neck band from becoming soiled.

3. Remove the inner cannula of the disinfected tracheostomy tube and insert the obturator. Check the cuff.
4. Lubricate the outer cannula and obturator tip with the water-soluble lubricant.
5. Unfasten the dirty tracheostomy tab holder that is around the patient's neck.
6. Be sure to deflate the cuff before removing the tracheostomy tube. Remove the tube from the patient's neck by pulling it steadily downward and outward. The patient may begin coughing while the tracheostomy tube is being withdrawn. Wait until the patient stops coughing before continuing to pull out the tube.
7. Remove the dirty gauze dressing.
8. Tell the patient to take a deep breath as you insert the lubricated tracheostomy tube and obturator. If the patient begins to cough, hold the tube in place until the coughing stops.
   NOTE: If you are unable to insert the new tracheostomy tube, reposition the patient's head and try again. If still unsuccessful, try to insert the tube you removed. If unable to do this, insert a suction catheter into the tracheostomy stoma (hole) and cut the catheter off about 6 inches above the stoma. *DO NOT LET GO OF THE CATHETER.* Get the patient to the emergency room. Do not leave the patient alone.
9. Remove the obturator.
10. Secure the wide tab to the soft material for proper length. Cut off excess material. There should be enough space for one finger between the tape and the patient's neck.
11. Insert the inner cannula and lock it in place.
12. Apply a fresh gauze dressing under the tracheostomy faceplate by folding it as shown below.

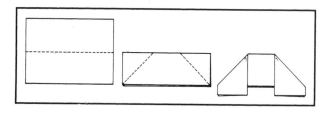

13. Discard the old tracheostomy tube holder and gauze dressing.

Next Steps

1. Wash the tracheostomy tube with soap and water. Store it with the other equipment that needs

to be disinfected. If you are using a disposable set, properly dispose of the tube.
2. Help the patient into a comfortable position.
3. Wash your hands.

Changing a Child's Tracheostomy Tube

1. Two people are needed when changing the tracheostomy tubes of infants and small children.

When Using Tracheostomy Ties

One person is responsible for holding the old tracheostomy tube in place after the ties are cut, removing the old tube, and securing the new ties. The other person is responsible for cutting the old ties, inserting the new tube, and holding the new tube in place until its ties are secured.

When Using a Tube Holder

1. One person is responsible for holding the old tracheostomy tube in place after the tube holder is removed, removing the old tube, and securing the new tube holder. The other person is responsible for unfastening the old holder, inserting the new tube, and holding the new tube in place until the new holder is secured. Children should be monitored to prevent unintentional unfastening of the holder.
2. Placing a rolled towel under the infant's or child's neck will make insertion of the tracheostomy tube easier.
3. Most tracheostomy tubes used for infants and children do not have inner cannulas.

TRACHEOSTOMY CARE

Routine tracheostomy care should be done once a day.
1. Gather your equipment. You need
   - Two nonsterile gloves,
   - A clean basin,
   - Hydrogen peroxide,
   - Normal saline or boiled tap water that is cooled to room temperature,
   - Clean 4×4 gauze pads,
   - Clean cotton-tipped swabs,
   - Clean pipe cleaners or a small brush,
   - Tracheostomy ties or tube holder
   - A clean towel,
   - A clean washcloth,
   - Clean scissors.
2. Wash your hands.

3. Help the patient into a comfortable sitting position.
4. Put on the gloves.
5. Suction the tracheostomy.
6. Remove the inner cannula. (If the tracheostomy tube does not have an inner cannula, go to step 12.)
7. Hold the inner cannula over the basin and pour the hydrogen peroxide over and into it.
8. Clean the inner cannula with the pipe cleaners or small brush.
9. Thoroughly rinse the inner cannula with normal saline or boiled tap water.
10. Dry the inner cannula completely with a clean 4×4 gauze. Make sure it is dry inside and out.
11. Reinsert the inner cannula and lock it in place.
12. Remove the soiled gauze dressing and throw it away.
13. Inspect the skin around the tracheostomy stoma for redness, hardness, tenderness, or a foul smell. If you notice any of these, call the nurse after you finish routine tracheostomy care.
14. Soak the cotton-tipped swabs in hydrogen peroxide. Use the swabs to clean the exposed parts of the outer cannula and the skin around the tracheostomy stoma.
15. Wet the washcloth with normal saline or boiled tap water. Use it to wipe away the hydrogen peroxide and clean the skin.
16. Dry the exposed outer cannula and the skin around the tracheostomy stoma with a clean towel.

When Using Tracheostomy Ties

1. Change the tracheostomy ties.
   a. Measure and cut a piece of tape long enough to go around the patient's neck twice.
   b. Lace the tape through one hole of the tracheostomy faceplate, around the back of the patient's neck, through the other hole of the faceplate, and again around the back of the patient's neck.
   c. Pull the tape snugly and tie a square knot on one side of the patient's neck. There should be enough space for one finger between the tape and the patient's neck.
   d. Cut, remove, and discard the old ties. (Do not cut the old ties until the new ones are in place and securely fastened together.)
2. Apply a fresh 4×4 gauze dressing under the tracheostomy ties and faceplate by folding it as shown in the illustration.
3. Wash the basin and small brush with soap and warm water. Dry them and put them away.
4. Remove the gloves. Throw them away.

5. Put the used washcloth and towel in the laundry.
6. Help the patient into a comfortable position.
7. Wash your hands.

When Using a Tube Holder

1. Change the tracheostomy tube holder.
   a. Thread the long narrow fastener strips through the openings on the sides of the tracheostomy faceplate.
   b. Bring the strips over the flange on the faceplate and secure the rough side of the strip to the soft material on the band. Allow a longer loop on the fastener tabs to keep the neck band from becoming soiled.
   c. Secure the wide tab to the soft material for proper length. Cut off excess material. There should be enough space for one finger between the tape and the patient's neck.
   d. Do not remove the old holder until the new one is in place and securely fastened together.
2. Apply a fresh 4×4 gauze dressing under the tracheostomy tape and faceplate by folding it as shown in the illustration.
3. Wash the basin and small brush with soap and warm water. Dry them and put them away.
4. Remove the gloves. Throw them away.
5. Put the used washcloth and towel in the laundry.
6. Help the patient into a comfortable position.
7. Wash your hands.

CARE OF TRACHEOSTOMY EQUIPMENT

1. Keep enough supplies on hand and ready for use.
2. Throw away collection canisters, connecting tubes, and suction catheters that are hard or cracked.
3. Attach a clean connecting tube to the suction machine every day.
4. Empty the collection canister once a day.
5. Disinfect reusable equipment (collection canister, connecting tubes, suction catheters, basins) at least once a week.
   a. Thoroughly wash the equipment in warm soapy water. Rinse completely.
   b. Boil the equipment in tap water for 15 minutes.
   c. Let the equipment cool.
   d. Dry the equipment with clean towels.
   e. Store the equipment in clean plastic bags, fresh jars, or freshly laundered towels.
6. Disinfect tracheostomy tubes at least once a week.
   a. Metal tubes—Wash with soap and warm water, using a pipe cleaner or small brush. Remove any tarnish with silver polish. Rinse the tube pieces well with running tap water and pipe cleaners. Boil the clean tracheostomy tube pieces in tap water for 15 minutes. Drain the water and let the pieces cool. Dry the pieces with a clean lint-free towel. Store them in a clean container with a lid.
   b. Plastic tubes—Wash with soap and warm water, using a pipe cleaner or small brush. Rinse the tube pieces well with running tap water. Soak the tube pieces for 8 hours in hydrogen peroxide. Rinse the tube pieces with rubbing alcohol. Rinse them well with boiled tap water. Dry the pieces with a clean lint-free towel. Store them in a clean container with a lid.
   c. Disposable equipment—Follow the instructions given by your nurse or doctor.

OTHER INSTRUCTIONS

Ventilator Care

GUIDELINES

Use the following guidelines to help you remember how to take care of the ventilator and the patient and how to respond to the ventilator's alarms.

The Ventilator

1. Do not reset the ventilator controls. Make a sign with the settings prescribed by the doctor. Put it on or near the ventilator. The settings prescribed by your doctor are
   - _____ Ventilator mode
   - _____ Airway pressure limit
   - _____ Positive end-expiratory pressure (PEEP)
   - _____ Respiratory rate
   - _____ Inspiratory time or inspiratory flow rate
   - _____ Expiratory time
   - _____ Tidal volume
   - _____ Heated humidifier setting
   - _____ Oxygen

   (*NOTE:* Not all settings above are found on all ventilators.)
2. Routinely check the ventilator throughout the day and before bedtime to make sure
   a. The settings are correct,
   b. The alarm lights are turned on,
   c. The humidifier is filled,
   d. The connections are secure,
   e. The tube is not filled with water,
   f. The tube is not kinked.
3. Position the ventilator close to the patient.
4. Make sure there is enough slack in the ventilator lines so that the patient can move his or her head without disconnecting the tube.
5. Keep the ventilator out of the reach of children. A childproof panel is recommended.
6. Use a grounded outlet or a grounding adapter.
7. Do not use an extension cord with the ventilator.
8. Keep enough extra supplies on hand. An extra tracheostomy tube with ties attached, a tracheostomy tube one size smaller, a manual resuscitator bag with an attached tracheostomy adapter, oxygen equipment, suctioning equipment, and a backup power source (12-volt batteries or an electric generator) are recommended.
9. Store extra supplies near the patient.
10. Keep the manufacturer's manual and troubleshooting guide near the ventilator.
11. Empty water out of the ventilator tube. Drain the water away from the cascade every 2 hours and as needed.
12. Clean the ventilator equipment (humidifier jar, tube, water traps, exhalation valve, tracheostomy swivel) every 2 to 3 days. Wash the equipment thoroughly with warm soapy water. Disinfect with appropriate solution. Rinse thoroughly with running tap water. Air-dry.

The Alarms

1. When an alarm sounds, check the patient.
   a. If the tracheostomy tube is out, replace it.
   b. If the tracheostomy tube is plugged, suction it. If suctioning is unsuccessful, change the tracheostomy tube.
   c. If there are air leaks, reinflate the cuff or change the ventilator tube, as necessary.
   d. If the patient shows signs of respiratory distress (restlessness, bluish lips and fingertips, yawning, sweating), remove the patient from the ventilator. Ventilate the patient with a manual ventilation bag until the reason for the alarm is corrected.
2. When an alarm sounds, check the ventilator.
   a. If the tubes are disconnected, reconnect them.
   b. If the nebulizer hood is off, replace it.
   c. If the ventilator has an internal mechanical problem, call the equipment supplier.
   d. If the oxygen or power sources are depleted, replace them.
3. Respond immediately to ventilator alarms.
4. It is important to be able to hear the alarms throughout your home.

CRITERIA FOR CONCERN
(to be filled in by the nurse):

When any of the following occur, call the nurse:

1.

2.

3.

Ventilator Care

When any of the following occur, call the doctor:

1.

2. ˙

3.

When any of the following occur, call the ambulance:

1.

2.

3.

OTHER INSTRUCTIONS

Ways to Save Your Energy

GUIDELINES

1. Pace your activities. Plan your day so you know what you are going to be doing at any given point of the day. Try not to fit everything into one day. Schedule only one big activity per day. (A big activity is one that tires you a lot.) Include "fatigue time" in your daily schedule. Fatigue time is a rest period and is an important part of saving your energy.

2. Sit instead of standing. Put chairs along the routes you most often walk in your home. Sit down when you feel like sitting: sit to sort through the mail, sit when you fold the laundry, and sit when you want to take a rest. Change your position often to relieve muscle strain.

3. Move slowly. Take your time and do not rush to get things done. Put a terry-cloth robe on after bathing and air-dry yourself instead of towel-drying. Wear loose, lightweight clothing and slip-on shoes to save energy when dressing and undressing.

4. Work at a comfortable height. This uses less energy than working at a height that is too high or too low. If you must bend down to do something, keep your back straight, flex your knees, place your feet apart, and use your thigh muscles to pull your body up and down.

5. Roll, push, or pull an object to save energy. If you must lift an object, pull in your abdominal muscles and squeeze your buttocks together. Straighten your back, place your feet apart, flex your knees, and use your thigh muscles to pull your body down. Bring the object toward you. Holding the object closer to you uses less energy than holding it away from your body. Use the muscles of your thighs to raise your body upward.

OTHER INSTRUCTIONS

Mental Health Alterations

Anxiety: How I Can Help Myself

1. Use relaxation techniques: deep breathing, muscle relaxation, imagery, meditation, reading, listening to soothing music, lying/resting quietly, limiting contact with others while anxious, taking a warm bath, listening to relaxation tapes.
2. Keep a log of events that come before, during, and after times of anxiety to identify anxiety patterns or themes of life associated with anxiety.
3. Set long- and short-term goals to get things done. Do only the important things. Break large tasks down into small manageable tasks.
4. Change your thinking by saying "stop" when you start to feel anxious.
5. Do your best to get regular exercise.
6. Take your medication as prescribed.
7. Don't stop taking your medication without checking first with your nurse or doctor.
8. Share your feelings with family members or friends.
9. Don't expect to get well overnight.
10. Be kind to yourself. Respect who you are.

OTHER INSTRUCTIONS

Anxiety Symptoms

1. Increased heart rate
2. Insomnia
3. Voice and hand tremors
4. Decreased ability to concentrate
5. Narrowed vision
6. Loss of appetite
7. Muscle tension
8. Dry mouth
9. Lack of coordination
10. Inability to move or make a decision
11. Frequent urination
12. Sense of impending doom
13. Cold and clammy skin
14. Easily startled
15. Headache, nausea, and vomiting

OTHER INSTRUCTIONS

Depression: How I Can Help Myself

1. Keep your appointments with your nurse and doctor.
2. Take your medications as prescribed.
3. Don't stop taking your medications without first checking with your nurse or doctor.
4. Try to get regular physical exercise.
5. Tell your nurse if your appetite decreases, you have less energy, or you are unable to sleep.
6. Avoid being alone too much. Share your feelings with family members or friends.
7. Telephone one friend or family member a day to discuss social things.
8. Change your negative thinking to positive. For instance, use the word "stop" when your thinking is negative, or make a list of five positive things about yourself.
9. Postpone making any major life decisions until you're feeling better.
10. If you are having thoughts of harming yourself or ending your life, call your nurse or doctor immediately.
11. Don't expect to get well overnight.
12. Be kind to yourself. Respect who you are.

OTHER INSTRUCTIONS

Nutritional Suggestions for Good Mental Health

RECOMMENDATION	EFFECT
1. Small frequent meals.	1. Stabilizes blood glucose with constant source of energy.
2. High carbohydrate intake.	2. Replenishes stored glucose and helps increase metabolism.
3. Moderate fat intake.	3. Helps possible weight loss.
4. Five fruits and vegetables/day.	4. Provides fiber and antioxidants.
5. Six to eight 8-ounce glasses of fluid/day.	5. Helps intestinal motility and prevents dehydration.
6. Nutritional supplements, especially B-vitamins.	6. Necessary for energy and metabolism.
7. Vitamin C.	7. Helps increase the immune response to colds.

OTHER INSTRUCTIONS

Reality Orientation

GUIDELINES

Reality orientation helps the confused person strengthen contact with the environment and improves the quality of interactions with others. The following are methods of reality orientation:

1. Identify the person's strengths and weaknesses; in this way you can adjust your expectations and efforts to his or her actual abilities.
2. Use nonverbal communication. Touching, stroking, and hand holding are especially useful for reminding a confused person that he or she is with people who care and are protective.
3. Make sure the person's eyeglasses, hearing aids, and other prosthetic devices are the correct prescription, are in good working order, and are being used.
4. Add memory-joggers to the environment.
   a. Use simple clocks with large numbers on the face.
   b. Hang calendars with large printing.
   c. Note the current day and special days by using brightly colored stickers on the calendar and wearing clothing or jewelry appropriate for the holiday.
   d. Keep window curtains and blinds open to see day and night.
   e. Use enough light in the person's room at night so that shadows are minimal and objects can be easily identified.
   f. Label cabinets, drawers, and appliances with identifying pictures, words, or both.
   g. Make a photograph album of clearly labeled pictures of family members, friends, pets, etc.
   h. Keep the person's personal belongings where they can be seen and where they are easily accessible.
   i. Help the person maintain a regular routine for meals, hygiene, and elimination.
   j. Include the confused person in family activities.

5. Keep your conversations focused. For example,
   a. Use your name and the person's name often during the conversation.
   b. Do not agree with inaccurate statements. Instead, describe the reality. Do not argue with the person.
   c. Talk about seasonal events during their particular time of year, for instance, Christmas caroling, Labor Day picnics, etc.
   d. Phrase your questions so that they only need a "yes" or "no" answer.
   e. Talk about the here and now, related past events, and the person's interests or hobbies.
6. Look directly at the person when talking to him or her.
7. Use very simple explanations when giving directions to the person.
   a. Break tasks down to their simplest steps.
   b. Use very specific and simple words.
   c. Allow the person time to finish each step before giving further instructions.
   d. When repeating instructions, use the same words.
8. Restrict the number of people who are with the person at any one time, but try to have at least one caring friend or family member with him or her as much as possible.
9. Provide diversionary activities for the person.
   a. Play memory games. Games for young children and those designed for playing while traveling in a car are especially good.
   b. Play the person's favorite records or tapes.
   c. Read aloud favorite books.
   d. Read the daily newspaper together.
   e. Listen to the radio or watch television together.
   f. Dance together.
   g. Paint or color.
   h. Write a journal, letters, stories, or poetry.
10. Create and maintain a safe environment. (The nurse can teach you how to do this.)

OTHER INSTRUCTIONS

When Sleep Is Not Restful

Here are some helpful hints if you are having trouble sleeping:

1. Avoid foods and drinks with caffeine (chocolate, cola soda, tea, coffee).
2. Do not take naps in the afternoon.
3. Do not eat or drink 2 to 3 hours before bedtime.
4. Create an evening ritual.
5. Use relaxation techniques at bedtime: deep breathing, muscle relaxation, imagery, meditation, listening to soft music, limiting contact with others, taking a warm bath.

OTHER INSTRUCTIONS

When To Call For Help

Living with someone who has a mental illness can be difficult. Often, family members are embarrassed by or ashamed of their situation. They are unsure of how others will react to hearing about the problems of living with a mentally ill person and so hesitate to share their feelings. Sometimes, even when they see worrisome changes in the person's behavior, family members are reluctant to reach out for help. They are afraid people will say they are overreacting or that they are not capable care givers. It is common for the family of a mentally ill person to feel isolated and alone.

However, help and support are available. The nurse can teach you about the mental illness and can help you deal with your feelings in a constructive way. When you are concerned about the way the mentally ill person is acting, you can ask yourself the following questions. If you answer "yes" to any of these questions, call _____, and tell them you need help.

QUESTIONS

1. Are the person's behaviors changing? Is the person acting differently than usual?
2. Is the person increasingly unable to cope with school, work, or personal needs?
3. Is the person unable to concentrate?
4. Is the person very anxious or fearful?
5. Is the person talking about fears that are not realistic?
6. Is the person withdrawing from usual activities? Is the person spending more and more time alone?
7. Does the person cry a lot and claim to have no energy?
8. Is the person unable to sleep?
9. Does the person claim to no longer have an appetite?
10. Does the person complain frequently about headache, indigestion, or constipation?
11. Does the person talk frequently about suicide or death-related topics?
12. Is the person a danger to self or to others?
13. Does the person express strange or outlandish ideas?
14. Does the person repeatedly express beliefs that are not true or that are impossible?
15. Does the person talk about hearing voices that no one else can hear? Does the person talk about seeing things that no one else can see?
16. Does the person constantly show anger that is out of proportion to the situation?
17. Is the person suspicious of others?
18. Does the person constantly and loudly blame others when things go wrong?
19. Is the person confused about his or her identity or where he or she is?
20. Is the person abusing drugs or alcohol?

OTHER INSTRUCTIONS

Cerebral Sensory Alterations

Range of Motion Exercises

General Information

Range of motion exercises can keep joints moving freely and fully. Exercise can also prevent deformities and loss of full motion of a joint. You can do the exercises yourself (active exercise) or you can exercise someone else (passive exercise). The drawings will help you do the exercises the way you were shown by the nurse.

Points to Remember

1. If you are exercising someone else, firmly hold the joint being exercised with one hand and use your other hand to create the movement you want.
2. Do all exercises in a slow, smooth motion.
3. Stop the exercise when you *feel* that the joint is no longer moving freely or when the person tells you he or she feels pressure or discomfort.
4. These exercises should be done _____ times per _____ .

Exercises

Shoulder and Arm Exercise (Over the Head)

1. *Starting position.* Place the patient's arm straight at the side, with the thumb up. Stand at the patient's side by the shoulder.
2. *Your hand position.* Place one hand above the patient's elbow. Hold the patient's hand with your other hand.

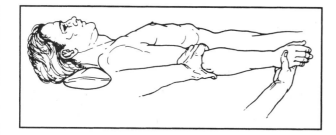

3. *Movement.* Lift the patient's arm over the head, toward the ear. Keep the patient's elbow straight.

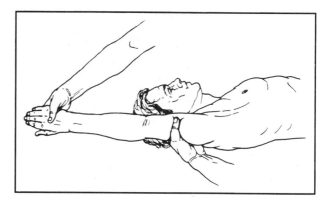

4. Return the patient's arm to the starting position.

Shoulder and Arm Exercise (to the Side)

1. *Starting position.* Place the patient's arm straight at the side, with the palm up. Stand by the patient's shoulder.
2. *Your hand position.* Place one hand above the patient's elbow and hold the patient's hand with your other hand.

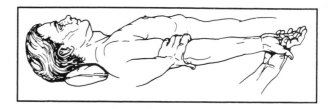

3. *Movement.* Move the patient's arm away from the side, around toward the ear. Keep the patient's elbow straight, the palm up, and the arm parallel to the floor.

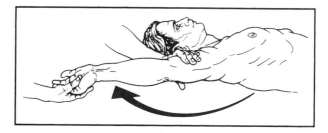

4. Return the patient's arm to the starting position.

Shoulder and Elbow Exercise

1. *Starting position.* Place the patient's arm at the side, with the elbow bent so the fingers are pointing toward the ceiling. Stand by the patient's elbow.
2. *Your hand position.* Place one hand above the patient's elbow and hold the patient's hand with your other hand.

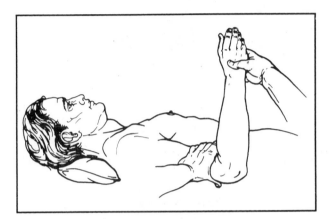

3. *Movement.*
   a. Lift the patient's upper arm so the hand moves across the chest.

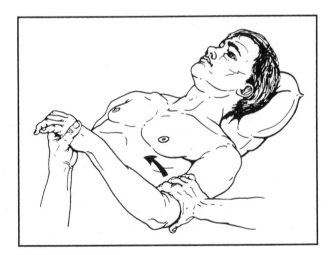

b. Turn the patient's upper arm out so the hand moves away from the chest.

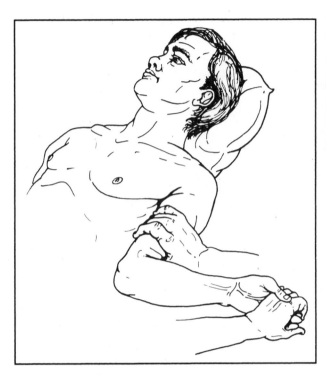

4. Return the patient's arm to the starting position.

Elbow Bending Exercise

1. *Starting position.* Place the patient's arm straight at the side, with the thumb up. Stand by the patient's elbow.
2. *Your hand position.* Place one hand above the patient's elbow and hold the patient's hand with your other hand.

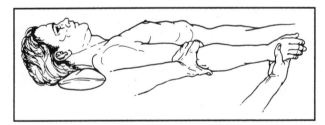

3. *Movement.* Bend the patient's elbow so that the hand goes toward the shoulder.

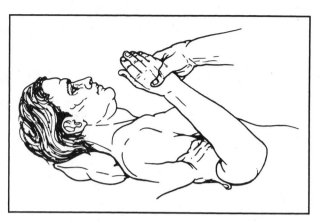

4. Return the patient's arm to the starting position.

Elbow Forearm-Turning Exercise

1. *Starting position.* Place the patient's arm on the bed at the side, with the elbow bent so the fingers are pointing toward the ceiling. The patient's thumb points toward the shoulder. Stand by the patient's elbow.

2. *Your hand position.* Hold the patient's hand with one hand and the patient's arm with your other hand.

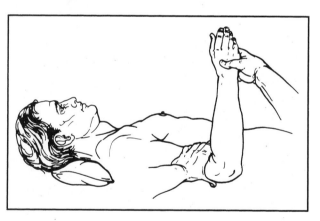

3. *Movement.*
  a. Turn the forearm so the palm faces toward the patient.

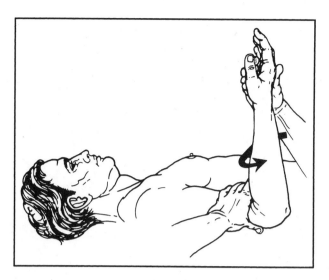

b. Turn the forearm so the palm faces away from the patient.

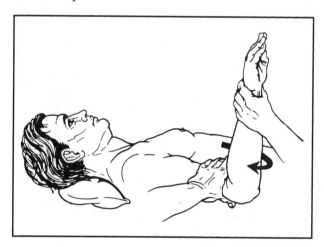

4. Return the patient's forearm to the starting position.

Wrist Bending Exercising

1. *Starting position.* Place the patient's arm at the side, with the elbow bent so the fingers point toward the ceiling. Stand by the patient's elbow.

2. *Your hand position.* Hold the patient's hand with one hand and hold below the patient's wrist with your other hand.

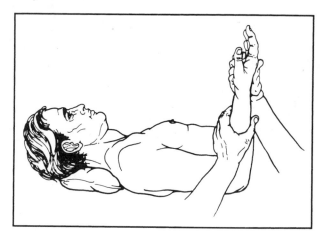

3. *Movement.*
   a. Bend the patient's hand backward.

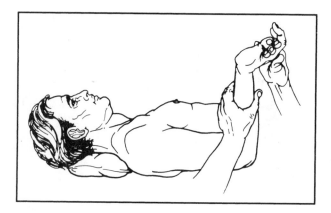

   b. Bend the patient's hand forward.

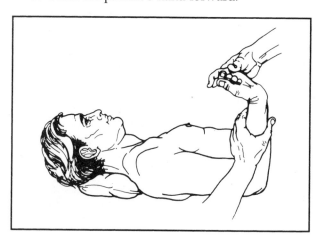

4. Return the patient's hand to the starting position.

Wrist Side-Bending Exercise

1. *Starting position.* Place the patient's arm at the side, with the elbow bent so the fingers point toward the ceiling. Stand by the patient's elbow.
2. *Your hand position.* Hold the patient's hand with one hand and hold below the patient's wrist with your other hand.

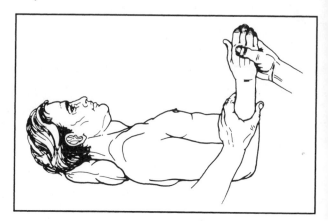

3. *Movement.*
   a. Bend the patient's hand sideways in the direction of the thumb.

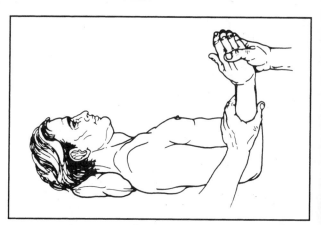

   b. Bend the patient's hand sideways toward the little finger.

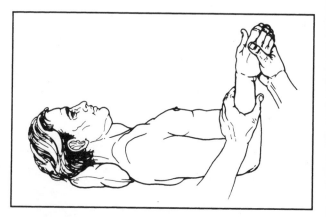

4. Return the patient's hand to the starting position.

Finger Bending and Straightening Exercise

1. *Starting position.* Place the patient's arm at the side, with the elbow bent and the fingers pointing toward the ceiling. Stand by the patient's elbow.

2. *Your hand position.* Place one hand palm down over the back of the patient's hand and support the patient's wrist with your other hand.

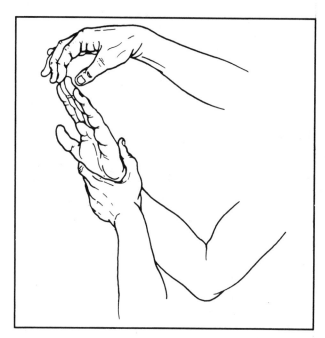

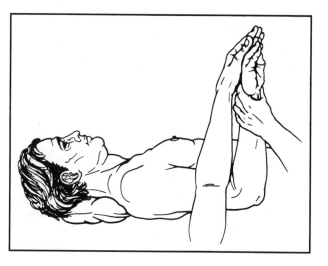

4. Return the patient's hand to the starting position.

Thumb Bending and Straightening Exercise

1. *Starting position.* Place the patient's arm straight at the side, with the palm up.

2. *Your hand position.* Hold the patient's hand with one hand and the patient's thumb with your other hand.

3. *Movement.*
   a. Help the patient make a tight fist.

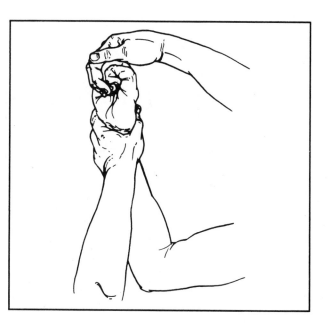

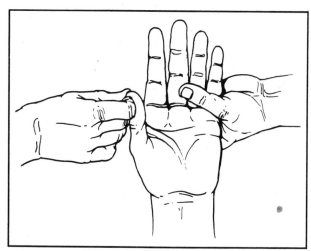

3. *Movement.*
   a. Bend the patient's thumb down into palm of the hand.

   b. Straighten the patient's fingers so the hand is flat.

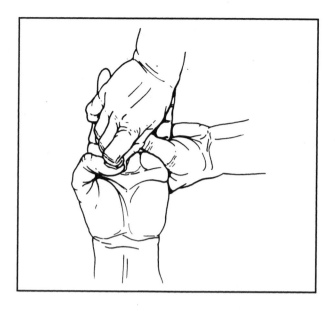

b. Straighten the patient's thumb to the "hitch-hike" position.

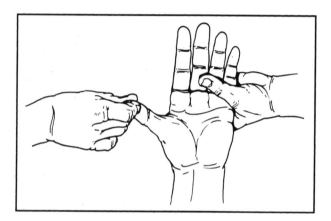

4. Return the patient's hand to the starting position.

Hip and Knee Bending Exercise

1. *Starting position.* Place the patient's leg out straight on the bed, with the kneecaps pointing toward the ceiling. Stand by the patient's knee.
2. *Your hand position.* Place one hand under the patient's knee and your other hand under the heel.

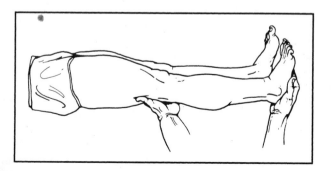

3. *Movement.* Bend the patient's knee toward the chest.

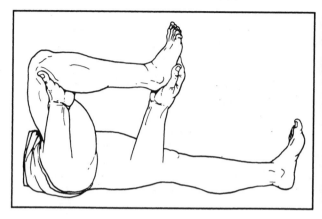

4. Return the patient's leg to the starting position.

Leg Exercise (to the Side)

1. *Starting position.* Place the patient's leg out straight on the bed, with kneecap pointing toward the ceiling. Stand by the patient's knee.
2. *Your hand position.* Place one hand under the patient's knee and your other hand under the heel.

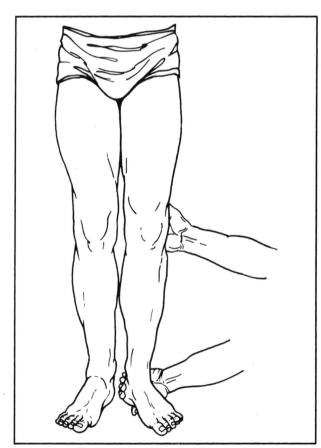

3. *Movement.* Move the patient's leg away from the other leg. Keep the knee straight and the toes pointed up. (To move the patient's leg all the way out to the side, you may have to take a step backward.)

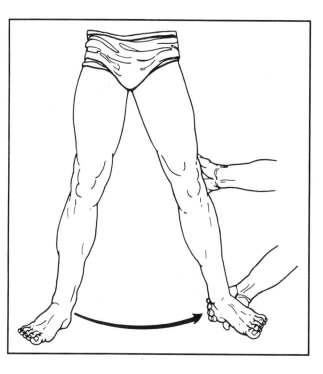

4. Return the patient's hand to the starting position.

Leg Raising Exercise

1. *Starting position.* Place the patient's leg out straight on the bed, with the kneecap pointing toward the ceiling. Stand by the patient's knee.
2. *Your hand position.* Place one hand under the patient's knee and one hand under the heel.

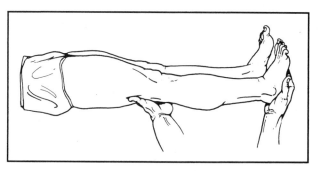

3. *Movement.* Lift the patient's leg up toward the chest while keeping the knee straight.

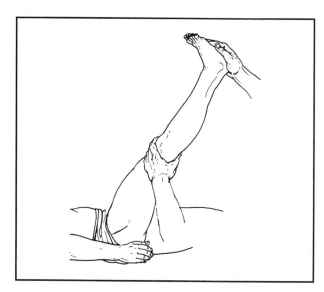

4. Return the patient's leg to the starting position.

Foot Exercise

1. *Starting position.* Place the patient's leg out straight on the bed, with the toes pointing upward. Stand by the patient's foot.
2. *Your hand position.* Cup the patient's heel in the palm of your hand, with ball of the foot resting against your arm. Place your other hand on top of the ankle.

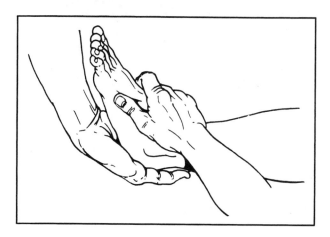

3. *Movement.*

    a. Bring the patient's foot up by pulling down on the heel and pressing up on the ball of the foot with your arm.

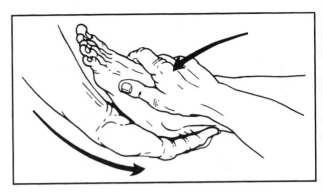

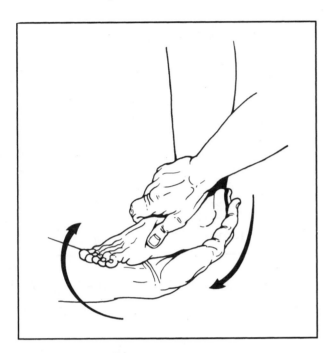

    d. Bring the patient's foot back to the starting positions, with the toes pointing toward the ceiling.

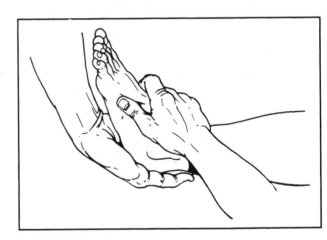

    b. Relax your arm and allow the foot to return to the starting position.

    c. Point the patient's foot down by pressing up on the heel and down on the foot.

OTHER INSTRUCTIONS

Warning Signs of a Stroke

GENERAL INFORMATION

A stroke is caused when the brain does not get enough blood. The stroke may be mild or severe and may last for a short time or be permanent. What the stroke does to the body depends on the size of the area and the place in the brain where the nerve cells die. A stroke can affect your movements, speaking, sight, reading, and ability to understand others.

Any of the following factors can increase the risk of a stroke:

- High blood pressure,
- High blood cholesterol,
- Heart disease,
- Diabetes,
- Cigarette smoking,
- Overweight,
- Relatives who have had strokes.

WARNING SIGNS

"Little strokes" may be warnings of a big stroke. Only a small area of the brain is involved. These "little strokes" may last only a few minutes or a couple of hours. They can have the same signs as a mild stroke.

Learn the warning signs of a stroke:

- Sudden weakness or numbness of the face, arm, or leg.
- Trouble with moving arms and legs, walking.
- Dizziness, tripping, or falls.
- Trouble swallowing.
- Loss of bowel and bladder control.
- Trouble talking or trouble understanding someone talking.
- Sudden change, loss or darkening of vision; you see double for a while.
- Sudden headaches for no reason; your headaches feel different.
- Change in your personality or ability to think.

If you have one or more of these signs, someone should call an ambulance or take you to the emergency department right away. Your body may be telling you something.

OTHER INSTRUCTIONS

Endocrine Alterations

Blood Glucose Monitoring

Blood glucose monitoring can help you better control your blood sugar (glucose) level.

EQUIPMENT

The equipment needed depends on the way you test for blood glucose. The equipment you need has been checked off by your nurse.

_____ Lancet (finger sticker)
_____ Test (reagent) strips
_____ Watch or clock that shows seconds
_____ Cotton (optional for some brands)
_____ Alcohol (optional)
_____ Automatic lancet device (optional)
_____ Blood glucose (reflectance) meter (optional)
_____ Log book
_____ Soap, water, and towel

STEPS

1. Gather the equipment and read the directions. Different brands may have different directions.
2. Look at the date on the test strip container.
   a. Throw out any out-of-date or discolored strips.
   b. When not in use, keep the container closed. Protect the strips from light, moisture, and heat.
3. Take out one test strip. Do not cut strips in half.

Obtaining a Drop of Blood

1. The earlobes and sides of the finger tips (not the pads) are sites that can be used to obtain a drop of blood. Change the site regularly.
2. Wash the site with soap and warm water. Dry the site completely.
   a. Warm water increases the blood flow.
   b. Careful drying keeps the test accurate.

   c. Wipe the site with alcohol *only* if you have been instructed to do so by your nurse or doctor.
3. When using the finger, hang your hand down by your side and gently "milk" the finger tip (squeeze and release) for 30 seconds. This will ensure a good drop of blood.
4. Twist off the cap on the lancet. Do not touch the sterile point.
5. If using an automatic lancing device, insert the lancet following your brand's directions.
   a. You can use alcohol to wipe the part of the device that touches the skin.
   b. Firmly hold the device against the site.

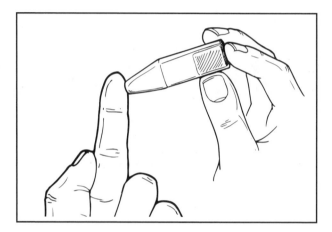

6. Puncture the skin.
7. Gently massage the site to get a large drop of blood.
   a. The drop of blood should hang from the finger (or earlobe).
   b. The drop of blood must be big enough to cover all of the test pad.
   Note: If you do not get a large enough drop of blood, repeat steps 2 to 6.

Performing the Test: Visual Method

Follow the directions on *your brand* for these steps.

1. Hold the test strip level and touch the blood drop to the pad.
  a. The blood must cover all of the pad.

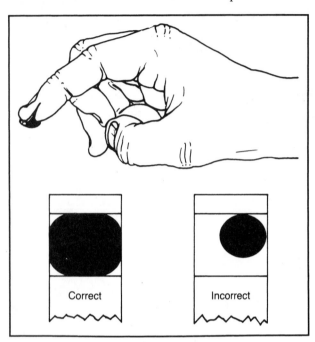

Correct   Incorrect

  b. Some brands do not allow you to smear blood on the pad.
2. Start timing as soon as the blood touches the test pad. The right timing is important.
3. Wipe or blot off the test strip.
4. Wait the amount of time prescribed in the directions to finish the test.
5. When timing is done, match the color of your test strip to the color scale on the container. The color that matches is your blood glucose (sugar) reading.

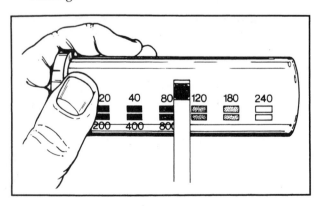

6. If the color of your test strip falls between two colors, the blood glucose is read as the range between the two numbers (for example, between 80 and 120).

Performing the Test: Meter Method

Since every meter is different in terms of the amount of blood needed, strip insertion, and timing, it is important to follow the steps in the educational pamphlet included with the meter.

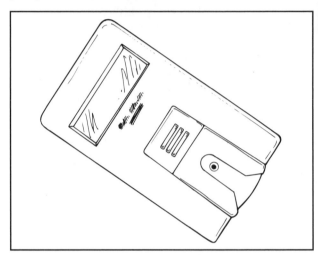

After the Test

1. Put the used lancet into a sharps container—a hard-plastic or metal container with a tight lid (such as a coffee can or laundry detergent bottle). Dispose of full container according to your local requirements.
2. Write your blood glucose reading, date, and time in your log book. Your nurse or doctor may tell you to write other things about your diet, exercise, and medication in your log book.
3. Look at any directions your nurse or doctor has given you about adjusting your medication, diet, or exercise. Discuss questions with your nurse or doctor.
4. If your nurse or doctor directs you, visually read test strips can be saved in a closed container for a few days. Write the date and time on each strip.

CARE OF EQUIPMENT

1. Store all equipment in a clean, dry place.
2. Wipe off any blood before storing the equipment. Use a damp, clean cloth or an alcohol wipe. If there is blood on the meter, follow manufacturer's recommendations for cleaning.
3. Check your meter for accuracy. Follow your brand's directions.

OTHER INSTRUCTIONS

Date	Insulin Type	BREAKFAST			LUNCH			DINNER			BEDTIME			Notes
		Insulin Dose	Blood Glucose Testing	Urine Glucose/ Ketone Testing	Insulin Dose	Blood Glucose Testing	Urine Glucose/ Ketone Testing	Insulin Dose	Blood Glucose Testing	Urine Glucose/ Ketone Testing	Insulin Dose	Blood Glucose Testing	Urine Glucose/ Ketone Testing	
	R N/L													
	R N/L													
	R N/L													
	R N/L													
	R N/L													
	R N/L													
	R N/L													

Foot Care

GENERAL INFORMATION

Foot care is important, especially if you have diabetes or poor circulation. Signs to watch for are cold or swollen feet; painful, burning or tingling feelings; lack of sensation (feeling); and slow healing of sores on the feet.

GUIDELINES

Check Your Feet Daily

1. Look for any infection (redness, swelling, pus, or pain), dry skin, cracks, blisters, cuts, and any changes in skin color or temperature.
2. Look at the tops and bottoms, between the toes, and around the toenails. Use good light; a mirror or magnifying glass can be helpful.

Wash Your Feet Daily with Warm Water and Mild Soap

1. Test the water temperature with your wrist before putting your feet in the water.
2. Soaking your feet is not necessary. It can be harmful and cause skin to crack and dry.
3. Dry your feet well, especially between the toes. Be gentle.
4. Use a mild lotion or skin cream daily for dry skin. You may use lanolin, vegetable oil, Crisco, Vaseline, cold cream, Nivea, and Eucerin. Do not use creams or lotions between toes or on open cuts.
5. Use a little powder for sweaty feet. You may use nonperfumed powder, talcum powder, or cornstarch to help keep your feet dry. Do not let the powder cake, especially between toes.
6. Use a small piece of plain gauze, cotton, or lamb's wool between toes if your toes overlap or if you have trouble with wetness between toes.

Cut Your Toenails Straight Across with Nail Clippers

1. Toenails are softer after bathing.
2. Use a file (emery board) to remove sharp edges.
3. Do not treat ingrown toenails or corns yourself. Call your doctor, nurse, or foot specialist.
4. Do not use chemicals (like iodine) or corn and callus removers.
5. Do not use razor blades, scissors, or other tools to cut toenails, corns, or calluses.

Wear Proper Shoes and Socks

1. Wear shoes that are wide and long enough to allow toes to wiggle without pressure. Shoes should be comfortable, fit well, and have good support.
2. Avoid shoes with seams or buckles that rub on your feet. Open shoes and sandals should not be worn if you have foot problems.
3. Buy new shoes in the afternoon. Your feet will be larger after walking for a while. Break new shoes in gradually.
4. Do not go barefoot, especially on hot sand or concrete.
5. Shake out shoes (to remove small objects) before putting them on.
6. Wear clean, dry socks or stockings every day. Socks should be colorfast and fit well.
7. Avoid tight socks, stockings, or garters with elastic tops.

Exercise Your Feet

1. Walking or doing other exercises your doctor or nurse has shown you can help your circulation.
2. Wear sturdy, comfortable shoes when walking.
3. Check your feet after exercise (for blisters, cuts, or redness).
4. Do not walk if you have pain or an open sore that rubs the shoe.

General Reminders

1. If you need help in caring for your feet, ask family or friends for assistance.
2. Do not put heat or cold packs directly on your feet (no heating pads, hot water bottles, or ice packs). Your feet may not have enough feeling to warn you of injury. Wear extra cotton socks or use a blanket to keep your feet warm at night.
3. No smoking. It is bad for your circulation. Crossing your legs also cuts down the circulation to your feet.
4. Eat a balanced diet. Limit the amount of cholesterol, saturated fat, and caffeine in your diet.
5. First aid for minor cuts and scratches:
   a. Wash the area with warm water and mild soap.

b. Dry your foot.

c. Cover the area with a dry, sterile bandage.

d. Use paper tape instead of adhesive tape.

6. Call your doctor or nurse if you have a foot infection (pain, tenderness, swelling, redness, pus, or a warm/hot area), an ingrown toenail, a problem cutting your toenails, or any foot problems or questions. Remember: early treatment can prevent major foot problems.

OTHER INSTRUCTIONS

How To Take Insulin

GENERAL INFORMATION

Insulin helps glucose (sugar) go from the blood into the body cells. The body uses glucose for energy. Insulin cannot be taken by mouth. It must be injected.

Insulin is made

- In different types: immediate-acting (lispro), short-acting (regular), intermediate-acting (NPH or Lente), long-acting (Ultralente or Protamine zinc), and pre-mixed (70/30, 50/50)
- In different strengths: U100 is common. The dose is measured in units.
- From different sources: human, beef, or pork.

GUIDELINES

It is very important to take *only* the type, strength, dose, and source your doctor has prescribed.

Your insulin is _____ .

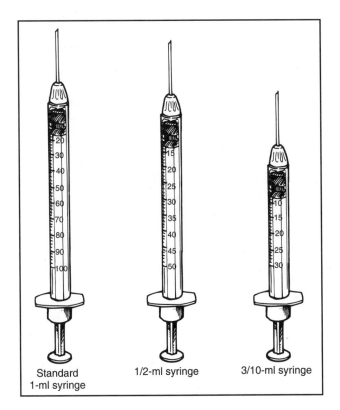

Standard
1-ml syringe

1/2-ml syringe

3/10-ml syringe

Learning about Syringes

1. Insulin syringes are made in 1-ml, 1/2-ml, and 3/10-ml sizes. The markings on each syringe scale are different. Use the syringe size your nurse or doctor has instructed you to use.
   Your syringe size is _____ .
2. To measure the insulin dose, look at the ring closest to the needle on the plunger tip. Your nurse will show you how to measure your dose.

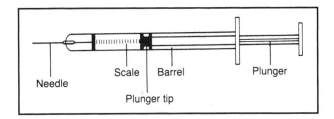

Needle   Scale   Barrel   Plunger
Plunger tip

Preparing the Insulin

Gather your equipment. You need

- Insulin,
- Needle and syringe,
- Alcohol wipe (or cotton ball moistened with isopropyl alcohol),
- Record of injection sites.

1. Wash your hands.
2. Check the insulin bottle for
   a. The right strength and type of insulin on the label,
   b. The expiration date on the label,
   c. Any floating objects or cracks in the bottle.
3. For an unopened bottle, flip off the plastic cap.

4. Roll the insulin bottle back and forth between your palms to mix the insulin. Do not shake the bottle.

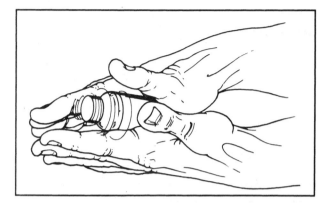

5. Clean the top of the insulin bottle with an alcohol wipe.
6. Draw air into the syringe by pulling back on the plunger. The amount of air should be the same as your insulin dose.
7. Take off the needle cap. Do not allow the needle or insulin bottle top to touch anything. Push the needle through the center of the rubber top of the insulin bottle. Push the plunger in.

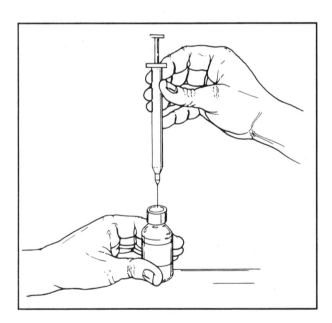

8. Turn the syringe and bottle upside down.
   a. Keep the needle tip covered by insulin. This prevents air bubbles from entering the syringe.
   b. Hold the syringe and bottle in one hand.
9. With your other hand, pull back slowly on the plunger until the right dose of insulin is in the syringe.

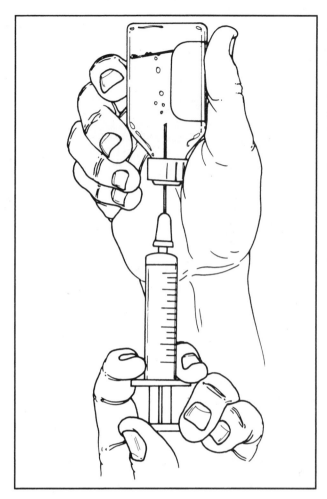

10. Check for air bubbles in the syringe.
    a. To remove air bubbles, lightly tap the syringe and then push in the plunger until the bubbles are gone.
    b. If you need to, pull the plunger down until you have the right dose of insulin in the syringe again.
11. Double check the insulin dose in the syringe.
12. Pull the needle and syringe out of the bottle. Put on the needle cover.

Sites for Injection

1. Use the areas marked on the body drawing (pp. 117 and 118). Follow your nurse's or doctor's directions for other areas and for rotation patterns.
2. Change (rotate) the site according to the instructions your nurse or doctor gives you. Don't stay in one area for more than a week.
3. Keep a record of your injection sites (include the date and time). You may use the body drawing to keep a record of injection sites by filling in the date in the appropriate box.

4. Use as many sites as possible.
   a. Avoid skin that is raised, thickened, very thin, or infected.
   b. Use the stomach sites on days when you will be doing activities that involve exercising the legs and arms.
   c. Remember that hot packs or hot baths can increase the rate insulin is absorbed.

Injecting Insulin

1. Check your injection site record to choose a new site.
2. Clean the injection site with an alcohol wipe and allow it to air dry. Keep the alcohol wipe within reach.
3. Hold the syringe like a pencil. Remove the needle cap without touching the needle.
4. With the other hand, pinch up about a 2- to 3-inch area of cleaned skin. Do not touch the skin where the needle will go.
5. Quickly push the needle into the skin (45–90 degree angle).

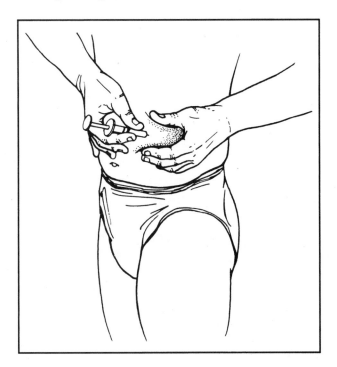

6. With one free finger, push the plunger all the way down.
7. Pull out the needle and press lightly on the site for a few seconds with the alcohol wipe.
8. Put on the needle cap or use the needle clippers.
9. Put used needles/syringes into a sturdy container such as a coffee can or laundry detergent bottle with a tight lid. Keep this container away from children.
10. Dispose of full container according to your local requirements.
11. Write the date, time, and site used in your record book.

Other Insulin Delivery Systems

1. Devices such as the insulin pen and insulin pump require specific training according to the individual manufacturer's recommendations.

Special Note: Reusing Syringes

Some patients are able to use the needle and syringe more than once to save money. Talk to your doctor or nurse about syringe reuse *before* you try it. Do not reuse bent needles or syringes that have fallen on the floor.

Safety Precautions

1. The insulin bottle you are now using should be kept at stable room temperature.
2. Keep your extra insulin bottle(s) refrigerated.
3. Keep insulin out of heat, sunlight, or freezing cold. Throw away insulin if it freezes.
4. When you are traveling, keep your insulin and syringes with you. Ask your physician for a prescription for syringes and your type and dose of insulin (in case you lose your supplies).
5. Never switch insulin without consulting your doctor.
6. Always carry some form of medical identification with you.

OTHER INSTRUCTIONS

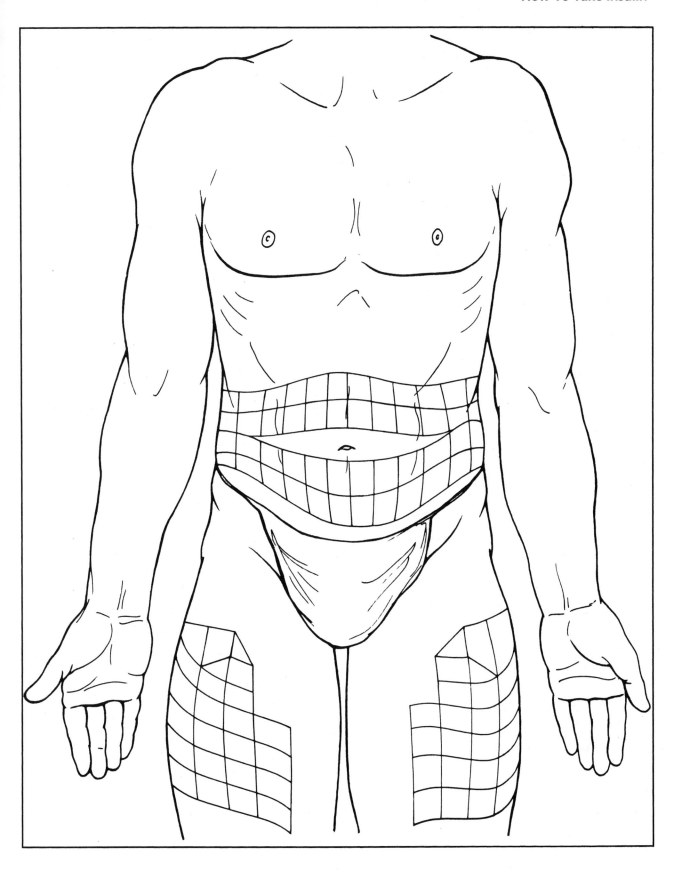

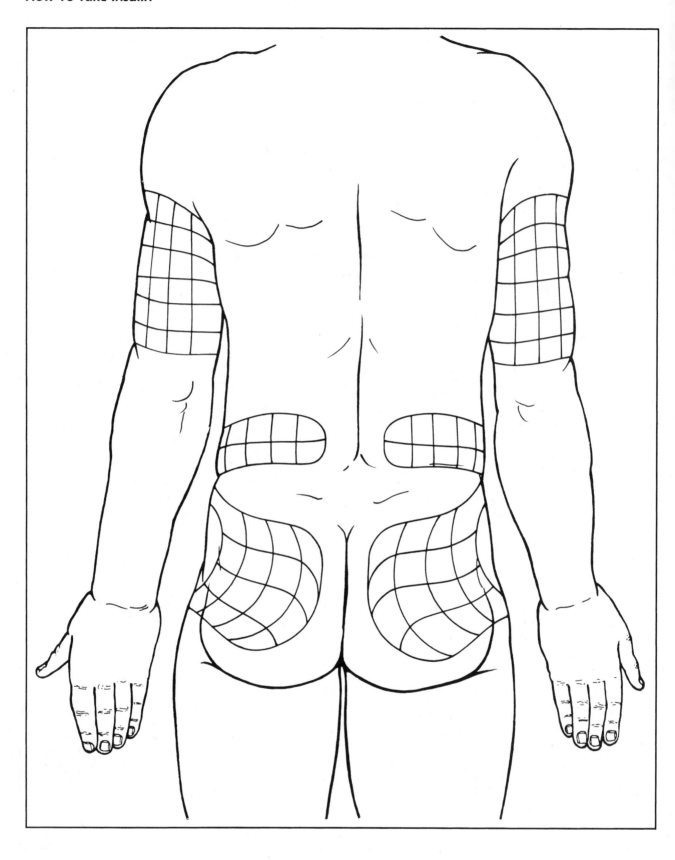

Hyperglycemia

GENERAL INFORMATION

A high blood glucose (sugar) level is called hyperglycemia. It develops when there is not enough insulin. If not treated, hyperglycemia can lead to complications known as ketoacidotic coma and hyperosmolar coma.

Ketoacidosis is most common in people with type 1 (insulin-dependent) diabetes. This type usually develops over a few hours or days. Urine tests show moderate to high levels of ketones. Hyperosmolar coma occurs in people with type 2 (non–insulin-dependent) diabetes. This type is more common in the elderly, especially during illness. It may take days or even weeks to develop.

GUIDELINES

It is important to learn how your body feels with high blood sugar so that you can take action right away (see table below).

PREVENTION

1. Follow your diet, medication, activity, and blood or urine testing plan properly.
2. Tell any new doctor or dentist that you have diabetes before you have any procedure or operation done.
3. Sick-day guides:
   a. Check with your doctor or nurse for specific directions.
   b. Treat all illness seriously.
   c. Take insulin or diabetes pills as directed.
   d. Test your urine or blood for sugar. Test your urine for ketones if instructed to do so by your doctor or nurse every 4 hours and if your blood sugar is over 240 milligrams / deciliter. Record the results.
   e. Drink fluids often. Drink about half a cup of water, tea, or broth every hour.
   f. Try to eat normally.
4. Remember, call your doctor or nurse if:
   a. You are sick more than 24 hours and are not getting better.

	High (250–350 mg/dl)	Very High (over 350 mg/dl)
WHAT IT FEELS LIKE (SYMPTOMS)	Increased urination Increased thirst Tiredness, weakness Blurred vision	Same as for high blood sugar but with Loss of appetite, feeling ill Nausea, vomiting Stomach pain Dehydration (dry mouth and skin) Fruity, acetone breath Deep, rapid breathing Drowsiness, mental dullness Unconsciousness Ketones in urine
WHAT CAUSES IT	Too little insulin or diabetes pills Too much or the wrong type of food Infection, illness, injury, or operation Emotional stress Decreased activity (without adjusting food intake) Previously undiagnosed diabetes Pregnancy	Same as for high blood sugar Ignored or not properly treated high blood sugar
WHAT TO DO (TREATMENT)	Follow your meal, medication, and activity plan properly Follow the sick-day guides your doctor or nurse has given you Test your urine for ketones Call your doctor or nurse when you have an infection or have been sick more than 24 hours (without getting better) Call your family or friends for help if you cannot take care of yourself	Call your doctor or nurse immediately. You need treatment quickly Call your emergency number if you cannot reach your doctor or nurse Test your urine for ketones

b. Your blood sugar is over 240 milligrams/deciliter for two tests in a row.

c. Your urine shows moderate to high levels of ketones.

d. You have symptoms of very high sugar levels.

e. You are not able to eat.

SPECIAL NOTES

If you have experienced low blood sugar levels within the past 24 hours, your body may release a hormone that may make your blood sugar levels high for several readings. This is called rebounding. The blood sugar level should return to normal after several readings. If you call your doctor or nurse, inform him or her you experienced low blood sugar levels *before* having high blood glucose levels.

OTHER INSTRUCTIONS

Hypoglycemia

GENERAL INFORMATION

Low blood glucose (sugar) is known by several names: hypoglycemia, insulin reaction, or insulin shock. Hypoglycemia has many causes (see table below). It can occur quickly, especially if you are taking insulin.

GUIDELINES

It is important to learn how your body feels with low blood sugar so that you can take action right away.

Special Note

Once the symptoms are gone, if you must wait more than 30 minutes until your next meal; eat a snack (half a sandwich, cheese and crackers, or a banana and half a cup of skim milk). Any food used to treat reactions is in addition to your regular meal plan; do not subtract this food from your next meal.

IF THE SYMPTOMS ARE NOT GONE WITHIN 30 MINUTES, CALL A FRIEND OR THE EMERGENCY NUMBER FOR HELP.

PREVENTION

Follow your doctor's or nurse's instructions:

1. Eat your snack before vigorous exercise.
2. Be alert for low blood sugar signs before meals, during and after exercise, and during your medication's peak action (especially with insulin).
3. Stay on your diabetic plan for food, medication, and exercise.
   a. Be alert for changes in your daily routine that can affect your blood sugar levels.

	Very Low (under 40 mg/dl) Severe Reaction	Low (40–65 mg/dl) Mild Reaction
WHAT IT FEELS LIKE (SYMPTOMS)	Confusion Personality changes, acting differently than usual Poor coordination, clumsiness Slurred speech Twitching muscles Pounding heart Increased weakness Convulsions Drowsiness, loss of consciousness	Shakiness and nervousness Sweaty, cold and clammy skin Sudden hunger Rapid heart rate Feel weak or lightheaded Blurred or double vision Headache Tingling or numb lips or tongue Nausea Nightmares or crying out during sleep
WHAT CAUSES IT	Ignored or not properly treated mild hypoglycemia	Too much insulin or too many diabetes pills Too little food, the wrong type of food, late or missed meals Too much exercise without eating enough A combination of the above Vomiting your last meal Use of medicines that can lower blood sugar levels Alcoholic beverages (especially on an empty stomach)
WHAT TO DO (TREATMENT)	Eat one of the simple sugars listed for mild reaction but use up to twice the amount indicated *If* you *become unconscious*, your family or friends should: call the emergency number, rub a thick form of sugar on the inside of your cheek or under your tongue (Monogel, Cake-Mate, or Instaglucose), turn your face toward the floor with it resting on your arms, inject glucagon	Eat one of the following: simple sugars (15 grams of carbohydrate will relieve most symptoms): 6 lifesavers, jelly beans, or sugar cubes; 4 ounces (1/2 cup) of orange or grapefruit juice; 4 ounces (1/2 cup) of regular soft drink (not diet); 2–3 glucose tablets; 2 tablespoons (1 small box) of raisins Repeat one of the above if you still have symptoms after 10–15 minutes

b. Do not skip or delay meals.

4. Before taking any other medications, even non-prescription ones, check with your doctor or nurse.

5. Always carry medical identification and some form of simple sugar with you. Take the simple sugar as soon as symptoms are felt.

6. Show family members and friends where you keep your emergency glucagon kit and how to give glucagon.

7. When you have a low blood sugar reaction, write down the date and time of day as well as your diet, exercise, and medication. Call your nurse or doctor with this information if
   a. The symptoms stay the same or become worse after treatments,
   b. You have repeated hypoglycemic reactions,
   c. You have any reactions while you are taking pills for diabetes control.

8. Follow your plan for monitoring your blood sugar level or testing your urine.

9. Only blood sugar testing can show low sugar levels. Ask your doctor or nurse before using alcoholic beverages. Alcoholic beverages would need to be made part of your diet plan.

Special Note

After having hypoglycemia, the body sometimes tries to compensate by releasing a hormone that increases the blood sugar level. This is called rebounding (Somogyi effect). You may find your next few blood sugar readings may be high after you have had hypoglycemia. The sugar levels usually return to normal within 24 hours. If you have questions, call your doctor or nurse before adjusting your insulin levels.

OTHER INSTRUCTIONS

Insulin Action

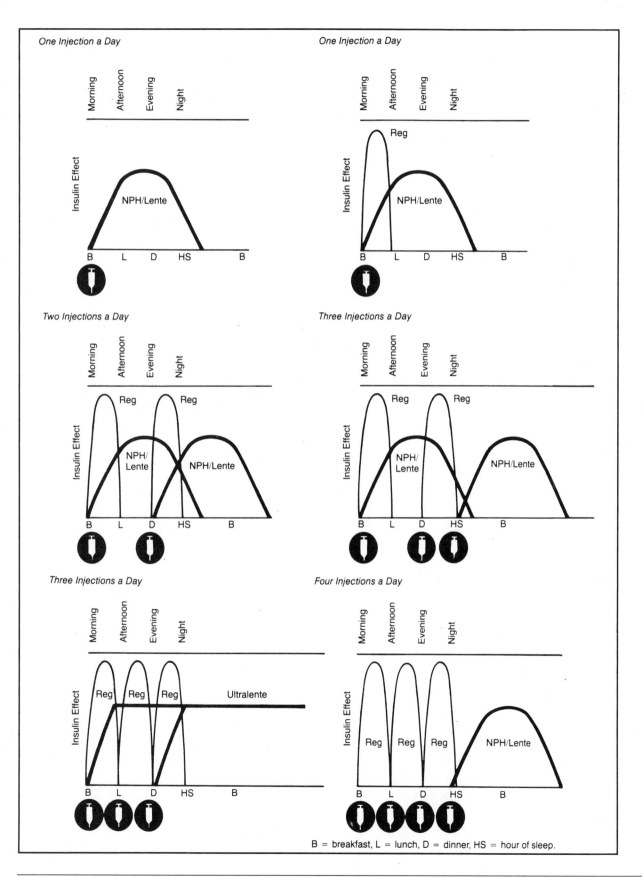

One Injection a Day

One Injection a Day

Two Injections a Day

Three Injections a Day

Three Injections a Day

Four Injections a Day

B = breakfast, L = lunch, D = dinner, HS = hour of sleep.

OTHER INSTRUCTIONS

Mixing Insulin

GENERAL INFORMATION

Your doctor may prescribe a combination of insulin types. By mixing the shorter-acting (regular) and longer-acting (NPH/Lente) insulins, you can give one injection.

EQUIPMENT

- Insulin: both shorter-acting (regular) and longer-acting (NPH/Lente)
- Needle and syringe
- Alcohol wipe or cotton ball moistened with isopropyl alcohol

STEPS

1. Wash hands.
2. Roll each insulin bottle back and forth between your palms to mix the insulin. Do not shake the bottle.

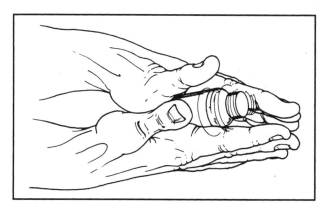

3. Clean the top of each insulin bottle with an alcohol wipe.
4. Draw air into the syringe equal to the dose of the longer-acting insulin by pulling back on the plunger.
5. Stick the needle through the rubber top of the *longer-acting* insulin bottle. Push the plunger in.
6. Pull out the *empty* needle and syringe *without* removing any insulin.
7. Draw air into the syringe again, equal to the dose of the *shorter-acting* insulin.
8. Stick the needle into the *shorter-acting* insulin bottle. Push the plunger in.

9. Turn the syringe and bottle upside down. Hold at eye level.
   a. Keep the needle tip covered by insulin to prevent air bubbles in the syringe.
   b. Hold the syringe and bottle in one hand.

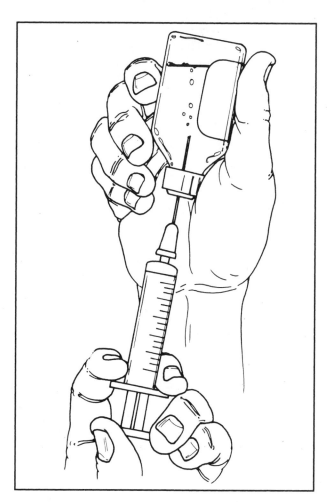

10. With your other hand, pull back slowly on the plunger until the right dose of the *shorter-acting* insulin is in the syringe.
11. Check for air bubbles in the syringe.
    a. To remove air bubbles, lightly tap the syringe and then push in the plunger until the bubbles are gone.
    b. Pull the plunger down until you have the right dose of insulin in the syringe again.

12. Double check the insulin dose in the syringe and pull the needle and syringe from the bottle.
13. Put the same needle and syringe into the bottle of *longer-acting* insulin.
14. Turn the syringe and bottle upside down.
15. Keep the needle tip covered by insulin to prevent air bubbles in the syringe.
16. *Slowly* pull down on the plunger to the number of units in the *total* dose:
    a. Do not go past the number of units in *your* dose.
    b. Do not push any insulin back into the bottle. *For example only*: if you wanted to take 6 units of regular (shorter-acting insulin) and 20 units of NPH/Lente (longer-acting insulin), your total number of units would be 26.
17. Always double check the insulin dose in the syringe.

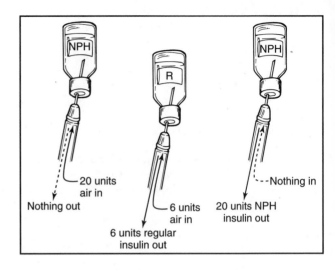

18. Pull the needle and syringe out of the bottle and put on the needle cap.

OTHER INSTRUCTIONS

Oral Hypoglycemic Medications

GENERAL INFORMATION

Oral (by mouth) hypoglycemic medications are sometimes called "diabetes pills." They are not oral insulin. Oral hypoglycemic medications help your body make better use of your own insulin. Insulin is important because it helps glucose (sugar) go from the blood into the body cells. The body uses sugar for energy.

These medications can be used only by some people who have type 2 (non–insulin-dependent) diabetes. People who have type 1 (insulin-dependent) diabetes and some who have type 2 must have insulin injections to control their blood sugar levels.

The several types of oral hypoglycemic medications differ in how quickly they work, how long they last in the body, and their side effects. The side effects of some of the medications could be an upset stomach, loss of appetite, or a skin rash. These side effects are usually not very serious. Ask your doctor or nurse if you have any questions about your medication. Remember to tell him or her if you have an allergy to sulfa medications (antibiotics). Take your medication as directed. Do not skip taking a dose and do not take an extra dose.

Medication helps, but it cannot replace diet and exercise in controlling your blood sugar level. Diet and exercise are the keys to success in diabetes control. Your doctor, nurse, or dietitian can plan a diet that is right for you. What you eat is as important as how much you eat. If you are overweight, your diet should help you lose weight. Follow your diet plan. Skipping meals and eating poorly can lead to a low blood sugar level (a reaction you want to avoid).

Regular exercise, like walking, helps your blood circulation and helps control your blood sugar level and weight. Check with your doctor or nurse before starting exercise. By following your medication, diet, and exercise plan, you can prevent complications.

IMPORTANT POINTS

Follow the directions of your doctor or nurse:

1. Know the signs and how to treat low blood sugar (hypoglycemia) and high blood sugar (hyperglycemia).
2. Check with your doctor or nurse before taking any medication.
   a. Even medications you can buy without a prescription, like aspirin, can cause side effects.
   b. Anticoagulants (blood thinners) and some heart and gout medications can cause low blood sugar (hypoglycemia).
   c. Steroids, some diuretics (water pills), and thyroid medications can cause high blood sugar (hyperglycemia).
   d. Alcohol can cause low blood sugar, face flushing, and other unpleasant reactions.
3. Always carry some form of simple sugar to take at the first signs of hypoglycemia. Many of the oral hypoglycemic medications last at least 12 hours in your body. You may need to take more a little later.
4. Test your urine or blood for sugar as directed. You may also be asked to test your urine for ketones. Keep a record of the date, time, and results of any tests you do.
5. Call your doctor or nurse if you:
   a. Are ill longer than 24 hours and are not getting better.
   b. Cannot eat or drink.
   c. Have an infection or are under extreme physical or emotional stress.
   d. Have frequent hypoglycemia or hyperglycemia.
6. If you are ill or are having an operation, your doctor may prescribe insulin. Always tell a new doctor or dentist you have diabetes before any procedure or operation.
7. Always carry or wear medical identification, including:
   a. Your medication's name and dose _____
   b. When to take it _____
8. You may get more information from
   American Diabetes Association, Inc.
   1701 N. Beauregard Street
   Alexandria, VA 22311
   1-800-DIABETES

OTHER INSTRUCTIONS

Viral and Communicable Disease Alterations

AIDS/HIV: Precautions for the Home

GUIDELINES

The following guidelines list factors that can spread the human immunodeficiency virus (HIV) and AIDS, as well as factors that can increase the risk of infection for the immunodepressed person or the person with AIDS. Next to each factor are precautions or corrective actions that specifically relate to the factor.

AIDS is a failure of the body's ability to defend itself against invading organisms; therefore, the person with AIDS is seriously threatened by infections that would not harm a person who does not have AIDS.

Factors That Increase the Risk of Infection

1. Poor personal hygiene.

2. Infrequent handwashing.

3. Superficial handwashing.

4. Inadequate household cleaning.

Precautions or Corrective Actions

a. Wash your body every day.
b. Wash your hair at least weekly.
c. Brush your teeth and rinse your mouth after every meal and at bedtime.
d. See your dentist at least twice a year and more often if needed.
e. Trim your fingernails and your toenails weekly.
f. Wear clean and laundered clothes.
g. Change dirty clothing and linens as soon as you notice soiling.

a. Wash your hands *before*
   • food preparation,
   • eating food,
   • serving food.
b. Wash your hands *after*
   • using the toilet,
   • contacting your own or another's body fluids,
   • blowing or wiping your nose,
   • outside activities.

a. Wet your hands with plenty of soap and water.
b. Work up a lather over your hands and wrists.
c. Rub the palm of one hand over the back of the other, and rub together several times; repeat for other hand.
d. Interlace the fingers of both your hands and rub back and forth.
e. Clean under your fingernails with a nail brush or orange stick.
f. Rinse your hands thoroughly under warm running water.
g. Dry your hands and wrists thoroughly.

a. Avoid household clutter.
b. Thoroughly air out the patient's room.
c. Clean the kitchen counter with scouring powder.
d. Dust and vacuum weekly.
e. Mop kitchen and bathroom floors weekly and when spills occur.
f. Clean the inside of the refrigerator weekly with soap and water.

Factors That Increase the Risk of Infection

Precautions or Corrective Actions

g. Add a teaspoon of bleach to each quart of water used for flower vases.

h. Add a teaspoon of vinegar to each quart of water or saline used for respiratory equipment, humidifiers, or dehumidifiers.

5. Inappropriate and inadequate food selection and preparation.

a. Use canned foods.
b. Cook all raw fruits and vegetables before eating them.
c. Peel fruits before eating them.
d. Cook meat well before eating it.
e. Use only pasteurized dairy products.
f. Avoid foods that make diarrhea worse.
g. Do not share food and drinks with others.
h. Do not lick your fingers or taste from a mixing spoon while cooking.

6. Exposure to people with infectious diseases.

a. Avoid crowds whenever possible.
b. Avoid people who have recently been vaccinated.
c. Avoid people with bacterial infections, cold sores, shingles, influenza, colds, chicken pox, measles, and the like.

7. Exposure to pet excreta.

a. Immunosuppressed people should not clean bird cages, aquariums, litter boxes, and so forth, and should avoid areas where dogs are walked.
b. When necessary, wear gloves when cleaning bird cages, litter boxes, aquariums, and so forth.

AIDS is caused by the human immunodeficiency virus (HIV). HIV is spread through blood and blood products, semen, vaginal secretions, and other body fluids; use caution with such fluids.

Factors That Can Spread AIDS

Precautions or Corrective Actions

1. Unsafe sexual practices and drug use.

a. Engage in safe sex (monogamy, body rubbing, massage, petting, hugging, and masturbation).
b. Use a latex condom when having intercourse.
c. Avoid questionably safe or unsafe sex (anal or vaginal intercourse with/without a latex condom, fellatio/orogenital contact, swallowing body secretions/excretions, anonymous sexual contacts, insertion of foreign objects into rectum, games/practices that cause mouth/genital trauma, wet French kissing).
d. Avoid use of recreational drugs.

2. Exposure to contaminated body fluids.

a. The patient should not donate blood, plasma, body organs or parts, and sperm.
b. Wear a mask if the patient has a productive cough.
c. Wear latex gloves when handling the patient's bedpan or urinal.
d. Cover your mouth with a tissue or your hand when sneezing or coughing.

Factors That Can Spread AIDS

3. Exposure to contaminated household or medical equipment.

Precautions or Corrective Actions

a. The AIDS virus is fragile and is easily destroyed on household and medical equipment by a mixture of bleach and water; scrub medical equipment with a 1:10 bleach-to-water solution.
b. Clean soap dishes, denture cups, and so forth weekly.
c. Do not use the same sponge to clean the bathroom and the kitchen.
d. Do not pour mop water down the kitchen sink.
e. Do not clean sponges and rags at the kitchen sink.
f. Disinfect mops and sponges weekly by soaking them in a 1:10 bleach to water solution for 5 minutes.
g. Flush the patient's body wastes down the toilet.
h. Do not clean bedpan, urinal, potty seats, and so forth in the kitchen sink.
i. Do not share towels, washcloths, lingerie, undergarments, and toothbrushes with the patient.
j. Wash dishes and utensils between use; do not share them until washed.
k. Launder the patient's clothes and bed linens separately from the rest of the family's; use household detergent.
l. Keep clothes and bed linens soiled by the patient in a plastic bag until laundered.
m. Double bag soiled dressings and trash and discard with household trash.
n. Put needles, syringes, and sharp items in a sturdy container such as a coffee can or laundry detergent bottle with a tight lid. Keep this container away from children. Dispose of full container according to your local requirements.
o. Flush used cleaning fluids down the toilet.
p. Use disposable items whenever possible and practical.

CALL YOUR NURSE OR DOCTOR

If any of the following happen, call your nurse or doctor:

1. Frequent cough
2. Sudden weight loss
3. Diarrhea
4. Vomiting
5. Increased redness of any wounds
6. Fever
7. Skin breakdown (no matter how small)
8. Lethargy
9. Night sweats
10. Aching
11. Rashes
12. Sore throat
13. Headache
14. Burning/pain during urination
15. Stiff neck

OTHER INSTRUCTIONS

Chickenpox

GENERAL INFORMATION

Symptoms

The symptoms of chickenpox are most likely to appear 10 to 21 days after exposure to a person with the disease. The symptoms are

- Slight fever,
- Fatigue,
- Loss of appetite,
- Small red spots.

The small red spots appear first on the front of the body and then spread to the face, neck, upper arms, and legs. The spots become little blisters filled with clear or yellowish fluid. They crust over in a few days, and the crusts fall off in 5 to 20 days. The spots and blisters are very itchy. The spots can also appear on the scalp, on the penis, and in the vagina, nose, mouth, and throat. Swallowing can be difficult. New spots appear every 3 to 4 days during the course of the disease.

How Chickenpox Spreads

Chickenpox spreads from an infected person to a noninfected person by droplets sprayed in the air when the infected person sneezes or coughs, by physical contact with the infected person, and by direct contact with items that have been freshly soiled by discharges from the infected person's nose and mouth or by open chickenpox blisters. Chickenpox is most likely to be infectious, or to spread, 5 days before the symptoms appear until 6 days after the last crop of spots disappears.

HOME CARE GUIDELINES

1. Warm cornstarch or baking soda baths, calamine lotion, and petroleum jelly relieve the itchiness.
2. Keep the patient's fingernails short. Put cloth mittens on small children. Scratching and breaking open the blisters may cause scarring.

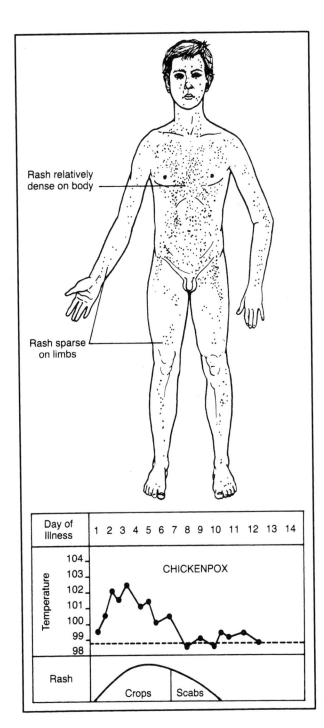

Rash relatively dense on body

Rash sparse on limbs

3. The patient and anyone who takes care of the patient should wash their hands frequently.
4. The patient's bed linens and clothing should be kept clean and fresh. They should be changed daily.
5. Have the patient wear light, loose-fitting clothes.
6. Keep the patient in bed until the fever is gone.
7. Provide the patient with quiet activities (simple board games, television, books, cards, radio) until all the blisters are crusted.
8. Offer the patient clear fluids throughout the day. Cool water is best. Avoid fruit juices and tart beverages, as these can be painful for the patient to swallow.
9. Serve soft foods (custards, eggs, Jell-O, ice cream), as these may be easier for the patient to swallow.

CALL YOUR NURSE OR DOCTOR

If any of the following happens, call your nurse or doctor:

1. The patient is very uncomfortable as a result of the itchiness.
2. The patient has a fever of 103°F or higher.
3. The patient has spots, blisters, or sores in the eye.
4. The patient's headache is constant and not relieved.
5. The spots look infected or become larger.

OTHER INSTRUCTIONS

Impetigo

GENERAL INFORMATION

Symptoms

The symptoms of impetigo are most likely to appear 2 to 10 days after exposure to a person with the disease. The symptoms are reddish lesions, which first appear on the face, usually around the mouth and nose. They become cloudy blisters and then straw-colored or brown crusts. The lesions spread to the arms and legs, forming patterns of arcs and circles as they spread. The lesions, blisters, and crusts are itchy.

How Impetigo Spreads

Impetigo spreads from an infected person to a noninfected person by physical contact with the infected person and by direct contact with items that have been freshly soiled by discharges from the blisters and crusts. Impetigo is infectious, or likely to spread, as long as the lesions remain unhealed.

HOME CARE GUIDELINES

1. Remove the crusts by soaking them or by using a lubricating skin ointment. Do this at least once a day.
2. Scrub the lesions gently and thoroughly at least three times a day with castile soap and warm water.
3. Keep the lesions dry and open to the air after scrubbing them.
4. Keep the patient's fingernails short. Put cloth mittens on small children.
5. The patient's bed linens and clothing should be kept clean and fresh. They should be changed daily. Good hygiene is an important part of the recovery from impetigo.
6. The patient should take antibiotics exactly as prescribed by the doctor.
7. Offer the patient fluids frequently throughout the day. Cool water is best, but any liquid is helpful.
8. Provide the patient with well-balanced meals. Nutrition is an important part of the recovery from impetigo.
9. All persons who take care of the patient should wash their hands frequently.

CALL THE DOCTOR

Call the doctor if the lesions, blisters, or sores become infected. Some signs of a possible infection are
- yellow, tan, or greenish drainage
- fever
- swelling
- increased redness of skin

OTHER INSTRUCTIONS

Infection Control for the Home

GENERAL INFORMATION

Illnesses that spread from one person to another are called infectious diseases. Each one has its own way or ways of spreading. Contact with infected body fluids (such as blood, urine, feces, mucus) or with the droplets that are sprayed into the air when an infected person sneezes or coughs is a way an infectious disease can spread. Sometimes, the illness can spread through an indirect link, such as having contact with items that have been freshly soiled by drainage from infected sores or discharges from the patient's body openings (nose, mouth, eyes, rectum).

Controlling the spread of an infectious disease means interrupting the way the illness travels from an infected person to a noninfected person. For example, if you have a cold and cover your mouth when you sneeze, you are stopping the spread of infected droplets.

Careful personal hygiene and household cleanliness are very effective in preventing the spread of disease. These and other helpful infection control measures are discussed below.

INFECTION CONTROL MEASURES

1. Maintain good personal hygiene.
   a. Wash your body every day.
   b. Wash your hair at least weekly.
   c. Brush your teeth and rinse your mouth after every meal and at bedtime.
   d. Trim your fingernails and toenails weekly.
   e. Wear clean and laundered clothes.
   f. Change dirty clothing and bedlinens as soon as you notice the soiling.
2. Wash your hands frequently.
   a. Wash your hands *before*
      • Food preparation,
      • Eating food,
      • Serving food.
   b. Wash your hands *after*
      • Using the toilet,
      • Contact with your own or another's body fluids,
      • Blowing or wiping your nose,
      • Outside activities.
3. Wash your hands thoroughly.
   a. Wet your hands with plenty of soap and warm water.
   b. Work up a lather over your hands and wrists.
   c. Rub the palm of one hand over the back of the other and rub them together several times. Repeat for the other hand.
   d. Interlace the fingers of both your hands and rub them back and forth.
   e. Clean under your fingernails with a nail brush or orange stick.
   f. Rinse your hands thoroughly under warm running water.
   g. Dry your hands and wrists thoroughly.
4. Clean your household thoroughly.
   a. Avoid household clutter.
   b. Thoroughly ventilate your home with fresh air.
   c. Clean the kitchen counter with scouring powder.
   d. Dust and vacuum weekly.
   e. Mop the kitchen and bathroom floors weekly and when spills occur.
   f. Clean the inside of the refrigerator weekly with soap and water.
   g. Add a teaspoon of bleach to each quart of water used for flower vases.
   h. Add a teaspoon of vinegar to each quart of water or saline used for respiratory equipment, humidifiers, or dehumidifiers.
   i. Wear gloves when cleaning bird cages, litter boxes, aquariums, and the like.
   j. Use exhaust fans vented to the outside.
5. Clean contaminated household and medical equipment thoroughly.
   a. Scrub medical equipment with a 70% alcohol solution or a solution of one part bleach to 30 parts water.
   b. Clean such articles as soap dishes and denture cups weekly.
   c. Do not use the same sponge to clean the bathroom and the kitchen.
   d. Do not pour mop water down the kitchen sink.
   e. Do not clean sponges or rags at the kitchen sink.
   f. Disinfect mops and sponges weekly by soaking in a one part bleach to nine parts water solution for 5 minutes.
   g. Flush body wastes down the toilet.
   h. Do not clean bedpans, potty seats, and urinals in the kitchen sink.
   i. Do not share towels, washcloths, lingerie, undergarments, and toothbrushes.
6. Decrease your exposure to people with infectious diseases.

a. Avoid crowds whenever possible.
b. Avoid people who have been recently vaccinated.
c. Avoid people with bacterial infections, cold sores, shingles, influenza, colds, chickenpox, measles.

d. Cover your mouth with a tissue or your hand when sneezing and coughing. Put the soiled tissue into waste bag. Wash your hands.
e. Do not share food and drink with others.
f. Do not lick your fingers or taste from the mixing spoon while cooking.

OTHER INSTRUCTIONS

Lice

GENERAL INFORMATION

Anyone can get lice (pediculosis). There are three types of lice: head, body, and pubic ("crab") lice. Lice are small bugs that are passed between people through body contact or sharing combs, hairbrushes, hats, scarves, clothes, and linens. Even holding hands or dancing can spread lice. This is why people who have had contact with the person with lice may need treatment.

If you think you or someone in your family has lice or has been with someone who has lice, get treatment right away. Call your doctor, nurse, or local health department. It may take days before any signs and symptoms appear. It is nothing to be ashamed of.

HOW TO LOOK FOR LICE

1. Before bathing, look for white eggs ("grains of sugar") stuck to the shafts of hairs.
   a. These eggs (nits) may be on clothes, too.
   b. Dandruff and hair spray drops are not the same. These are easy to remove. Lice eggs are hard to remove.
   c. Also look for small red bites.
2. Look closely at the hair, scalp, back of head and neck, shoulders, armpits, stomach, waist, lower thighs, and groin area.
   a. Use a strong light and, if needed, a magnifying glass.
   b. Use a comb so that you can see the hair shafts about 1/4 inch away from the skin.
3. Itching is very common and is often worse at night. Look for scratch marks on the skin.
4. Sometimes, mild fever or muscle aches are present.

TREATMENT

1. Follow the directions for the shampoo or cream you have been given. You will use _____ .
   a. Be sure to use the shampoo or cream *exactly* as directed.
   b. Cover all involved skin areas.
   c. Keep the shampoo or cream on the skin for _____ minutes.
2. After treatment,
   a. Put on just-washed clothes.
   b. Use freshly washed towels and sheets.
   c. Wash all clothes that have come in contact with the skin (underwear, pants, shirts, socks) right away.
   d. No one should use the same towels, clothes, or linens until these items have been washed.
3. A follow-up treatment may be needed.

PREVENTION

1. Follow these directions to prevent getting lice again:
   a. Soak hairbrushes and combs in very hot water for at least 10 minutes.
   b. Wash clothes you have worn lately right away. Keep those clothes away from other clothes.
   c. Items that can be washed (like clothes, shirts, and towels) can be cleaned by machine or hand washing them in hot water (so hot that you cannot keep your fingers in the water).
   d. Dry the clothes on the hot cycle, *or*
   e. Press the clothes with a hot iron.
   f. If clothes, blankets, or pillows cannot be washed, place them in a plastic bag and keep it sealed for 30 to 35 days. It is best to keep the bag at room temperature.
   g. Dry cleaning can also be used. Tell the dry cleaner to treat the clothes as possibly infected.
   h. Vacuum carpets, upholstery, and mattresses during treatment.

OTHER INSTRUCTIONS

Mumps

GENERAL INFORMATION

Symptoms

The symptoms of mumps are most likely to appear 12 to 26 days after exposure to a person with the disease. The symptoms are

- Sudden fever,
- Headache,
- Loss of appetite,
- Fatigue,
- Pain beneath the ear,
- Swelling and tenderness of the glands between the ear and the angle of the jaw. The swelling is at its worst by the third day.

How Mumps Spreads

Mumps spreads from an infected person to a noninfected person by droplets sprayed in the air when the infected person sneezes or coughs and by direct contact with the saliva of an infected person. After puberty, males who have not had mumps should avoid all contact with the infected person. Mumps is most likely to be infectious, or to spread, 5 days before the glands swell until 9 days after the swelling is gone.

HOME CARE GUIDELINES

1. Pack a hot towel, a hot water bottle, or an ice bag around the patient's swollen glands.

2. Serve soft foods to the patient. Chewing can be painful for the patient with mumps.
3. Offer the patient clear fluids often throughout the day. Cool water is best. Avoid fruit juices and tart beverages, as these can be painful for the patient with mumps.
4. Provide the patient with quiet activities (radio, television, books, cards, simple board games)
5. Help the patient brush his or her teeth and rinse his or her mouth with water after every meal and at bedtime. This helps prevent infections.

CALL YOUR NURSE OR DOCTOR

If any of the following happens, call your nurse or doctor:

1. The patient has a temperature of 104°F or higher.
2. The patient has abdominal pain and is vomiting.
3. The patient's headache is constant and not relieved.
4. The patient is very drowsy and unable to stay awake.
5. The patient's eyes are red.
6. The patient complains of dizziness.
7. The muscles of the patient's face begin twitching.
8. The male patient's testicles swell or are tender or painful.

OTHER INSTRUCTIONS

Otitis Media

GENERAL INFORMATION

Symptoms

Otitis media is an infection of the middle ear. It usually occurs when a child has a bad cold. The symptoms are

- Tugging the ear,
- Rubbing the ear,
- Rolling the head from side to side,
- Fussiness or irritability,
- Loss of appetite,
- Complaints of dull, throbbing earache,
- Dizziness,
- Nausea and/or diarrhea,
- Complaints of feeling of fullness in the ear.

You might notice that your child does not hear you when you speak or that your child is keeping the television set at a higher volume than usual. Otitis media takes about 1 week to resolve with treatment.

HOME CARE GUIDELINES

1. Give prescribed medications to your child as directed by your nurse or doctor.
2. Make sure your child is dressed properly in cold and rainy weather.
3. When your child blows his or her nose make sure he or she blows gently with the mouth slightly open. This prevents drainage from being forced into the middle ear.
4. Always hold your child's head up when feeding him or her. The child should not be fed with a propped bottle or when lying on the back. Proper positioning prevents fluid from getting into the middle ear and causing an infection.

CALL YOUR NURSE OR DOCTOR

If any of the following happens, call your nurse or doctor:

1. Fever 101°F or higher.
2. Crying even when comforted after the medication has been started.
3. Drainage of any type from the ears.

OTHER INSTRUCTIONS

Pertussis (Whooping Cough)

GENERAL INFORMATION

Symptoms

The symptoms of pertussis are most likely to appear 5 to 21 days after exposure to a person with the disease. The symptoms are

- Slight fever,
- Runny nose,
- Coughing eight to ten times in one breath and catching breath in one long noisy intake of air (whooping). Shortness of breath, extreme fatigue, or vomiting may follow the coughing bout. The coughing bout may cause the infected person's face to turn blue.

How Pertussis Spreads

Pertussis spreads from an infected person to a noninfected person by droplets sprayed in the air when the infected person sneezes or coughs and by direct contact with items that have been freshly soiled by discharges from the infected person's nose and mouth. Pertussis is infectious, or likely to spread, during all stages of the illness until antibiotics have been taken for 5 days.

HOME CARE GUIDELINES

1. Stay with the patient during coughing bouts. Keep the patient's head tilted downward to prevent the inhalation of vomitus or mucus. Watch the patient for signs of difficult breathing. Reassure the patient and remain calm.
2. Offer the patient fluids often throughout the day. This is especially important with children, because they can become dehydrated quickly.
3. Serve the patient small, frequent snacks throughout the day. Avoid foods that are dry and crumbly or peppery, as these might bring on a coughing bout.
4. Keep the patient in bed, because pertussis can cause extreme fatigue. If lying down starts a coughing bout, sit the patient up in bed, using a backrest and pillows for support.
5. Provide the patient with quiet activities (books, radio, television, simple board games, cards). Avoid active playing or excitement, as these may bring on a coughing bout.
6. Keep the temperature in the patient's room at a comfortable level. Avoid hot and cold extremes, as these may bring on a coughing bout.
7. Put a cool mist vaporizer or humidifier in the patient's room to help relieve the coughing.
8. Keep the patient's room free of dust and smoke.
9. The patient should take antibiotics exactly as prescribed by the doctor.
10. All persons who take care of the patient should wash their hands frequently.

CALL YOUR NURSE OR DOCTOR

If any of the following happens, call your nurse or doctor:

1. The patient has thick, discolored mucus either draining from the nose or brought up by coughing.
2. The patient is short of breath most of the time.
3. The patient has seizures.
4. The patient is confused.
5. The patient does not seem to be getting better.

OTHER INSTRUCTIONS

Rubella (German Measles)

GENERAL INFORMATION

Symptoms

The symptoms of rubella are most likely to appear 14 to 21 days after exposure to a person with the disease. The symptoms are

- Fever,
- Runny nose,
- Loss of appetite,
- Fatigue,
- Sore throat,
- Tender and slightly swollen glands in the neck,
- Sore or stiff neck when the head is moved,
- A rash first appearing as small pink spots on the face and along the hairline. The spots spread to the trunk of the body, the arms, and the legs. The rash lasts 3 to 7 days.

How Rubella Spreads

Rubella spreads from an infected person to a non-infected person by droplets sprayed in the air when the infected person sneezes or coughs, by physical contact with the infected person, and by direct contact with items that have been freshly soiled by discharges from the infected person's nose and mouth. Pregnant women should avoid all contact with the infected person. Rubella is most likely to be infectious, or to spread, 7 days before the rash appears until 4 days after the rash subsides.

HOME CARE GUIDELINES

1. Cornstarch baths, calamine lotion, and petroleum jelly relieve the itchiness.
2. Have the patient wear light, loose-fitting clothes.
3. Provide the patient with quiet activities (radio, television, books, cards, simple board games).

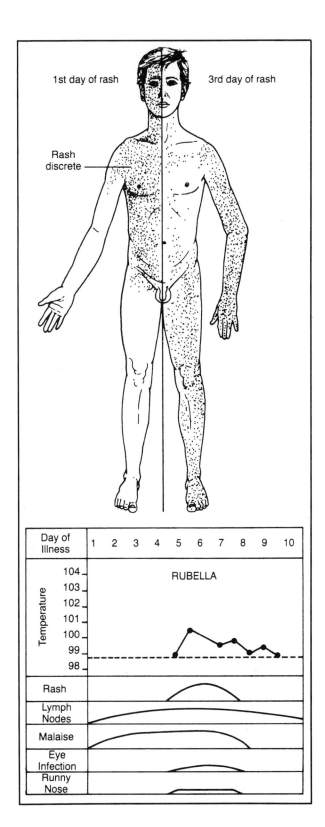

CALL YOUR NURSE OR DOCTOR

If any of the following happens, call your nurse or doctor:

1. The patient has a fever of 103°F or higher.
2. The patient's eyes are red.

OTHER INSTRUCTIONS

Rubeola (Measles)

GENERAL INFORMATION

Symptoms

The symptoms of rubeola are most likely to appear 8 to 20 days after exposure to a person with the disease. The symptoms are

- Fatigue,
- Runny nose,
- Red, sore eyes and sensitivity to light,
- Coughing or sneezing,
- Loss of appetite,
- High fever that climbs steadily until 2 to 3 days after the rash starts,
- A dark red, dry rash that first appears on the hairline and spreads to the rest of the face, the neck, the ears, the trunk of the body, and the arms and legs. The rash turns brown and scaly after 5 to 6 days. White spots surrounded by red (Koplik spots) can appear in the mouth after 3 to 7 days. Koplik spots usually disappear in 12 to 18 hours.

How Rubeola Spreads

Rubeola spreads from an infected person to a noninfected person by droplets sprayed in the air when the infected person coughs or sneezes, by direct contact with items that have been freshly soiled by discharges from the infected person's nose and mouth, and by physical contact with the infected person. Pregnant women and very young children (5 months to 2 years old) should avoid all contact with the infected person. Rubeola is most likely to be infectious, or to spread, at the time the runny nose or 4 days before the rash appears and until 7 days after the rash is gone.

HOME CARE GUIDELINES

1. Sponge-bathe the patient with cool water to decrease the fever.

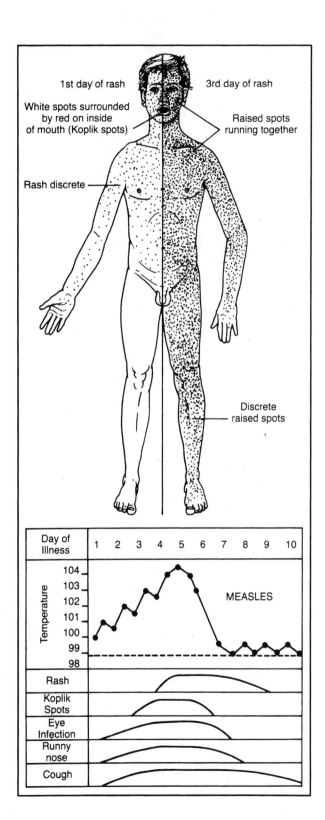

2. Keep the patient in bed until 2 days after the fever has gone down.
3. Provide the patient with quiet activity. Do not let the patient read or watch television until his or her eyes are no longer red or sore.
4. Keep the patient's room only dimly lit to avoid irritating the eyes. Offer the patient sunglasses.
5. Rinse the patient's eyes with cool to warm water to remove any crusts.
6. Discourage the patient from rubbing the eyes.
7. Put a cool moisture vaporizer in the patient's room to help relieve the coughing.
8. Offer the patient fluids often throughout the day. Cool water is best, but any liquid is helpful.

CALL YOUR NURSE OR DOCTOR

If any of the following happens, call your nurse or doctor:

1. The patient's temperature returns to almost normal and then rises over 101°F.
2. The patient has an earache.
3. The patient's cough lasts longer than 4 or 5 days.
4. The patient has thick, discolored mucus either draining from the nose or brought up by coughing.
5. The patient is short of breath.
6. The patient has a headache and a stiff neck.

OTHER INSTRUCTIONS

Scabies

GENERAL INFORMATION

Anyone can get scabies. Scabies are small bugs that are passed between people through body contact or sharing combs, hairbrushes, hats, scarves, clothes, and linens. Even holding hands or dancing can spread scabies. This is why people who have had contact with scabies may need treatment.

If you think you or someone in your family has scabies or has been with someone who has scabies, get treatment right away. Call your doctor, nurse, or local health department. It may take up to 30 days before any signs and symptoms appear. Only a skin test can confirm you have scabies. It is nothing to be ashamed of.

HOW TO LOOK FOR SCABIES

1. Look for very small, wavy, gray-white streaks ("threads") on the skin. There may be spots of redness along the streak.
2. Look closely at the skin before bathing, especially behind the knees, in the armpits, between and under the buttocks, along the waist, in the groin, under the breasts, around the wrists, and between the toes and fingers. For children, look at the face, palms of the hands, and soles of the feet.
3. Itching is very common and is often much worse at night. Look for scratch marks on the skin.

TREATMENT

1. Follow the directions for the cream or lotion prescription you have been given. You will use _____.

   a. Be sure to use the cream or lotion *exactly* as directed.
   b. Cover the body completely, from neck to toes, even under the fingernails.
   c. Keep the cream or lotion on the skin for _____ hours.
2. After treatment,
   a. Put on freshly washed clothes.
   b. Use freshly washed sheets and towels.
   c. Wash all clothes that have come in contact with the skin (underwear, pants, shirts, socks) right away.
   d. No one should use the same towels, clothes, or linens until these items have been washed.
3. A follow-up treatment may be needed.

CARE OF ITEMS

1. Soak hairbrushes and combs in very hot water for at least 10 minutes.
2. Wash all clothes that you have worn lately right away. Keep these clothes away from other clothes.
3. Items that can be washed (clothes, sheets, and towels) can be cleaned by machine or hand washing in hot water (so hot that you cannot keep your fingers in it).
   a. Dry the clothes on the hot cycle, or
   b. Press the clothes with a hot iron.
4. If the clothes cannot be washed,
   a. Put them (even blankets, pillows) in a plastic bag and seal it for 30 to 35 days. Keep the bag at room temperature.
   b. Dry cleaning can be used. Tell the dry cleaner to treat the clothes as possibly infected.
5. Vacuum carpets, upholstery, and mattresses during treatment.

OTHER INSTRUCTIONS

Scarlet Fever

GENERAL INFORMATION

Symptoms

The symptoms of scarlet fever are most likely to appear 1 to 6 days after exposure to a person with the disease. The symptoms are

- Sudden high fever,
- Headache,
- Fatigue,
- Nausea and vomiting,
- Sore throat,
- Strawberry-colored tongue,
- A rash of red raised spots that appears on the neck, chest, and groin. The spots turn white when pressed on. The rash lasts about 5 days. When the rash disappears, the skin may peel.

How Scarlet Fever Spreads

Scarlet fever spreads from an infected person to a noninfected person by physical contact with the infected person. Scarlet fever is most likely to be infectious, or to spread when fever or rash appear, from 2 days before the rash to 3 days after the rash is gone or after an antibiotic has been taken for at least 24 hours.

HOME CARE GUIDELINES

1. Keep the patient in bed until the fever is gone.
2. Provide the patient with quiet activities (simple board games, books, radio, cards, television).
3. Put a cool mist vaporizer or humidifier in the patient's room to help relieve the sore throat.

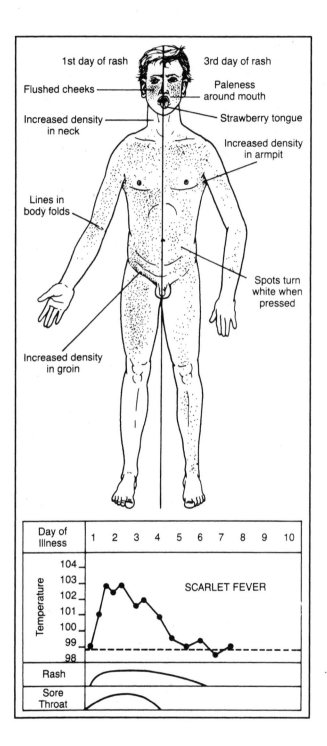

4. Serve liquid or soft foods (eggs, custard, Jell-O, milkshakes, ice cream), as these may be easier for the patient to swallow.
5. The patient's bedlinens and clothing should be kept clean and fresh. They should be changed daily.
6. The patient should take antibiotics exactly as prescribed by the doctor. The antibiotics are an important part of treating scarlet fever and preventing complications.

OTHER INSTRUCTIONS

CALL YOUR NURSE OR DOCTOR

If any of the following happens, call your nurse or doctor:

1. The patient's fever does not come down.
2. The patient has an earache.
3. The patient has a sore neck and a headache.
4. The patient does not seem to be getting any better.

Seborrheic Dermatitis (Cradle Cap)

GENERAL INFORMATION

Symptoms

Seborrheic dermatitis (cradle cap) is an inflammatory skin disease. Its cause is unknown. Thick yellow or pink crusted lesions appear on the scalp, eyelids, eyebrows, and external ear canal. They can also be found behind the ears, under the arms, and in the diaper area. The lesions are usually not itchy.

How Seborrheic Dermatitis Spreads

Seborrheic dermatitis spreads from an infected person to a noninfected person by physical contact with the infected person or with clothing or bed linens that have touched the infected areas of the body.

HOME CARE GUIDELINES

1. Shampoo the affected scalp once a day. Shampoo vigorously and thoroughly; your home care nurse can show you how.
2. Use two applications of shampoo each time.
3. Wash your hands after touching the affected parts of the body.
4. Change bed linens and clothing that touches the affected parts of the body at least once a day.

OTHER INSTRUCTIONS

Signs of a Possible Infection

1. Sore throat
2. Fever
3. Chills and/or sweating
4. Nausea and/or vomiting
5. Pain and/or burning with urination
6. Cloudy or very dark urine
7. Diarrhea
8. Red skin, skin rashes
9. Swelling near a cut or wound
10. Yellow, tan, or green drainage from a cut or wound
11. Stiff neck and/or headache
12. Difficulty breathing and/or wheezing
13. Persistent cough
14. Fast pulse rate

OTHER INSTRUCTIONS

Thrush

GENERAL INFORMATION

Symptoms

Thrush is an infection caused by the *Candida* fungus. It begins as tiny white spots in the mouth. These spots come together and form slightly raised patches on the tongue, gums, or sides and roof of the mouth. They look like curdled milk but you can't remove them. A child with thrush may have pain while sucking or drinking. Thrush can also cause the child to have a fever, stomach upset, or bowel discomfort or inflammation.

The *Candida* fungus can also infect the diaper area. It causes a red rash with tiny blisters. Your child may be very uncomfortable when the diaper is wet or during cleaning of the diaper area. The rash blisters usually dry up and fall off in about 2 weeks when treated with medicated ointment prescribed by your doctor.

How Thrush Spreads

Thrush spreads from an infected person to a non-infected person by physical contact with the infected person. It is infectious as long as the white patches remain.

HOME CARE GUIDELINES (INFECTION IN THE MOUTH)

1. Wash your hands after touching your child's mouth.
2. Do not let other children use the infected child's pacifier or drink from the infected child's cup or glass.
3. Sterilize baby bottle nipples after each use by placing them in boiling water for 20 minutes. Let the nipples cool before using them.
4. Change the child's pacifier several times a day. Sterilize them by placing them in boiling water for 20 minutes. Let the pacifiers cool before using them.
5. Make sure your child drinks plenty of fluids. Children with thrush may not drink as much as usual because of the mouth pain.
6. If you are breast-feeding, clean each breast with water and air-dry after each feeding.
7. Follow all feedings with water for your child.
8. Finish the medication as directed even if the white patches have cleared up.

HOME CARE GUIDELINES (INFECTION IN THE DIAPER AREA)

1. Wash your hands after changing your child's diapers.
2. With each diaper change, wash the diaper area with warm water and mild soap using a clean cloth. Wipe from front to back. Pat dry.
3. Apply the medicated ointment prescribed by the doctor.
4. Do not apply other ointments, oils, or powders unless directed by your nurse or doctor.
5. Change your child's diapers as soon as possible after soiling.
6. Check a newborn's diapers once every hour.
7. Take the child's diaper off for a few minutes several times a day. Air helps heal the *Candida* infection.
8. Wash cloth diapers with a simple laundry soap like Ivory, rinse them well using Diaparene to reduce ammonia residue.

CALL YOUR NURSE OR DOCTOR

If any of the following happens, call your nurse or doctor:

1. If you are breast-feeding and your breasts become red or sore.
2. The child's mouth becomes raw and/or bloody.
3. The child refuses to eat or drink.

OTHER INSTRUCTIONS

Tuberculosis

GENERAL INFORMATION

Symptoms

Tuberculosis (TB) infection begins in the lungs but can spread throughout the body. The TB germs can live in your body without making you sick. TB infection is not the same as TB disease. Your immune system traps the TB germs and limits their spread in your body. As a result, you

- Have a positive TB skin test,
- Do not feel sick, and
- Cannot give TB to others.

Sometimes, the TB germs break away from your immune system. This can happen months or years after the TB infection. Then the TB germs cause TB disease. The TB germs attack the lungs and other parts of the body. The person with TB disease needs medical treatment. If the person does not get medical help, he or she could die.

If you have TB disease, you may
- Feel weak,
- Lose your appetite,
- Lose weight,
- Have a fever, or
- Sweat a lot at night.

These signs of TB disease may last for weeks. Without medical help they usually get worse.

If the TB disease is in your lungs, you may
- Cough a lot,
- Cough up mucus or phlegm,
- Cough up blood, or
- Have chest pain when you cough.

If you have TB disease in another part of your body, the symptoms will be different. Ask your nurse to teach you about them.

How TB Spreads

TB is spread through the air. Infected persons produce infectious droplets when they speak, cough, sneeze, laugh, or sing. When air contaminated with infectious droplets is breathed, a person can become infected with TB. The chance of becoming infected with TB depends on the number of infectious droplets in the air, the length of time a person is breathing in the infected air, and whether or not a person is using protective equipment such as masks and exhaust fans.

HOME CARE GUIDELINES

1. TB infection and TB disease can be cured by using special drugs that kill TB germs. It takes at least 6 to 9 months of medication to wipe out TB germs. *It is very important that you take all of your medication as prescribed by your doctor.*
2. Do not stop taking your medications until your doctor tells you. If you stop taking your medication too soon, it will cause a big problem. The TB germs in your body will become even stronger. You will need stronger medications to wipe out these "new" TB germs.
3. Decrease the spread of TB infection and disease by using infection control measures in your home, wearing a surgical mask, and making sure exhaust fans are vented to the outside. Ask your home care nurse for more information about infection control measures in your home.
4. Wash your hands frequently.
5. Cough into a disposable tissue. Dispose of the tissue in a waste can. Do not reuse disposable tissues. Do not use cloth handkerchiefs.
6. Stay away from other people until your doctor tells you that you can't spread TB germs.
7. Maintain a nutritionally balanced diet to strengthen your immune system and recover from TB. Eat small frequent meals with foods high in protein and carbohydrate. Drink at least eight to ten 8-ounce glasses of fluid every day. This will help thin mucus and phlegm, making them easier to cough up. Ask your nurse for more information about a diet plan that will help you.

CALL YOUR NURSE OR DOCTOR

If any of the following happens, call your nurse or doctor:

1. Numbness or tingling in your hands or feet,
2. No appetite,
3. Nausea and/or vomiting,
4. Yellow skin or eyeballs (jaundice),
5. Very itchy skin,
6. Very dark urine,
7. Extreme fatigue,
8. Blurred vision,
9. Inability to see the colors red or green,
10. Dizziness,

11. Light-headedness,
12. Ringing in your ears,
13. Roaring or fullness in your ears,

14. Painful swelling in your joints,
15. Fever and/or chills.

OTHER INSTRUCTIONS

Impaired Comfort and Personal Care

Bathing the Person in Bed

GUIDELINES

Use this procedure for the patient who cannot get out of bed and who cannot bathe himself or herself.

1. Make sure the room is warm and that there are no drafts. Give the patient privacy by closing doors and curtains.
2. Place a table next to the patient's bedside. Choose a table that is a comfortable working height for you.
3. Wash your hands.
4. Gather your equipment. You need
   - A deep basin filled three-quarters of the way with warm water,
   - Soap or bath oil (if the patient's skin is dry, alternate soap one day and bath oil the next),
   - A washcloth,
   - Towels,
   - Clean clothes.
5. Put the equipment on the table. Make sure everything is within your reach.
6. Take the top linens off the bed and leave the patient covered by a single sheet.
7. Undress the patient. Keep the patient covered by a single sheet.
8. Put a towel over the patient's chest.
9. Make the washcloth into a bathmitt.
   a. Put your hand on the washcloth and fold one side over.
   b. Fold the other side over your hand.

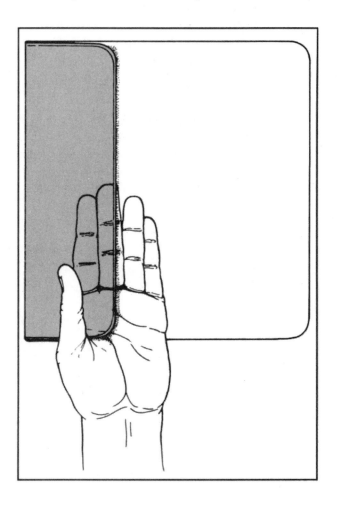

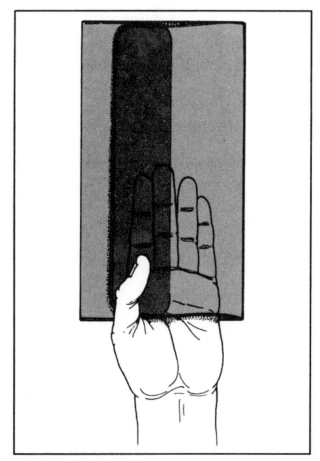

c. Fold the top down and tuck it in.

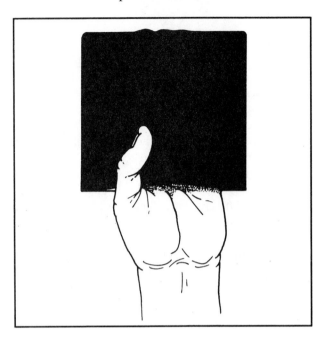

10. Wet and soap the washcloth. Wash the patient's face, neck, and ears. Rinse and dry them well.
11. Put a towel under one of the patient's arms. Wash the arm. Pay special attention to the underarm area. Rinse and pat the arm dry.
12. Do the same for the other arm.
13. Put the basin on a towel on the bed.
14. Soak and wash the patient's hands. Use a nailbrush or orange stick, if necessary, to clean the patient's fingernails. Dry the patient's hands and fingers thoroughly.

15. Pull down the sheet and towel to expose the patient's chest and abdomen. Wash, rinse, and dry these areas. Make sure all creases and folds in the skin are completely dry. Cover the patient.
16. Uncover one of the patient's legs. Put a towel underneath it. Wash, rinse, and dry the leg. Put the basin on a towel on the bed and soak the patient's foot. Use a nailbrush or an orange stick to clean the patient's toenails. Dry the patient's foot and toes thoroughly. Cover the patient.
17. Do the same for the other leg and foot.
18. Change the water in the basin.
19. Wash, rinse, and dry the patient's genital area. The patient may prefer to do this himself or herself, if capable.
20. Change the water in the basin.
21. Help the patient turn to one side. Place a towel beneath the patient's back and buttocks. Wash, rinse, and dry the back and buttocks. Help the patient turn to the other side, and repeat.
22. Gently massage lotion onto the dry areas of the patient's skin.
23. Help the patient get dressed in the clean clothes.
24. Help the patient complete (or do them for the patient) other personal hygiene tasks (mouth care, denture care, shaving, hair combing, putting on make-up, and the like).
25. Straighten and tidy the bed linens.
26. Help the patient to a comfortable position. Open the closed doors and curtains.
27. Clean the equipment and put it away.
28. Wash your hands.

OTHER INSTRUCTIONS

Bathing the Person in a Chair

GUIDELINES

Use this procedure to help the patient who is able to get out of bed and into a chair and who can stand a little but is unable to walk to the bathroom.

1. Make sure the room is warm and that there are no drafts. Give the patient privacy by closing doors and curtains.
2. Help the patient move from the bed to a chair. Make the patient comfortable.
3. Place a table in front of or next to the patient. Choose a table that is a comfortable working height for the patient.
4. Gather your equipment. You need
   - A deep basin filled three-quarters of the way with warm water,
   - Soap or bath oil (if the patient's skin is dry, alternate soap one day and bath oil the next),
   - A washcloth,
   - A towel,
   - Clean clothes.
5. Put the equipment on the table. Make sure everything is within the patient's reach.
6. Have the patient undress to the waist. If the patient is unable to do this alone, help him or her.
7. Ask the patient to wash the top half of his or her body. Leave the room to give the patient some privacy. Tell the patient to call you when he or she is done.
8. Have the patient lean forward. Wash, rinse, and dry the patient's back.
9. Ask the patient to wash his or her legs. If the patient is unable to do this, wash, rinse, and dry the patient's legs.
10. Soak and wash the patient's feet in the basin of water. Rinse and dry the patient's feet thoroughly.
11. Change the water in the basin.
12. Ask the patient to stand. Provide assistance if necessary.
13. Ask the patient to wash his or her genital and anal areas. Leave the room to give the patient privacy. (Do not leave the room if there is a possibility that the patient may fall.) Tell the patient to call you when he or she is done.
14. Help the patient get dressed in the clean clothes.
15. Help the patient complete other personal hygiene tasks (mouth care, denture care, combing hair, shaving, putting on make-up, and the like).
16. Help the patient to a comfortable position. Open the closed doors and curtains.
17. Clean the equipment and put it away.
18. Wash your hands.

OTHER INSTRUCTIONS

Care of the Patient Confined to Bed

GENERAL INFORMATION

The patient who is confined to bed is at risk of developing problems such as skin breakdown, breathing difficulties, and constipation. Use the following guidelines to help you remember how to care for the patient in bed and so lessen the chance of any new physical problems.

GUIDELINES

Relieve Pressure on the Patient's Body

Pressure causes skin damage and can lead to bedsores. The bony parts of the body are most likely to be affected by pressure. The circled areas in the drawings show the bony parts that are most affected for each position. Use an egg crate or air mattress, heel pads, ankle or elbow pads, sheepskin pads, and soft pillows to keep the patient's body from experiencing too much pressure. Elevate the lower extremities by putting pillows under the patient's calves so that the heels hang freely. A bed cradle is also helpful. It keeps the sheets and blankets off the patient's feet and legs. Check the bony parts of the patient's body at least twice a day for reddened areas. If you find a red area, reposition the patient. If the reddened area does not go away, you should call the nurse.

Change the Patient's Position at Least Every Hour

Changing the patient's position relieves the pressure on the bony parts, stops fluid from pooling in the patient's lungs, and is one way for the patient to get a little exercise. Change the patient's position to include lying on the back, lying on the stomach, lying on the right side, lying on the left side, and sitting up. Establish a turning schedule as a reminder of when and how to turn the patient. Use pillows to help support the patient in each position. The pictures on the next pages give you an idea of how to position the patient and how to place the pillows.

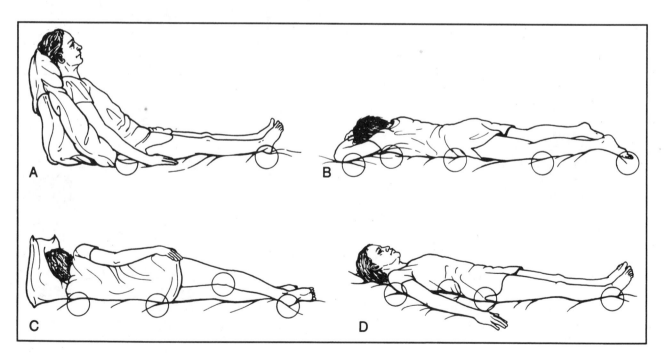

Position 1

Time: _____

Maximum time in this position: _____

Left side

Position 2

Time: _____

Maximum time in this position: _____

Back

Position 3

Time: _____

Maximum time in this position: _____

Right side

Position 4

Time: _____

Maximum time in this position: _____

Stomach

REMEMBER:
Only a 30 degree angle on the side position.
A pillow under the shoulders or hips to hold the position.
Pad all bony areas with pillows or rolled towels.
Never let the heels of the feet rest directly on the bed.

Lying on the Back

Put a flat, firm pillow under the patient's head. The patient's head and back should be in alignment. The patient's arms should be at his or her sides, with the palms up. Firm, flat pillows can be placed under the patient's arms and hands to support them. Straighten the patient's legs, point the patient's toes upward, and put a foot board at the end of the bed to support the patient's feet. Place a small, firm pillow beneath the patient's ankles to allow the heels to hang freely. Whenever possible use a draw sheet or transfer board to move the patient.

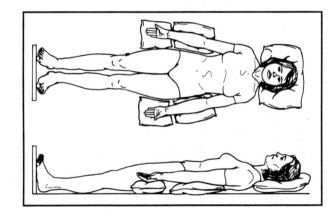

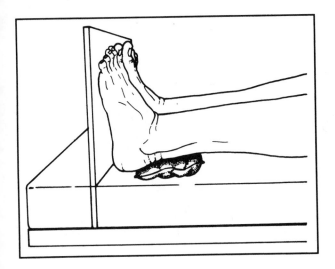

the top leg. Support the top leg and foot with a pillow. The patient's arms can be positioned as shown in the pictures.

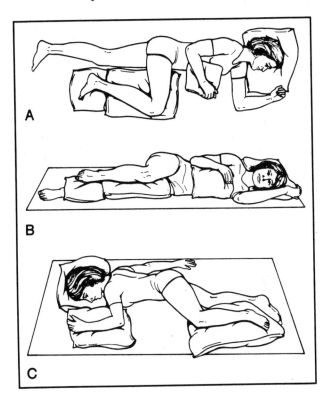

Lying on the Stomach

Put the patient on his or her stomach, with the face to one side and the arms bent at the elbows. Roll a small towel and place it under the patient's shoulder. Put a large pillow under the patient's legs from the knees to the ankles. Make sure the patient's feet hang from the pillow and that the patient's toes are not touching the bed. Place a small pillow under the patient's head for comfort.

Sitting Up

Help the patient to a sitting position. Put several pillows behind the patient to serve as a bolster. Put pillows under the patient's arms and legs to support them. A footboard with pillows in front of it will support the patient's feet and keep the patient from sliding down.

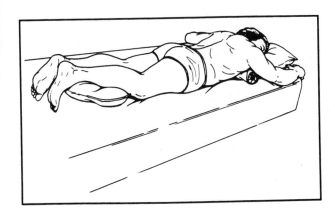

Lying on the Right or Left Side

Put the patient on one side, with the head and back in alignment. Tuck a pillow snugly behind the patient's back. Put a firm, flat pillow under the patient's head, making sure that the patient's neck is straight. Extend the patient's bottom leg and bend

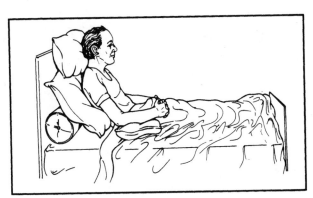

Turning

If the patient cannot turn without help, fold a sheet in half along its width and put it across the middle of the bed, under the patient. Roll the patient over the rolled section of the sheet. This is called a drawsheet. The drawsheet should extend from the patient's chest to the knees. To turn the patient, go to one side of the patient's bed, reach across the patient, and grab the end of the drawsheet on the

other side. Pull it toward you and use the drawsheet to turn the patient toward you. Prop the patient as described in the section *Lying on the Right or Left Side*.

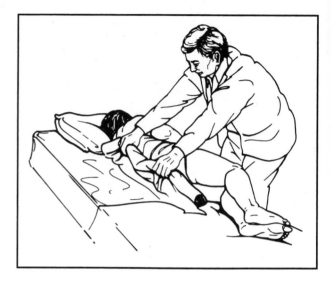

Schedule Exercises for the Patient at Least Every 2 Hours

Exercise helps prevent the pooling of fluids in the patient's lungs. It also helps keep the patient's bowels regular. Ask the nurse for a copy of the instruction sheet for range-of-motion exercises. The nurse can show you how to do exercises with the patient who is confined to bed.

Keep the Patient's Skin Clean

Skin that is not kept clean is more likely to develop problems. Ask the nurse for a copy of the instruction sheet for skin care. Even wrinkles or bumps in the bed linens or clothing can cause friction and skin irritation, so keep bed surfaces as smooth and clean as possible.

Make Sure the Patient's Diet Is Well Balanced

A well-balanced diet will help the patient maintain strength and well-being. Ask the nurse for a copy of the instruction sheet *A Healthful Eating Plan*.

OTHER INSTRUCTIONS

Care of Dentures

Dentures should be cleaned after every meal and at bedtime.

STEPS

1. Wash your hands.
2. Gather the equipment. You need
   - A basin,
   - A washcloth,
   - A denture cup with a top,
   - A toothbrush,
   - Toothpaste or dentifrice,
   - Mouthwash.
3. Remove the dentures.
   a. Grasp the front of the upper plate on either side with your thumbs and index fingers. Placing the washcloth or a gauze pad between your fingers and the dentures may make this easier.
   b. Use slight pressure and gently wiggle the denture to break its seal on the gum.
   c. When the seal breaks, pull the denture forward to remove it from the patient's mouth.
   d. Put the upper denture into the basin.
   e. Grasp the front of the lower denture between your thumb and index finger. Placing the washcloth or a gauze pad between your fingers and the dentures may make this easier.
   f. Turn the lower denture slightly (this breaks the seal).
   g. When the seal breaks, lift the denture out of the patient's mouth.
4. Take the basin with the dentures to the bathroom.
5. Put a washcloth on the bottom of the sink and fill the sink half way with warm water. The washcloth acts as a cushion if the dentures are accidentally dropped.
6. Put the dentures carefully into the sink.
7. Put toothpaste or dentifrice on the toothbrush.
8. Scrub both dentures carefully and thoroughly.
9. Rinse the dentures with cold running water.
10. Offer the patient mouthwash or help the patient gently brush his or her tongue and gums.
11. Rewet the dentures with cool water just before reinserting them. The water helps form a stronger seal between the dentures and gums than if the dentures were put in dry.
12. If the patient uses a dental adhesive, apply it to the dentures according to the directions on the package.
13. Insert the upper denture into the patient's mouth. Press the denture firmly in place with your fingers.
14. Insert the lower denture. Make sure the denture is properly aligned on the gum.
15. Wash your hands.
16. If the dentures are put into a denture cup for overnight storage, add water and a drop of peppermint oil, lemon juice, or vinegar. This will deodorize the dentures. Be sure to rinse the dentures well under cool running water before reinserting them into the patient's mouth.

OTHER INSTRUCTIONS

Changing Dressings

GENERAL INFORMATION

A dressing (bandage) is used to protect a wound from being hurt or getting dirty (infected). The wound heals better if the dressing is changed to keep the wound clean.

KEY POINTS

1. Wash your hands with warm water and soap (or a moist disposable towelette) before and after each dressing change.
2. Dressings are made in lots of shapes, sizes, and materials.
3. When changing the dressing, follow the steps as you were shown. Change the dressing as often as directed.
4. Call your nurse or doctor if
   a. There is more swelling of the skin and wound,
   b. There is more pain at the wound,
   c. There is more redness of the skin and wound,
   d. The skin around the wound is warm to the touch (do not touch the wound),
   e. There is a fever (an oral temperature over 100°F),
   f. Drainage occurs after the wound was dry,
   g. There are any openings in the wound after the skin has closed.

EQUIPMENT

You will need

- Dressings _____ ,
- Tape _____ ,
- A bag for old dressings to be thrown away (use a plastic bag if dressings are wet).

You may be told to use one or more of these:

_____ Gloves (unsterile),
_____ A cleaning solution,
_____ Medicine or ointment,
_____ A protective waterproof pad.

STEPS

1. Wash your hands with warm water and soap or use a moist disposable towelette. Dry your hands well.
2. Gather all equipment that will be used for the dressing change and place the supplies on a clean surface.
3. Open the bag for old dressings.
4. Change the dressing in a brightly lit, comfortable, private area.
   a. Do not change the dressing at mealtime.
   b. If the dressing smells bad, air out the room.
5. Remove the old dressing by
   a. Peeling back the tape's edge while holding the skin tight.
   b. If the edges of the tape do not pull away easily, use a little baby oil on a cotton-tipped swab to loosen them.
   c. Remove the tape by pulling slowly straight toward the wound.
6. Remove the old dressing with care.
   a. Put gloves on before touching the old dressing.
   b. Do not touch the wound.
   c. Try to remove the dressing by touching only the edges.
   d. Look for any drainage on the dressing.
7. Put the old dressing in the garbage bag.
   a. If the dressing is wet, use a plastic bag.
   b. If using gloves, place them in the bag also.
   c. Wash your hands.
8. Look at the skin and wound. Note
   a. Any changes in the skin or wound since you last changed the dressing,
   b. The color of the skin around the wound (the skin should not be red, swollen, or warm).

9. Look at the wound.
   a. If there is drainage, note
      • The color,
      • The odor,
      • The amount,
      • Whether this is new drainage in a wound that was dry.
   b. Note any swelling or more redness of the wound.
   c. Note any open place in a wound that looked like it had already healed or closed.
10. If you are told to clean the wound,
   a. You may need to place a waterproof pad under the patient to protect linens and clothes from spills.
   b. Put on clean gloves.
   c. Pour the solution onto the gauze pad or cotton-tipped swabs.

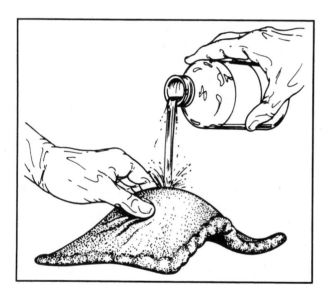

   • Do not touch the part of the pad or cotton that will touch the wound.
   • Do not reuse any pads or cotton-tipped swabs.

   d. Clean the wound by starting from the wound and moving outward. Do not return to an area you have already cleaned.

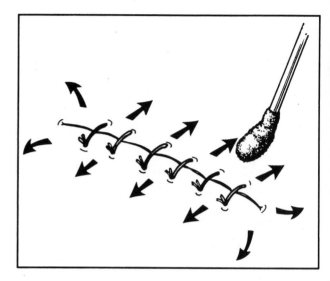

11. Apply the dressing so that it covers and protects the wound.
   a. Put on clean gloves.

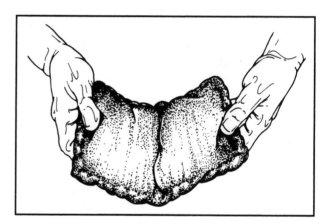

   b. Touch only the edges of the dressing. Do not touch the dressing where it will touch the wound.

c. If you are using a split dressing, place the slit carefully around the tube.

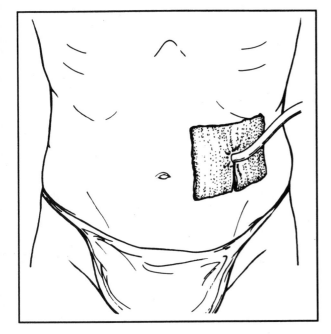

c. If you are using gloves, remove them and put them into the garbage bag.

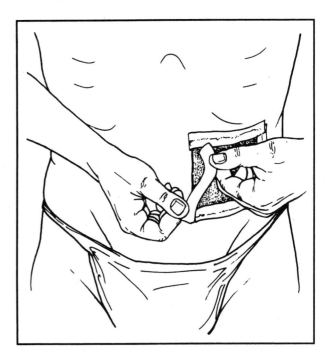

d. Change your dressing every _____
_____ .

e. If you are using a transparent dressing, follow the directions on the package.

12. Tape the dressing so it does not move.
   a. First tape the edge of the dressing.
   b. Gently press on each side to fasten the tape.

13. Close the garbage bag tightly and put it in a closed garbage can.
   a. Do not forget to use a plastic bag if the dressing is wet.
   b. Being careful to throw away the old dressing avoids the spread of disease.

14. Wash your hands well.

OTHER INSTRUCTIONS

Clinical Signs of Imminent Death

SIGNS

The following signs usually indicate that death can be expected within 48 hours:

1. Twitching of the arms or legs,
2. Aimless, and often unconscious, picking at the bed linens,
3. General restlessness,
4. Cold skin,
5. Mottling (blotching) or cyanosis (blue or blue-gray discoloration) of the feet, hands, lips, arms, and legs,
6. Blurred vision,
7. Hallucinations (particularly of a religious nature or of significant persons who are dead),
8. Difficulty speaking,
9. Relaxation of the facial muscles,
10. Cheyne-Stokes respirations (a cycle of breathing in which respirations become faster and deeper and are followed by a slower rate and periods of no breathing that may last up to 60 seconds),
11. Death rattle (breathing that is noisy, bubbling, or gurgling),
12. Statements by the patient such as, "I know I am going to die soon,"
13. Fever,
14. Little or no urinary output.

WHAT TO DO

Telephone the home care agency or hospice or the doctor when these signs appear. Follow-up instructions will be given to you.

The patient may or may not lose consciousness. In either case, you can help your loved one through the process of dying and the actual moment of death by touching, stroking, hand holding, expressing your feelings of love, speaking of shared memories, praying, and saying goodbye. Although it may be difficult, it is often reassuring to your loved one to hear that it is okay to let go or to take leave of this life.

Schedule a shift of persons special to the patient so that the patient has a constant companion during this time. With this approach, no one becomes overwhelmed, and the patient does not feel abandoned.

OTHER INSTRUCTIONS

Comfort Measures for Dehydration

GENERAL INFORMATION

The loss of necessary body fluids is called dehydration. A person can become dehydrated because of vomiting, diarrhea, excessive perspiration, or inadequate fluid intake.

HOME CARE GUIDELINES

The following guidelines are used to help a person who is dehydrated be more comfortable.

1. Encourage daily intake of at least ten 8-ounce glasses of fluid.
   a. Offer a range of fluids for selection.
   b. Offer fresh drinking water.
   c. Offer small drinks often (for example, 4 ounces of fluid every hour).
   d. Measure and record each day's fluid intake.

   e. Offer ice chips or cubes.
   f. Offer gelatin and popsicles.
2. Offer hard candy such as lemon drops or sugar-free mints.
3. Moisten food with gravies and sauces.
4. Use a humidifier.
5. Use artificial saliva and tears.
6. Do mouth care regularly and often throughout the day.
   a. Moisten lips with a wet washcloth.
   b. Apply bland lip cream.
   c. Avoid commercial mouthwashes.
   d. Rinse the mouth with a nonirritating solution you can make by mixing one teaspoon of salt, one teaspoon of baking soda, and one quart of water.
   e. Avoid toothpaste with rough grains in it.
   f. Choose a toothbrush with soft, rounded bristles.
7. Measure the individual's fluid intake and output.

OTHER INSTRUCTIONS

General Comfort Measures

The following are ways to help the patient feel better.

COMPANY

- Visits by family members and friends
- Telephone calls from family members and friends
- Cards, notes, and letters from family members and friends
- Being in the part of the home where family members spend most of their time
- Being by a window where the neighborhood activities can be seen

SURROUNDINGS

- A room that is not too hot or too cold
- Use of a humidifier or dehumidifier
- A room with good ventilation and fresh air
- A room that is not overcrowded and cluttered
- A room that is clean
- A noise level that is not loud and annoying
- No unpleasant odors in or near the room
- A natural or soft lighting
- A bed or chair that is clean and free of wrinkles
- Wall colors and decor that are pleasing to the patient
- A variety of textures (flannel, cotton, satin), prints, and colors for bed linens and pajamas
- Loose-fitting and comfortable clothing
- Needed things that are within the patient's reach
- A way the patient can call for help (bell, buzzer, telephone)

ACTIVITIES

- Read books and magazines.
- Play cards and board games.
- Play video or computer games.
- Watch television.
- Listen to the radio.
- Do crossword puzzles, find-a-word puzzles, and word jumbles.
- Draw, paint, or color.
- Listen to tape cassettes.
- Do arts and crafts.
- Do needlework.
- Keep a diary or journal.
- Snuggle with a loved one.

WAYS FOR THE PATIENT TO RELAX

- Tense up and relax your body parts from head to toe.
- Close your eyes and think about someplace you would rather be.
- Take slow deep breaths; keep your eyes closed.
- Have a back rub.
- Lie or sit in a comfortable position.
- Change your position at least once an hour.
- Snuggle under a quilt or afghan.
- Lie on a sheepskin pad or soft blanket that is fresh from the dryer.
- Drink a glass of warm milk, tea and honey, or a hot toddy.
- Lie next to a warm hot-water bottle.

OTHER INSTRUCTIONS

Hair Washing in Bed

STEPS

1. Wash your hands.
2. Gather your equipment. You need
   - A low chair or stool,
   - Two pitchers of warm water,
   - Shampoo,
   - A bucket for dirty water,
   - A shampoo basin,
   - Large plastic bags or sheets,
   - A pillow wrapped in plastic,
   - Towels,
   - A comb or brush.
3. Put the low chair or stool near the head of the patient's bed. Put the bucket on it.
4. Help the patient into a comfortable position, with his or her shoulders on the pillow.
5. Place the shampoo basin under the patient's head. Make sure the spout of the basin extends past the edge of the bed to over the bucket. (If you don't have a shampoo basin, use a regular wash basin. Use extra pillows to prop the patient's head high enough to let the rinse water go into the basin without difficulty.)
6. Place the plastic bags around and under the edges of the shampoo basin.
7. Wet the patient's hair with warm water.
8. Apply a little bit of shampoo to the patient's hair.
9. Work the shampoo into a lather. Massage the patient's scalp gently with your fingertips. Start at the patient's hairline and move to the back of the head.
10. Rinse the patient's hair with warm water. Make sure all the shampoo is rinsed out.
11. If necessary, repeat steps 8 through 10.
12. Squeeze the excess water out of the patient's hair.
13. Wrap a towel around the patient's head.
14. Remove the equipment from the bed and help the patient to a comfortable position.
15. Dry the patient's hair. If the towel becomes saturated, use another one.
16. Help the patient comb his or her hair.
17. Change any wet bed linens or wet clothing.
18. Clean the equipment and put it away.
19. Wash your hands.

OTHER INSTRUCTIONS

Hand Washing

The friction of rubbing your hands together with soap and water is adequate for removing almost all germs that can cause disease.

Wash your hands often.

- Wash before you touch or eat foods.
- Wash before you touch your eyes or mouth.
- Wash before you touch a cut or a bandage.
- Wash after you go to the bathroom.
- Wash after you blow your nose, cough, or sneeze.
- Wash after you touch an animal, even your own pet.

Use this technique when you wash your hands.

1. Use warm water and a mild soap.
2. Wash for a at least a half-minute.
3. Wash all parts of your hands, including the back of your hands, between your fingers, and under your fingernails.
4. Rinse all the soap off.
5. Dry your hands with a paper towel or a clean cloth towel. Do not share your towel.

OTHER INSTRUCTIONS

Mouth Care

GENERAL INFORMATION

Mouth care prevents bad breath, tooth decay, gum disease, and infections of the oral cavity. It should be done at least after each meal and at bedtime.

STEPS

1. Wash your hands.
2. Gather your equipment. You need
   - Mouthwash,
   - A cleansing solution of sodium bicarbonate and water or of hydrogen peroxide and water,
   - Mouth-care applicators (bought or made by wrapping several gauze pads around the end of a tongue blade) or a soft toothbrush,
   - Petroleum jelly,
   - Towels,
   - A basin.
3. Have the patient sit up. If the patient is unable to sit up, place the patient on his or her side, facing you.
4. Put a towel under the patient's chin.
5. Soak an applicator or a soft-bristled toothbrush in the cleansing solution.
6. Gently insert the applicator or toothbrush into the patient's mouth and clean the patient's tongue from the back to the tip.
7. Wipe the gums, teeth, roof of the mouth, floor of the mouth, and inside of the cheeks with soaked applicators or toothbrush. If you are using applicators, change to a new one often.
8. Repeat steps 4 through 6 with mouthwash or cool water. If the patient is able, let him or her gargle with the mouthwash or water. Orange juice diluted with water is also a refreshing mouth rinse.
9. Dry the patient's mouth and chin.
10. Put a small amount of petroleum jelly on the patient's lips and gums.
11. Wash your hands.
12. Help the patient to a comfortable position.

LET THE NURSE KNOW

If any of the following happens, tell the nurse:

1. The patient's gums bleed during mouth care.
2. The patient develops very bad breath.
3. The patient's gums are red, swollen, or tender.
4. Pus comes out between the patient's teeth and gums during mouth care or when they are pressed.
5. The patient has or develops loose teeth.
6. The patient's gums begin to shrink away from the teeth.
7. There is a change in the way the patient's teeth come together when biting.
8. The patient's dentures fit differently.

OTHER INSTRUCTIONS

Muscle Relaxation Technique

Relaxation is an important part of your lifestyle. It makes you feel good and is also helpful in

- Decreasing heart rate,
- Decreasing blood pressure,
- Slowing down the body so it can recharge,
- Releasing muscle tension and relieving body aches.

The following technique may be helpful when you need to relax. Read each step and follow the instructions and see if it works for you.

1. Sit quietly in a comfortable position.
2. Close your eyes. *Do not fall asleep.*
3. Tighten all muscles in your body as tight as possible to the count of 10, then relax them all at once.
4. Breathe through your nose—deep breathe in, then as you breathe out, say the word *one* silently to yourself as you continue to breathe out. Example: breath in . . . out, *one,* in . . . out, *one.* Breathe easily and naturally.
5. Continue to do this for 10 to 20 minutes. You may open your eyes to check the time, but do not use an alarm. When finished, sit quietly for a few minutes before opening your eyes and getting up.
6. Do not worry about whether you are successful in achieving a deep level of relaxation. Let relaxation occur at its own pace.
7. When distracting thoughts occur, try to ignore them and return to repeating *one.*
8. Make this technique a part of your daily routine. Practice once or twice a day.

OTHER INSTRUCTIONS

Skin Care

GENERAL INFORMATION

Keeping the skin in good condition is most important. By following the guidelines for good skin care, you can prevent most pressure sores (bedsores). Pressure sores can develop quickly in people who

- Are very thin,
- Are obese,
- Collect fluid in their tissues (have edema),
- Have poor nutrition,
- Are elderly,
- Already have skin damage or an infection,
- Are mentally confused,
- Are bed-bound or cannot turn from side to side (at least every 1 to 2 hours),
- Suffer from bowel and or bladder incontinence.

GUIDELINES

Healthy skin can be broken by pressure, moisture, and shearing (friction). Follow these guidelines to prevent problems.

Pressure

1. Turn the patient *at least* every 1 to 2 hours to avoid pressure on bony areas of the body.
2. Massage reddened skin gently at least three or four times daily. Use lotions like Keri, Uni-Derm, or Vaseline Intensive Care.
3. Use pillows to support the patient who is lying on his or her side. Ask your nurse or doctor for a copy of *Care of the Patient Confined to Bed.*
4. Use a pressure-relief device (like a 4-inch foam pad) for the bed or chair. Your nurse or doctor will discuss which is best for your situation.

Moisture (Skin that Is Often Wet)

1. Keep the skin clean and dry.
2. Soap and alcohol can dry out the skin. Soap also leaves a film unless it is carefully rinsed off.
3. For patients who cannot control their bladder or bowels, wash the genital area (from front to back) after each urination or passage of stool. Use neutral skin cleansers like Peri-Wash or Uni-Wash.

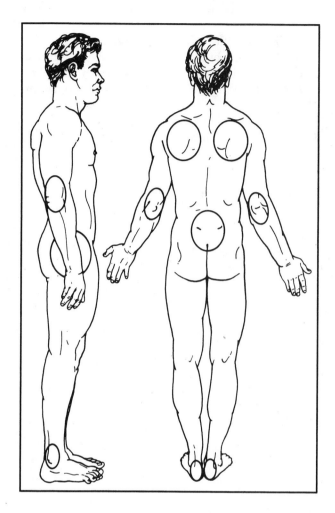

4. After the skin is cleaned and dried, use a protective ointment or spray such as A&D ointment, Uni-Derm, Peri-Care, or Sween Cream, if so instructed.
5. Keep linens dry, with the bottom sheet tightly tucked in.

Shearing (Friction)

1. Use sheepskins or turning sheets for turning and moving the patient. Do not drag or pull the patient for positioning.
2. Heel and elbow protectors are helpful.
3. Keep the surface of the bed smooth and clean.
4. If the patient is bed-bound, raise the foot of the bed slightly (no more than 30 degrees) and support him or her with pillows to reduce the chance of sliding down in the bed.

CARE OF THE SKIN

1. Provide privacy and uncover only the body area you are washing.
2. Place a towel under the body area that will be washed.
3. Wash the skin with warm water. If soap is needed, use a brand like Dove, Basis, or Purpose or use a castile soap. These soaps are nonalkaline and nondrying. Rinse well with warm water. Pat dry.
4. Massage red skin areas gently.
5. Use protective ointment or medicated ointments, if instructed.
6. Cornstarch can be sprinkled lightly between the patient and the linens, if needed. Avoid using powders, since they harden and cake.
7. Turn and position the patient every _____ hours. Post a turning schedule. Ask your nurse for a copy of *Care of the Patient Confined to Bed.*
8. Call your nurse or doctor if
   a. The patient develops an open skin area,
   b. The open skin area/sore is getting bigger,
   c. The open skin area feels warm, is red, and has an odor or drainage.
9. Encourage the patient to eat a well-balanced diet.

OTHER INSTRUCTIONS

12 Steps for Mastering Pain

The following will help you take an active role in the control and management of pain.

1. Accept the pain.
2. Plan activities that distract from the pain.
3. Take your medicine on a schedule. Discuss with your nurse the amount of medication you take and how it should be used.
4. Keep a written log of your pain: what causes the pain, when the pain is increased, and what things relieve the pain.
5. Exercise daily.
6. Practice relaxation techniques regularly.
7. Keep busy and do not allow your pain to determine your plans.
8. Pace yourself to avoid getting overtired and run down.
9. Share your feelings with family members, friends, or others who have pain.
10. Tell your nurse or doctor about the pain. Be honest about whether or not the pain is relieved by your pain medications.
11. Remain hopeful.

OTHER INSTRUCTIONS

UNIT 9

Neurologic and Musculoskeletal Alterations

Arthritis

GENERAL INFORMATION

Arthritis is a general name used to describe almost 100 diseases that result in pain, stiffness, and swelling in one or more joints. It can affect people of all ages. The different types of arthritis call for different treatments.

It is most important that you follow only the treatments your doctor and nurse have discussed with you. The treatment plan may be made up of medicine and an exercise and joint protection plan, as well as ways to help you adjust to this disease.

GUIDELINES

These suggestions are meant to help you adjust to arthritis. Your nurse can explain each of them.

1. Follow only the treatments in your treatment plan.
   a. Keep your appointments with your doctor, nurse, or clinic.
   b. Avoid promises of "miracle cures" and fads. There is no cure for arthritis.
   c. Use of herbal and alternative medications or treatments should be discussed with your nurse or doctor.
2. Eat a well-balanced diet.
   a. The nurse can teach you the basics of good nutrition.
   b. Ask the nurse or doctor about weight loss if you are overweight.
   c. Your nurse or doctor will give you a copy of your diet.
3. Follow your activity, exercise, and rest program.
   a. Exercise is the key to keeping good joint motion.
   b. Alternate work and rest periods.
      • Work at an even pace.
      • Avoid fatigue.
   c. Do the range-of-motion exercises as you have been shown.
      • Plan your exercise for those times when your joints are less stiff.
      • Exercise can be easier in water (a pool or bathtub).
   d. Your nurse or doctor will tell you about your activity and exercise plan.
4. Ask about self-help devices that can help you with daily activities. The nurse, therapist, or doctor can suggest specific devices that will be best for you. Some common self-help devices are

• Bath and toilet grab bars,
• Long-handled combs and shoe horns,
• Bath brushes,
• Devices for putting on socks,
• Eating utensils with large, easy to hold handles,
• Velcro fasteners for clothes and shoes.
5. Follow energy- and joint-saving guidelines.
   a. Take a warm shower or bath for 15 to 20 minutes.
      • In the morning, to relieve morning stiffness and allow more free exercise of joints,
      • Before bedtime, to help with sleep.
      • Use a shower stool to save energy.
   b. Avoid standing or sitting for long periods.
      • Change position as often as possible (at least every 30 minutes).
      • Always use good posture when lying down, standing, or sitting. Your nurse can teach you.
   c. Raise the height of items, if needed.
      • Use raised chair and toilet seats.
      • The bed can be raised on blocks.
      • The height of electric outlets can be raised or an extension cord can be secured at the right height.
   d. Wear tieless or Velcro-fastened shoes.
   e. Wear clothes that fasten in the front or that do not have small buttons.
   f. Build ramps to replace stairs.
6. Take your medicine as instructed.
   a. Do not take any medicine without checking with the nurse or doctor first.
   b. Call the nurse or doctor if you have any of the side effects that were discussed with you.
   c. Keep handy accurate information about your medicine:
      • Your medicine's name,
      • When to take,
      • Possible side effects,
      • Special notes.
7. The nurse can teach you about resources that can help you learn to live with arthritis.
   a. A social worker or a family service agency in the community can help with
      • Financial aid to meet your long-term health needs,
      • Household help for care of children or for an elderly family member.
   b. The State Division of Vocational Rehabilitation and State Employment Services may help with job retraining and employment.

c. Sexual counseling may be useful (position and techniques) if joint pain and stiffness affect sexual satisfaction.

d. Self-help groups such as the Arthritis Club can be a source of support.

e. You may get more information from

The Arthritis Foundation
PO BOX 19000
Atlanta, Georgia 30326

- Your local chapter _____

_____ .

OTHER INSTRUCTIONS

8. Signs and symptoms to report to your nurse or doctor:

a. Stiffness and swelling that is getting worse,

b. Skin breakdown,

c. Falls,

d. Unusual bleeding (bleeding gums, skin bruises),

e. Medicine side effects.

Cast Care

GENERAL INFORMATION

A cast is used to keep a part of the body from moving until the bones or ligaments can heal. Protecting the skin inside the cast is cotton padding. Casts are made of different materials. They can be used on almost any part of the body.

GUIDELINES

Cast Care

1. For a plaster cast, keep the cast clean and dry.
   a. White shoe polish can be used for touch-ups (do not paint the cast).
   b. Using a washcloth and basin may be the easiest way to bathe.
   c. If your nurse or doctor allows you, cover the cast with a waterproof sleeve or a plastic bag before you take a shower or bath. Tie the bag securely above the cast. Do not wet the cast. It can cause skin rashes.
   d. If the cast becomes wet, dry it with a hair dryer.
2. With a fiberglass cast, you may be allowed to wet the cast.
   a. Dry the cast following your nurse's or doctor's directions.
   b. Dampness should not be felt under the cast after drying.
3. Carefully check the skin at the edges of the cast for redness. Cover rough edges on the cast with mole skin. Do not use oils, lotions, or powders on the skin under the cast.
4. Do not scratch the skin under the cast. Do not stick anything down into the cast to scratch the skin. Be careful to keep crumbs and small objects from falling inside the cast.
5. Do not wear rings on the fingers of your casted arm. Support the casted arm in a sling, if given one. Use an old hat or a sock to keep your fingers or toes warm.

Activity

1. Follow your nurse's or doctor's directions for exercise and diet.
2. Do not walk on a leg cast unless your doctor approves.
3. Follow your nurse's or doctor's directions for the use of cast aids (crutches or a sling).

4. Avoid activities that could damage the cast like hard sports or swimming.

Elevation

1. Keep the cast raised (elevated) above the level of your heart, when possible.
2. Minor swelling, discomfort, and change in skin color (blue tinge) are common for the first few days after the cast is put on. This is normal when the casted limb is not raised.
3. Using pillows under and around the cast, especially while sitting, may help to make you feel better.
4. Raise the casted leg on pillows for at least the first 24 hours and when sitting.
5. Support the casted arm in a sling, if given one.
6. Wiggle your fingers or toes occasionally to prevent swelling.

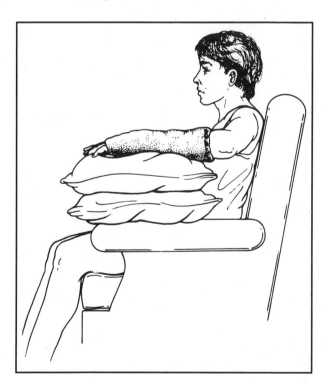

Pain Relief

1. Follow your doctor's directions for medications.
2. If allowed, your doctor may also recommend taking acetaminophen or ibuprofen.

REPORT TO YOUR NURSE OR DOCTOR IMMEDIATELY

If any of the following happens, call your nurse or doctor immediately:

1. Any break or crack or softness in the cast,
2. Any very red skin areas or any break in the skin,
3. Signs of a tight cast,
   a. Extreme redness, coldness, or increased swelling of fingers or toes after the casted limb is raised above the level of your heart,
   b. Fingers or toes that remain discolored (pale) or blue-tinged after the casted limb is raised above the level of your heart,
   c. Numbness, tingling ("pins and needles") or burning of fingers or toes,
   d. Pain that is not relieved by medication or pain that is getting worse,
4. The cast feels too loose or too tight.
5. Unusual or bad smell or drainage from the cast,
6. Fever higher than 101°F (39.3°C),
7. New problems with moving fingers or toes,
8. A child with a cast who is fussy for no reason.

OTHER INSTRUCTIONS

Type of cast _____

Use of cast aids _____

Activity _____

Diet _____

Guidelines for Describing Seizure Activity

A seizure is caused by abnormal electrical activity in the brain. Depending on the area of the brain and the amount of abnormal activity, the seizure can range from mild twitching to major body muscle spasms. The following questions are useful for organizing your observations of a seizure. Become familiar with them, and you will be able to recall important details of a seizure for the nurse or doctor.

	Yes	No	Comments

PRESEIZURE FACTORS

1. Did the patient have some kind of emotional upset?
2. Was the seizure started by some kind of environmental stimulus (for example, flashing lights or screechy noises)?
3. Did the patient forget to take his or her medication?
4. Did the patient have a temperature (convulsions with fever can occur with a temperature of 104°F or 40°C)?

AURA

1. Did the patient know he or she was going to have a seizure? How did the patient know?
2. Did the patient have any unusual taste, smell, or visual change before the seizure occurred?

INVOLVEMENT

1. Was there body rigidity (tonic) at the start of the seizure? How long did it last?
2. Was there tingling and twitching of one part of the body?
3. Was there muscle spasms and jerking (clonic) of one part of the body?
4. Did the twitching spread from one body part to another?
5. Was the seizure localized (confined to one part of the body) or generalized (involved the whole body)?
6. Did the position of the body change?
7. Were the teeth clenched?
8. Was there foaming from the mouth?
9. Did the lips or face change color?

EYE CHANGES

1. Did the eyes move to either side, upward, or downward?
2. Were there any involuntary rapid eye movements?
3. What were the size and reactions of the pupils?

ELIMINATION	Yes	No	Comments

1. Did the patient lose control of his or her bowels or bladder?

RESPIRATORY PATTERN

1. Was there any difficulty breathing?
2. Did the patient stop breathing?
3. Was there any irregular breathing, loud breathing, or snoring?

CONSCIOUSNESS CHANGES

1. Was there a loss of consciousness?
2. How long was the patient unconscious?
3. Could the patient be roused to the point of response?
4. Was the patient sleepy or confused during the seizure?
5. Was there an intense feeling of fear?
6. Did the child become confused, become difficult to wake up, or start to act very sick?

AFTER THE SEIZURE

1. Was the patient able to move all the extremities?
2. Did the patient experience any weakness or did the caregiver notice any weakness?
3. Did the patient have any complaint of discomfort or unusual sensations after the seizure?
4. Did the patient have any changes or peculiarities of speech?
5. Was the patient confused? How long did the confusion last?
6. Did the patient have any other behavioral change?
7. Did the patient complain of a headache?
8. What was the patient's level of consciousness?

FREQUENCY AND DURATION

1. How long had it been since the last seizure?
2. How long did this seizure last?

OTHER INSTRUCTIONS

SEIZURE RECORD

Date	Time	How Long Seizure Lasted	Description of Seizure Activity

Management of Seizure Activity

STEPS

The following steps will maintain the comfort and safety of a person who is experiencing or states he or she is about to experience a seizure.

1. Gently lower the person to the floor.
   - The floor is preferable to a bed or couch, since there is no chance of falling.
2. Clear the area around the person.
   - Move furniture and other objects that would cause injury if hit by the person during seizure activity.
3. Place something soft under the person's head.
   - A flat pillow or a rolled sweater or coat is usually enough to protect the person's head.
4. Insert a mouth gag, a padded tongue blade, or an oral airway into the person's mouth, *if the jaws are not clenched*.
   - Do not attempt to insert anything into the person's mouth if the jaws are clenched. Doing so could cause great injury.
5. Loosen tight clothing around the person's head, neck, and chest.
6. Do not restrain (hold the person still) or interfere with the person's movements.
   - Interference or restraint could worsen the seizure activity.
7. Turn the person onto his or her side after the seizure.

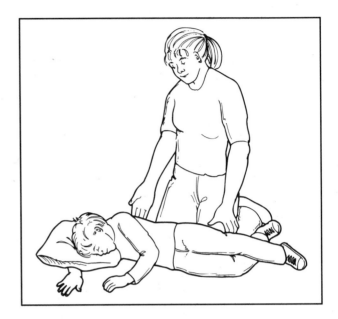

8. Give artificial respiration, if needed.
9. Remain with the person during and after the seizure.
10. Tell the person where he or she is and what happened, after the seizure.
11. Time how long the seizure lasts.
    - Call for emergency services if the seizure lasts more than 3 to 5 minutes.

OTHER INSTRUCTIONS

Seizure Precautions

GUIDELINES

The following suggestions can help reduce the chance of seizure activity and protect you from injury when seizures do occur.

Reducing the Chance of Seizure Activity

1. Take your medications as prescribed.
2. Do not discontinue your medications unless told to do so by your doctor.
3. Try to keep a regular daily schedule.
4. Do not physically overexert yourself. Know your limits.
5. Avoid emotional stress. The nurse can teach you stress-management techniques.
6. Get at least 8 hours of rest a day or the amount that you need to feel refreshed.
7. Make sure your diet is well balanced. Avoid eating or drinking too much. The nurse or dietitian can teach you how to do this.
8. Avoid coffee and tea or switch to decaffeinated brands. Abrupt withdrawal from caffeine can provoke seizure activity.
9. Avoid alcoholic drinks, as the alcohol can affect your medications.
10. Avoid smoking.
11. Avoid using herbal or alternative medications or treatments, stimulants, and sedatives without prior approval from your doctor.
12. Fever control

   a. For adults: take aspirin or acetaminophen and use cool compresses.
   b. For children: check with your doctor about taking acetaminophen or ibuprofen, encourage drinking plenty of fluids, use only one blanket for a cover to prevent overheating, and use cool compresses to reduce fever.

13. Identify and avoid things that provoke your seizure activity (for example, flashing lights or screechy noises).
14. Be aware that fever and infection can provoke seizure activity.

Protecting Yourself from Injury

1. Wear an emergency medical identification bracelet or tag.
2. Take your temperature under your arm, rectally, or use an ear thermometer. The nurse can teach you how to do this. Avoid taking your temperature by mouth.
3. Do not swim alone.
4. Do not take a bath in a tub until you have been free of seizures for the amount of time specified by your doctor (_____ months).
5. Do not operate heavy equipment until you have been free of seizures for the amount of time specified by your doctor (_____ months).
6. Do not drive until you have been free of seizures for the amount of time specified by the state division of motor vehicles (_____ months).

OTHER INSTRUCTIONS

UNIT 10

Elimination Alterations

Bladder Retraining

GENERAL INFORMATION

The goal of bladder retraining is to train your body to pass urine at regular and predictable times. A consistent schedule and practice of certain exercises will strengthen your bladder's muscle tone and help achieve this goal.

Retraining can take weeks, or even months, to complete; you might become frustrated. You might be afraid to go out because of the possibility of an accident. You might become irritated at having to follow a rigid schedule closely. You might feel embarrassed because your family is focusing so much attention on one of your personal body functions. These emotions are a normal and expected part of the retraining process.

Talk to the nurse about how you feel. The nurse will help you deal with your feelings in a constructive way.

The nurse will also teach you about bladder retraining and how to cope with the changes it makes in your life. The following information will help you remember what the nurse teaches.

INSTRUCTIONS

Your Toileting Schedule

_____

_____

_____

_____

_____

General Guidelines for Bladder Retraining

1. Learn to recognize when your bladder needs to be emptied. The signs of a full bladder are restlessness, a feeling of fullness in the lower abdominal region, chills, excessive perspiration, and headache.
2. Go to the bathroom as soon as you feel the urge to pass urine.
3. A high intake of fluid is necessary to produce enough urine to stimulate the voiding reflex (your body's signal to you that it needs to pass urine). Drink at least _____ glasses of water each day. Plan a regular schedule of fluid intake (for example, one 6-ounce glass of water every hour). This will make it easier to establish a predictable

routine for urinating. Limiting your fluid intake when away from home and increasing it when you return will help prevent accidents.
4. Strengthen the muscles that are used during urination by stopping the urine stream, holding back a few seconds, and starting the stream again. Women should also do Kegel exercises (tense up your buttocks, hold for 3 seconds, and relax) 15 to 20 times each hour.
5. Call the nurse or doctor if you develop a fever, have pain when you urinate, or notice that your urine is cloudy or smells bad.

Ways to Stimulate Urination

1. Think about rain, flowing rivers, dripping faucets, and waterfalls.
2. Turn on the faucets in the bathroom sink.
3. Pour warm water over your genitals.
4. Put your hands into warm water.
5. Gently press a warm or cold washcloth over your lower abdominal area.
6. Rock back and forth.
7. Rhythmically stroke your lower abdomen and upper thighs.
8. Use a circular motion to apply gentle pressure over your bladder.
9. Apply gentle pressure with your index finger to one side of your urinary meatus.
10. Inhale oil of peppermint.

Ways to Control Odor

1. Maintain good personal hygiene. Wash with soap and water after urinating and dry the skin gently but thoroughly.
2. Keep underclothing and bed linens as fresh as possible. Change them when wet and launder frequently.
3. Use disposable absorbent pads. The pads provide protection when accidents occur and can be quickly changed and easily disposed of.
4. Use personal hygiene deodorant sprays (follow the manufacturer's directions). Talcum powder and cornstarch, if used, should be dusted on sparingly.
5. The following is a list of foods that may make controlling your urine more difficult.
   • Alcoholic drinks, beer, wine
   • Coffee
   • Chocolate

- Soda
- Fruit and juice (citrus)
- Honey
- Sugar
- Tea
- Products and medications with caffeine.

6. Resources:

HIP (Help for Incontinent People)
P.O. Box 544
Union, South Carolina 29379

National Kidney Foundation, Inc
Two Park Ave
New York, New York 10016

National Association for Continence
P.O. Box 8306
Spartanburg, South Carolina 29305

National Kidney and Urologic Diseases
Information Clearing House
P.O. Box NKUDIC
Bethesda, Maryland 20892

National Institute on Aging
Information Center
P.O. Box 8057
Gaithersburg, Maryland 20898-8057

OTHER INSTRUCTIONS

Colostomy Care

GENERAL INFORMATION

An ostomy is a created opening into the body. The new opening is called a stoma. A colostomy is formed from a part of your colon (large intestine). The purpose of a colostomy is to allow stool to bypass a diseased or damaged part of the colon.

GUIDELINES

These guidelines will help you in caring for your colostomy.

1. Gather all supplies.
2. Gently remove the soiled pouching system. Use one hand to press down against the skin. Use the other hand to peel away the system.

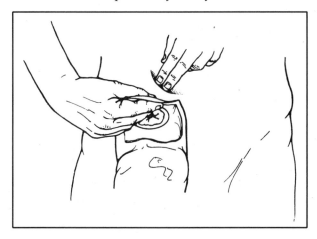

3. Measure your stoma with a measuring guide. Compare the measured stoma size with the size of the pouching system you are using. The size of the pouch opening should be no more than ½ inch larger than the stoma.

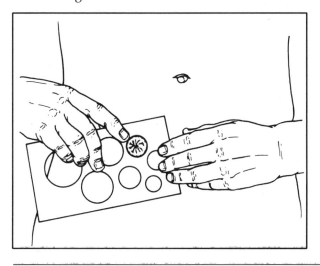

4. Clean the skin around the stoma with warm water and a paper towel or a soft white washcloth. Do not use toilet paper, because it breaks apart when wet. There is no need to scrub the skin.

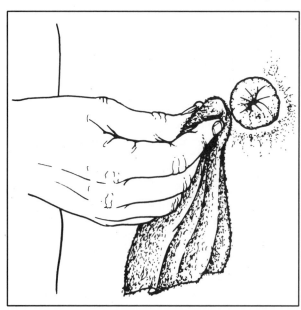

5. Using soap is not necessary. Soap can leave a residue and lead to skin irritation and poor pouch bonding. If soap is used, be sure it is nonalkaline and nondrying (such as Dove, Basis, Purpose, or a castile soap).
6. Rinse well with warm water. Pat the skin dry. Never rub your skin, as it may become irritated. Dry skin helps pouch adherence.
7. Look for any redness or rash on the skin around the stoma. For irritated skin, follow the skin care directions given by your nurse or doctor.
8. Apply your pouching system by following the instructions for your system (see *Pouching System Instructions*).
9. For odor control, squeeze 8 to 10 drops of ostomy deodorizer into the pouch between emptying or complete changes. Do not use aspirin in the pouch, as it can irritate the stoma and cause bleeding. You may also try soaking a cotton ball with pure vanilla extract and placing it in the pouch after each emptying. This will also absorb odor.

Pouching System Instructions
One-Piece Precut Pouching System

1. Remove any protective papers or backing from the pouch adhesive.

2. Carefully center the pouch opening over the stoma.
3. Press the adhesive gently but firmly onto the skin.

Two-Piece Snap-On Pouching System

1. Use a pencil to trace the stoma outline onto the backing of the adhesive wafer.
2. Using small scissors, cut out the pattern as evenly and smoothly as you can. By placing some of your fingers inside the bag once a small hole is made, you can keep the bag open to prevent cutting a hole through the bag.
3. Peel the paper backing off the adhesive wafer.
4. Place the adhesive side toward your skin. Center the opening over the stoma.
5. Press the adhesive gently but firmly onto the skin.
6. Center the pouch over the wafer. Align the snap seals.
7. Firmly press in a circular motion until the pouch is completely snapped on.

Two-Piece System with an Adhesive Wafer and Adhesive-Backed Pouch

1. Remove the backing paper from the adhesive pouch. Lay the pouch flat, with the adhesive side up.
2. Leave the backing paper on the wafer. Hold the wafer paper side up. Center the wafer over the adhesive area of the pouch. Press into place, aligning the edges of each as best as you can.
3. Use a pencil to trace the stoma outline onto the backing paper of the adhesive wafer.
4. Cut out the pattern as evenly and smoothly as you can. Use small scissors.
5. Peel the paper backing off the adhesive wafer.
6. Place the adhesive side toward your skin. Center the opening over the stoma.
7. Press the adhesive gently but firmly onto the skin.

Faceplated System with Three or More Pieces (Reusable Faceplate and/or Gasket, Wafer, Pouch)

1. Use a pencil to trace the stoma outline onto the backing of the adhesive wafer.
2. Using small scissors, cut out the pattern as evenly and smoothly as possible.
3. Peel the paper backing off the adhesive wafer.
4. Place the adhesive side toward your skin. Center the opening over the stoma.

5. Press the adhesive gently but firmly onto the skin.
6. Peel off one side of the paper backing of the double-sided adhesive gasket.
7. Place the back of the reusable faceplate onto the adhesive gasket. Be very careful to fit the faceplate to the gasket to avoid wrinkles. Wrinkles may cause leakage.
8. Peel off the remaining paper backing from the gasket. Center the faceplate over the stoma.
9. Press onto the wafer already on your skin.
10. Attach the pouch to the faceplate. Depending on the brand, you may need to stretch the pouch collar over the faceplate or to use an adhesive ring.
11. Place the belt onto the faceplate (if desired). You should be able to slip two fingers between your skin and the belt.

Pouches

Drainable Pouch

1. Be sure to close it tightly at the bottom with the clips.
2. Empty the pouch when it is ⅓ full.
3. Waiting too long between emptying may loosen the seal between your skin and the pouch. Leakage may occur.
4. Each person's "wearing time" is different.
5. You should plan to change your system at least every 7 days.
6. Do not put pin holes in the pouch. This will defeat the odor properties of the pouch.
7. Some pouches have filters in them to allow gas to escape.

Closed-Ended Pouch

1. Change the pouch when it is ⅓ to ½ full.
2. Changing the pouch more than twice a day may irritate your skin.

Removable Reusable Pouch

1. Remove the pouch every day (morning).
2. Replace it with a clean pouch.
3. Wash soiled pouches in dish detergent or mild soap. Rinse them well with warm water and hang them to dry.

IMPORTANT POINTS

1. Keeping your skin healthy is most important.
   a. Always remove a leaking pouch system as soon as possible. This prevents skin irritation.

b. If the skin around the stoma has a rash or sore or is red and weepy, call your nurse or doctor immediately.

c. Be sure your pouch system is the right size. Your size may change, especially in the first 12 weeks after the operation. If you have questions before you buy a system of a different size, call your nurse or doctor.

d. If the pouch opening is too large, leakage and skin irritation may occur. If the pouch opening is too small, stool may not be able to get through the stoma, and leakage may occur.

2. With a colostomy you can shower or bathe just as you did before. Soap and water will not get into your stoma or hurt it in any way. You may choose to shower or bathe with your pouch on or off. You should be able to return to your usual activities. Check with your nurse or doctor for any special instructions.

3. There are no nerve endings in the stoma, so the stoma (opening into the body) is not painful. The stoma is always red and moist just like the inside of your mouth. The stoma may also bleed, especially if it is hit or rubbed. This type of minor temporary bleeding of the stoma is normal. If the bleeding continues, you should call your nurse or doctor.

4. Eat a well-balanced diet.

a. Limit the amounts of or stop eating foods that upset your regular bowel pattern.

b. You may want to limit foods that may increase stool odor, such as fish, eggs, onions, peas, cabbage, broccoli, asparagus, cheese, and some vitamins. Foods that reduce fecal odor are parsley, yogurt, buttermilk, and cranberry juice.

c. You may want to limit foods that may increase gas, such as mushrooms, beer, carbonated drinks, onions, eggs, cabbage, beans, and milk. Chewing gum may also increase gas.

d. The bulk and residue in your diet affect the consistency of the stool. It may take a few weeks for you to learn what is best for you.

e. It's important to remember that each person with a colostomy is an individual and some of the foods mentioned may not affect him or her in that specific way. Experiment with a different food every 2 or 3 days. If you have any questions call your nurse or doctor.

5. Call your nurse or doctor if your ostomy stops working.

6. You can obtain free information from your ostomy supply company and from

United Ostomy Association
36 Executive Park, Suite 120
Irvine, California 92714-6744.

OTHER INSTRUCTIONS

Colostomy Irrigation

GENERAL INFORMATION

Regular colostomy irrigation can help to control the passage of stool. Success depends on:

- Irrigating at the same time regularly. How often you irrigate depends on your body. It can be every day or every 2 or 3 days.
- Eating a well-balanced diet.
- Regular exercise.

Irrigate when you will regularly have 30 to 40 minutes of bathroom time. Plan to be comfortable and relaxed. A padded toilet seat, a comfortable table chair next to the toilet, a foot stool, a cushion for back support, a sweater for warmth, a radio, or a magazine may help.

Use the supplies you have been instructed to use by your nurse or doctor.

STEPS

1. Gather your supplies.
2. Attach the irrigation tube to the irrigation bag (fluid container).
3. Attach the cone or catheter tip to the irrigation tube. Fill the irrigation bag with lukewarm tap water. Never use hot or cold water. This could cause burning or cramping.
4. Open the regulator clamp on the irrigation bag tube. Let the water run through the tube until all air is out. Reclamp the tube.
5. Remove your colostomy pouch.
   a. For a one-piece system, remove the entire pouch.
   b. For a system with two or more pieces, remove only the pouch. Leave the wafer or faceplate on.
6. Put the irrigation drainage sleeve over the stoma. The sleeve attaches with a belt, adhesive, or a "snap-on seal."

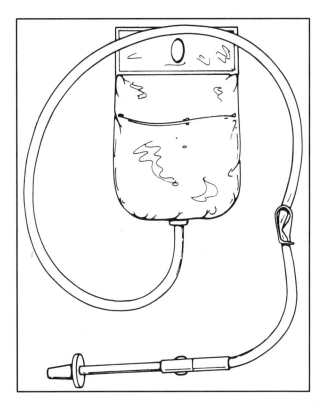

7. Hang the irrigation bag on a hook. Line up the bottom of the bag with your shoulder when you are seated. Holding the bag is tiring, but it can be done.
8. Cover the cone or catheter tip with water-soluble jelly.
9. Sit comfortably on the toilet or on a chair next to the toilet.
10. Place the open end of the irrigation drainage sleeve into the toilet.
11. Gently put the cone or catheter tip into the stoma.
    a. With a cone tip, insert it until it fits snugly.
    b. With a catheter tip, insert it 2 inches.
    c. Never force the tip into the stoma if it will not go in easily. Take a deep breath to relax your abdomen and try again.

12. Hold the tip in place with one hand. Use the other hand to open the clamp for the water to flow.

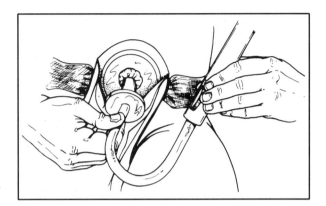

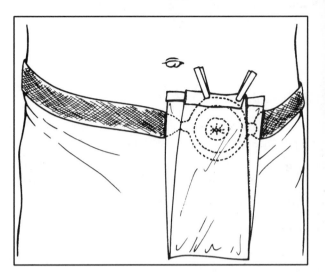

13. The water should flow in slowly, for about 10 to 15 minutes.
    a. Adjust the clamp to slow the water flow if the water is running too fast. If your clamp does not adjust, shut the clamp off and wait a minute or so before restarting.
    b. Gently turn the tip slightly if the water flow stops. A piece of stool may be blocking the flow.
    c. Slow the water flow or shut off the clamp if water leaks out around the tip. Wait until the leaking stops before restarting.
14. Once the amount of water needed has flowed in, clamp the tube. Remove the cone or catheter tip from your stoma. Place the tip aside.
15. Close the top of the irrigation sleeve securely.
16. Sit patiently and allow the returns to flow into the toilet.
    a. Most of the returns are expelled in 15 to 20 minutes.
    b. The rest of the returns may take another 15 to 20 minutes. You can fold and clamp the bottom of the irrigation sleeve and use this time to walk around and do other things.

17. Once the returns are completed, remove the irrigation sleeve.
18. Clean the skin. This may be a good time to bathe or shower.
19. Apply the colostomy pouch or dressing as usual.
20. Wash all reusable equipment with mild dish detergent and warm (never hot) water.
21. Rinse equipment well and hang it to dry.
22. Store equipment in a clean container between uses.

IMPORTANT POINTS

1. Do not irrigate if you have diarrhea.
2. Call your nurse or doctor if
    a. Diarrhea persists more than 72 hours,
    b. You have questions or problems with irrigation.
3. If you are receiving radiation treatments, call your doctor before you irrigate.

OTHER INSTRUCTIONS

Constipation

SYMPTOMS

Constipation exists when the following changes persist for at least 3 days:

- Your stools are harder, dryer, and smaller than usual.
- You experience a decrease in the frequency of your bowel movements.
- You feel that your rectum has not completely emptied after a bowel movement (you still feel a slight rectal pressure).
- It is harder than usual for you to have a bowel movement; you have to strain.

Additional Signs for Infants and Children

- Stools change from their usual type. They are less frequent, hard, large, wide, or can range from soft to diarrhea.
- The stomach area may become swollen with gas, causing cramping.
- Straining or pain can occur when having a bowel movement.

GUIDELINES

The following suggestions will help you regain your normal bowel function. Improvement is usually noticed within 3 weeks. If constipation has been your normal pattern for months or years, it may take longer for you to achieve a more comfortable bowel function.

1. Increase your fluid intake to at least eight to ten 8-ounce glasses of fluid each day. Fresh drinking water is an especially good choice.
2. Increase the daily crude fiber in your diet by adding bran, whole- and cracked-wheat cereals, fresh fruits (especially those with skin), fresh vegetables (especially green, leafy vegetables and root vegetables), nuts, prunes, and prune juice.
3. Increase your daily activity with a mild exercise such as walking. The nurse or physical therapist can teach you other exercises that are most suitable for you.
4. Establish a regular time for defecation. Go to the bathroom the same time every day. If you do not have a bowel movement, do not strain. Try again about 30 minutes after your next meal. In this way, your body develops the habit of having a bowel movement.
5. Drink decaffeinated coffee or tea or hot cocoa 1 hour before the scheduled defecation time. The warm liquid helps relax your bowels and can stimulate a movement.
6. Defecate when you first feel the urge.
7. Spend at least 15 minutes on the toilet. Do not strain. Sit so your thighs can be bent against your abdomen. A footstool can help you achieve this position. Relax while you are sitting on the toilet.
8. Do not routinely use laxatives to help you produce a bowel movement. It is possible for your body to become dependent on them and for you to lose the natural urge to defecate.
9. Do not use enemas, purgatives, and cathartics unless prescribed by your doctor. They can be harmful to your bowels if used incorrectly.

Your doctor has prescribed the following for you:

- Medication/enema: _____

  _____

- Directions: _____

  _____

- Purpose and side effects: _____

  _____

10. If your rectum becomes irritated, cool washcloth compresses and petroleum jelly will ease the discomfort. The nurse can teach you how to give yourself a sitz bath, which will also relieve the irritation.

Additional Guidelines for Infants and Children

1. Diet suggestions for infants
   - If you are nursing, give fruit juices (prune, apple, or pear).
   - If your infant is eating baby food, give fruits and vegetables.
   - Check with your nurse or doctor before making changes.
   - If stools become too loose, give fewer fruits or vegetables.

- Rice cereal can be constipating; try oatmeal or barley cereal.
2. Diet suggestions for children
   - Be sure your child eats fruits, vegetables, and whole grain cereals every day.
   - Bran cereal may help with constipation.
   - Encourage drinking fruit juices and water between meals; a serving of prune juice daily may help.
   - Check with your nurse or doctor before making changes.
3. Helping your child with constipation
   - Try to create a relaxed approach to having a bowel movement.
   - Allow enough time, perhaps 10 minutes of sitting on the toilet; use a foot stool to prevent your child's feet from dangling.
   - Try to be positive and reward your child for such things as
     - Following diet changes,
     - Using the toilet when he or she has the urge,
     - Trying to sit on the toilet for 10 minutes.
4. Do not give laxatives, an enema, or suppositories unless ordered by your doctor.
5. Call your nurse or doctor with any of the following:
   - Stomach or rectal pain that continues with the constipation,
   - Constipation that continues for _____ days,
   - Bright red streaks of blood in the stool.

OTHER INSTRUCTIONS

Continuous Ambulatory Peritoneal Dialysis: Special Conditions

The kidneys work to remove waste from the body. When the kidneys are not working, peritoneal dialysis helps rid the body of wastes. Special dialysis fluid passes into the open space in your abdomen (the space outside your digestive system). The dialysis fluid enters your body through a tube called a catheter. Waste and excess water are drawn through the lining of the abdomen into the dialysis fluid, similar to the way tea flows out of a tea bag into hot water. The dialysis fluid is drained out of the abdomen. The fluid carries out the waste with it. Ask your nurse if you have questions about how to use the peritoneal dialysis equipment. The following instructions will help you to learn how to manage special conditions if you experience them.

LOW BACK PAIN

What Causes It

Pressure and weight of the dialysis fluid in the abdomen.

What to Do

If instructed to do so,

1. Exercise to strengthen your stomach muscles.
2. Take a pain reliever if your doctor permits.
3. Sit with a pillow behind the low part of your back or place the pillow under your abdomen.

SHORTNESS OF BREATH

What Causes It

Too much fluid (volume) or large exchange.

What to Do

1. Call your nurse or doctor. The fluid amount at each exchange may need to be adjusted.
2. Sit upright.
3. Wear loose fitting clothing around your waist and abdomen.

PRESSURE IN THE BLADDER, RECTUM, OR STOMACH

What Causes It

Catheter position, large exchange, or full bowel.

What to Do

1. Call your nurse or doctor. The position of the catheter may need to be adjusted.
2. For a full bowel, a bowel movement is needed. If you have trouble with constipation, tell your nurse or doctor.

INFLOW PAIN OR CRAMPING (SHOULDER PAIN MAY OCCUR)

What Causes It

Usually this discomfort decreases in the first 2 weeks.

1. Cold dialysis fluid
2. Too rapid inflow
3. Stretching and irritation inside the abdomen

What to Do

1. For cold dialysis fluid, warm the fluid to body temperature (98.6°F or 37°C) with a heating pad or a microwave oven (check the temperature carefully before using the fluid).
2. Slow the inflow rate.
3. For stretching and irritation of the abdomen,
   a. Be sure to drain the abdomen completely at each exchange.
   b. During inflow, clamp off the tubing while fluid is still in the bag. This prevents air from getting into the abdomen.
   c. Your nurse or doctor may need to adjust the amount of fluid used during exchanges.

OUTFLOW FAILURE OR POOR OUTFLOW

What Causes It

1. Bowel full of stool
2. Catheter blockage

3. Bed or chair not high enough
4. Misplaced or chinked catheter

What to Do

1. For a full bowel, a bowel movement is needed, If you have trouble with constipation, tell your nurse or doctor.
2. For catheter blockage, change positions or stand up and walk.
3. If the bed or chair height is too low, raise the height. Blocks can be used for the bed and chair.
4. For a misplaced or kinked catheter,
   a. Changing positions may help.
   b. If changing your position does not work, your nurse or doctor may need to check the catheter's position.

DIALYSIS FLUID LEAKING AROUND THE CATHETER

What Causes It

1. Too much fluid during the exchange
2. Catheter blockage
3. Tunnel infection
4. Catheter position problems (displacement or problems with healing after placement)

What to Do

1. For too much fluid, your nurse or doctor may need to adjust the amount of fluid at each exchange.
2. For catheter blockage,
   a. Change positions.
   b. If changing positions does not work, your nurse or doctor may need to test the catheter by pushing fluid through it.
3. For tunnel infection,
   a. Look for redness, swelling, and tenderness around the exit site.
   b. If any of these are seen, call your nurse or doctor immediately.
4. For catheter position problems,
   a. Change positions.
   b. If changing positions does not work, your nurse or doctor may need to check the catheter's position.

HERNIA (MUSCLE BULGE ON STOMACH)

What Causes It

A weakness in the muscle wall and an increase in pressure in the abdomen.

What to Do

1. Tell your nurse or doctor when you first notice it.
2. You may be instructed to avoid overexertion.
3. Avoid constipation. If you have trouble with constipation, tell your nurse or doctor.

SIGNS AND SYMPTOMS TO IMMEDIATELY REPORT TO YOUR NURSE OR DOCTOR

Prompt treatment can save the catheter and prevent serious complications.

1. Peritonitis (infection of the lining of the abdomen)
   a. Persistent pain in the abdomen
   b. Abdomen fullness
   c. Fever
2. Cloudy outflow
3. Bright yellow or bright red outflow
4. Problems with outflow
5. Feeling ill
6. Redness, swelling, and tenderness around the catheter
7. Inflow problems (catheter kinking)
8. Dialysis fluid leaking around catheter
9. Chest pain during dialysis
10. Shortness of breath
11. Swelling of ankles
12. Cramps
13. Nausea or vomiting
14. Constipation
15. Itching
16. Numbness or burning of the feet or legs
17. Scrotal edema

IMPORTANT POINTS

1. Good hand washing, careful tube changing, and good skin care are important to prevent infection.
2. Take your medication as directed.
   a. Learn the name, action, dose, and side effects of all medications. Know when and how you should take them.
   b. Check with your nurse or doctor before taking any new medication, even ones you can buy without a prescription.
   c. Learn how to and when to add medications to the dialysis fluid. It is very important to add medications properly to avoid infection.
3. Follow your diet and salt limitations.
4. Learn to sleep in a position so that you do not kink the catheter.
5. Keep your bowels moving regularly.
   a. Your nurse or doctor can help you with ways to keep your bowels regular.

b. Do not take laxatives or use other bowel medications unless your nurse or doctor tells you to do so.

6. Keep the emergency services number by your phone.

RECORDS

1. Weigh yourself daily at the same time during the same phase (dwell or empty) _____
2. Take your temperature daily _____ and whenever you feel like you have a fever.
3. Take your pulse _____
4. Take your blood pressure _____
5. Take respirations (breathing rate) _____
6. Type of dialysis fluid: _____
7. Medications added to dialysis fluid: _____
8. Total number of exchanges: _____
9. Length of inflow: _____
10. Length of dwell: _____
11. Length of outflow: _____
12. Amount of dialysis fluid inflow: _____
13. Amount of fluid inflow: _____
14. Outflow (color, clearness, anything floating in the fluid. Note: any cloudiness is unusual after the first week and should be reported): _____

15. Anything unusual before, during or after dialysis
    a. Problems with inflow or outflow _____
    b. Stopping dialysis for any reason—include reason and length of time: _____
16. Condition of exit site and tunnel (redness, drainage around exit site): _____
17. Exit site care: _____

QUESTIONS

Discuss any questions with your nurse or doctor.

OTHER INSTRUCTIONS

Diarrhea

GENERAL INFORMATION

Diarrhea can be caused by many reasons. Some people have cramping and nausea in addition to the loose watery bowel movements. Diarrhea can be caused by a change in routine or diet, a minor infection, medications, surgery, or radiation treatments. For both adults and children, having diarrhea can lead to dehydration (a loss of too much fluid from the body).

GUIDELINES

1. Cut down on solid foods for 24 to 48 hours.
2. Drink more fluids.
   - For adults, sport electrolyte drinks like Gatorade may be helpful.
   - For children, in addition to popsicles or Gatorade, special drinks, such as Pedialyte, may be recommended by your doctor or nurse.
   - Do not give infants or children soups or broth
3. Take oral or axillary (under the arm) temperature regularly.
4. Antidiarrhea medications may help.
   - Do not use these medications for children unless your doctor directs you to.
   - These medications should be used only for 24 to 48 hours.
5. Wash your hands carefully after using the toilet.
6. Treat rash and skin irritation.
   - Your nurse or doctor can suggest an ointment to place on the skin around the rectum
   - For diaper rash
     - Change the diaper as soon as it is wet or has stool,
     - Wash the baby's bottom every time you change the diaper,
     - Use mild soap and water to clean the skin and skinfolds,
     - Rinse the skin well and gently pat the skin dry,
     - Lay your baby on his or her stomach on a towel or diaper for a short time (by leaving the diaper off, the air will help healing of the skin),
     - Your doctor may order an ointment for the skin,
     - Do not use diaper or skin wipes; they can irritate the skin,
     - Do not use baby powder,
     - Call your nurse or doctor if the rash does not improve.
7. Call your nurse or doctor
   - Immediately with signs of dehydration
     - Decreased amount and numbers of urination; for children no urination for 5 to 6 hours,
     - Dry mouth,
     - Eyes that look sunken with dark circles,
     - Feeling weak, tired, and listless; children may be less active and very sleepy.
   - If diarrhea continues for more than 48 hours; for infants and children you may be directed to call after 24 hours.

OTHER INSTRUCTIONS

Ileostomy Care

GENERAL INFORMATION

An ostomy is a created opening into the body. The new opening is called a stoma. An ileostomy is formed from a part of your ileum (the last part of the small intestine).

GUIDELINES

These guidelines will help you in caring for your ileostomy.

1. Gather all supplies.
2. Gently remove the soiled pouching system. Use one hand to press down against the skin. Use the other hand to peel away the system.

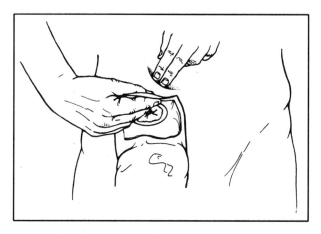

3. Measure your stoma with a measuring guide. Compare the measured stoma size with the size of the pouching system you are using. The size of the pouch opening should be no more than ⅛ inch larger than the stoma.

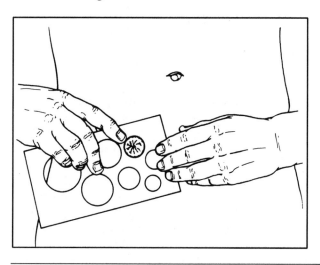

4. Clean the skin around the stoma with warm water and a paper towel or a soft white washcloth. Do not use toilet paper, since it breaks apart when wet. There is no need to scrub the skin.

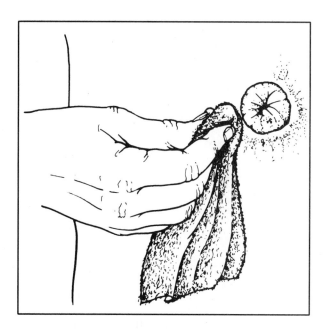

5. Using soap is not necessary. Soap can leave a residue and lead to skin irritation and poor pouch seal. If soap is used, be sure it is nonalkaline and nondrying (such as Dove, Basis, Purpose, or a castile soap).
6. Rinse well with warm water. Pat the skin dry. Never rub your skin, as it may become irritated. Dry skin helps pouch bonding.
7. Look for any redness or rash on the skin around the stoma. For irritated skin, follow the skin care directions as instructed by your nurse or doctor.
8. Apply your pouching system by following the instructions for your system (see *Pouching System Instructions*).
9. Close the drainage spout at the bottom of the pouch with the clip included with your pouch (tail closure).
10. Ileostomy pouches should be emptied every 2 to 3 hours. Stand or sit near the toilet, release the clip, empty the contents into the toilet, and reapply the clip.
11. If you are using a reusable pouch, you should remove the pouch every morning only and re-

place it with a clean one. Pouches should be washed with liquid dish soap and warm water and hung to dry.

12. The entire system is changed at designated intervals. Each person's "wearing time" is different and should average 5 to 7 days. It is advisable to change the entire system at least every 7 days.

13. If odor control is necessary, squeeze 8 to 10 drops of commercially available ostomy deodorizer directly into the pouch or onto a cotton ball and drop it into the pouch once a day. Do not use aspirin in the pouch, as it can irritate the stoma and cause bleeding.

Pouching System Instructions

One-Piece Precut Pouching System

1. Remove any protective papers or backing from the pouch adhesive.
2. Carefully center the pouch opening over the stoma.
3. Press the adhesive gently but firmly onto the skin.

Two-Piece Snap-On Pouching System

1. Use a pencil to trace the stoma outline onto the backing of the adhesive wafer.
2. Using small scissors, cut out the pattern as evenly and smoothly as you can. By placing some of your fingers inside the bag once a small hole is made, you can keep the bag open to prevent cutting a hole through it.
3. Peel the paper backing off the adhesive wafer.
4. Place the adhesive side toward your skin. Center the opening over the stoma.
5. Press the adhesive gently but firmly onto the skin.
6. Center the pouch over the wafer. Align the snap seals.
7. Firmly press in a circular motion until the pouch is completely snapped on.

Two-Piece System with an Adhesive Wafer and Adhesive-Backed Pouch

1. Remove the backing paper from the adhesive pouch. Lay the pouch flat, with the adhesive side up.
2. Leave the backing paper on the wafer. Hold the wafer with the paper side up. Center the wafer over the adhesive area of the pouch. Press it

into place, aligning the edges of each as best as you can.
3. Use a pencil to trace the stoma outline onto the backing paper of the adhesive wafer.
4. Cut out the pattern as evenly and smoothly as you can. Use small scissors.
5. Peel the paper backing off the adhesive wafer.
6. Place the adhesive side toward your skin. Center the opening over the stoma.
7. Press the adhesive gently but firmly onto the skin.

Faceplated System with Three or More Pieces (Reusable Faceplate and/or Gasket, Wafer, Pouch)

1. Use a pencil to trace the stoma outline onto the backing of the adhesive wafer.
2. Using small scissors, cut out the pattern as evenly and smoothly as possible.
3. Peel the paper backing off the adhesive wafer.
4. Place the adhesive side toward your skin. Center the opening over the stoma.
5. Press the adhesive gently but firmly onto the skin.
6. Peel off one side of the paper backing of the double-sided adhesive gasket.
7. Place the back of the reusable faceplate onto the adhesive gasket. Be very careful to fit the faceplate to the gasket to avoid wrinkles. Wrinkles may cause leakage.
8. Peel off the remaining paper backing from the gasket. Center the faceplate over the stoma.
9. Press the faceplate onto the wafer already on your skin.
10. Attach the pouch to the faceplate. Depending on the brand, you may need to stretch the pouch collar over the faceplate or use an adhesive ring.
11. Place the belt onto the faceplate (if desired). You should be able to slip two fingers between your skin and the belt.

IMPORTANT POINTS

1. Keeping your skin healthy is most important.
   a. Always remove a leaking pouch system as soon as possible. This prevents skin irritation.
   b. If the skin around the stoma has a rash or sore or is red and weepy, call your nurse or doctor immediately.
   c. Be sure your pouch system is the right size. Your size may change, especially in the first 12 weeks after the operation. If you have questions before you buy a system of a different size, call your nurse or doctor.

d. If the pouch opening is too large, leakage and skin irritation may occur. If the pouch opening is too small, stool may not be able to get through the stoma, and leakage may occur.

2. Eat a well-balanced diet.
   a. Limit the amounts of or stop eating foods that upset your regular bowel pattern.
   b. You may want to limit foods that may increase stool odor, such as fish, eggs, onions, peas, cabbage, broccoli, asparagus, cheese, and some vitamins. Foods that reduce fecal odor are parsley, yogurt, buttermilk, and cranberry juice.
   c. You may want to limit foods that may increase gas, such as mushrooms, beer, carbonated drinks, onions, eggs, cabbage, beans, and milk. Chewing gum may also increase gas.

3. To prevent food blockage,
   a. Eat slowly and chew food very well.
   b. Drink plenty of fluids with meals.
   c. Avoid foods such as cheese, lima beans, nuts, corn, orange pulp, celery, pineapple, seeds, popcorn, coleslaw, Chinese vegetables, coconut, and fruit skins, which may bind together in the bowel and form a food blockage.

4. To prevent dehydration,
   a. Drink at least 10 to 12 glasses of water or fluid daily.
   b. Drink tea, chicken broth, carbonated drinks, or Gatorade if you have diarrhea or vomiting.

c. Dehydration can be caused by fever, vomiting, diarrhea, too much exercise (excessive sweating), decreased humidity, or increased temperature.

5. Ask your nurse or doctor before taking any medication.
   a. Certain medications will not dissolve properly before reaching the stoma. Avoid taking medications that are enteric-coated tablets or time-released spansules.
   b. Do not use laxatives.

6. Do not allow anyone to attempt to take your temperature rectally or to give you an enema.

7. With an ileostomy you can shower or bathe just as you did before. You should be able to return to your usual activities. Check with your nurse or doctor for any special instructions.

8. Call your nurse or doctor if your ostomy stops working.

9. You can obtain free information from your ostomy supply company and from

United Ostomy Association (UOA)
36 Executive Park, Suite 120
Irvine, California 92714-6744

Crohn's Colitis Foundation of America, Inc. (CCFA)
386 Park Avenue South
New York, NY 10016-8804

OTHER INSTRUCTIONS

Intermittent Self-Catheterization (Female)

GENERAL INFORMATION

Catheterization is a procedure in which a small plastic or rubber catheter is placed into the bladder to drain the urine. Intermittent catheterization is placing a catheter into your bladder on a regular schedule to prevent too much urine from collecting or to help with incontinence.

EQUIPMENT

- Number _____ straight catheter (plastic or rubber)
- Soap, water, and a washcloth or moist disposable towelettes
- A plastic bag or glass jar for the used catheter
- A container for collecting urine (if a toilet is not available or the urine is to be measured)
- Two clean towels
- A mirror
- Optional: lubricant

STEPS FOR CATHETERIZATION

1. Try to urinate before catheterizing yourself.
2. Wash your hands with soap and warm water. If no soap and water are available, use a moist disposable towelette.
3. Organize your equipment within easy reach.
4. Get into a position that is as comfortable and natural as possible. Sit on the edge of the toilet or a chair, or stand with one foot elevated on a stool (as if inserting a tampon).
5. The mirror can be positioned between your legs to help you find your urinary meatus (opening). However, you should also learn to find the meatus without the mirror, because a mirror may not always be available.
6. Separate your vaginal folds with the thumb and middle finger of your nondominant hand.
7. Wash the vaginal area with warm water and soap. If soap and water are not available, wash with a moist disposable towelette. Use downward strokes from front to back.

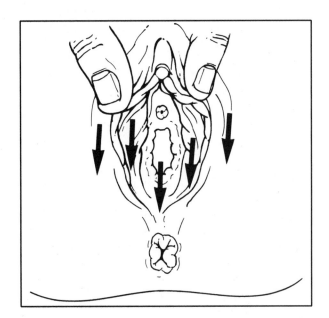

8. Keep your vaginal folds separated.
9. Hold the catheter about ½ inch from the tip, using your dominant hand. You may be instructed to use a lubricant on the tip to help with insertion.
10. Position the draining end of the catheter so that the urine can flow into the toilet or the collection container.
11. Slowly insert the catheter into the urinary meatus.

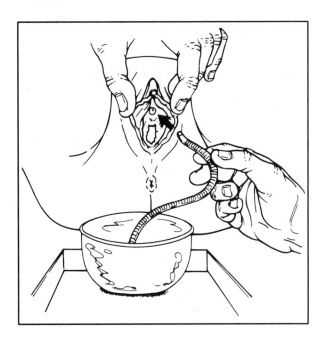

12. When the urine begins to flow, insert the catheter 1 inch more. This is to make sure the catheter is in your bladder.
13. When the urine stops flowing, change your position or press (strain) your stomach muscles. This helps to empty your bladder completely.
14. Withdraw the catheter slowly. Keep the catheter tip pointed up to avoid dribbling urine.
15. Wash your hands and get dressed.
16. Complete your *Self-Catheterization Log*.
17. Follow the steps for catheter care.

Catheter Care

1. Wash the dirty catheter with warm water and soap. (If there is no soap and water, wipe it with a moist disposable towelette and put it into the bag or jar. Complete total catheter care when soap and water are available.)
2. Rinse the catheter (inside and out) with clear clean water.
3. Dry the catheter completely with a clean towel.
4. Put the catheter in a plastic bag or glass jar.
5. When all of the catheters are used (or once a week), boil them for 20 minutes in water.
6. Store the boiled catheters in clean towels, clean glass jars, or fresh plastic bags. KEEP BOILED CATHETERS IN A SEPARATE LOCATION FROM USED CATHETERS.
7. Use each catheter only once after it has been boiled.
8. Buy new catheters to replace ones that crack or become hard.

IMPORTANT POINTS

1. Follow your catheterization schedule at all times.

2. Take your medications as prescribed.
3. Take liquid refreshments at evenly spaced times between the time you get up and 2 hours before you go to bed. Do not drink large amounts in short periods of time.
4. Avoid caffeine (coffee, tea, cocoa, cola, and chocolate).
5. Limit the calcium-rich foods in your diet (milk, milk products, eggs, green leafy vegetables, broccoli, legumes, nuts, and whole grains).
6. Limit the phosphorus-rich foods in your diet (milk, milk products, lean meats, processed foods, and soft drinks).
7. Be accurate when recording information on your *Self-Catheterization Log*.
8. Keep extra supplies for catheterization at home and work.
9. If you are incontinent (have uncontrolled urination) between catheterizations,
   a. Wash the wet skin with soap and water,
   b. Dry the skin completely,
   c. Expose the skin to the air for as long as possible,
   d. Use powder or cornstarch sparingly,
   e. Change into dry underwear and clothes,
   f. Consider the use of an external urine collection device.
10. Ask the nurse or doctor anything you are unsure of or have questions about.
11. Urine is usually a light yellow color with little odor. Dark urine with a strong odor may be a sign of not drinking enough fluids or of a urinary tract infection. Some foods and medications can cause a urine odor. Call your nurse or doctor if you notice dark, strong-smelling urine.

OTHER INSTRUCTIONS

			Changes in Urine		
Date	Time	Amount of Urine Returned	COLOR	ODOR	CLARITY

Self-Catheterization Log

Intermittent self-catheterization (female).

Intermittent Self-Catheterization (Male)

GENERAL INFORMATION

Catheterization is a procedure in which a small plastic or rubber catheter is placed into the bladder to drain the urine. Intermittent catheterization is placing a catheter into your bladder on a regular schedule to prevent too much urine from collecting, or to help with incontinence.

EQUIPMENT

- Number _____ straight catheter (plastic or rubber)
- Soap, water, and a washcloth or moist disposable towelettes
- Water-soluble lubricant
- Paper towels
- A plastic bag or glass jar for the used catheter
- A container for collecting urine (if a toilet is not available or the urine is to be measured)
- Two clean towels

STEPS FOR CATHETERIZATION

1. Try to urinate before catheterizing yourself.
2. Wash your hands with soap and warm water. If soap and water are not available, use a moist disposable towelette.
3. Organize your equipment within easy reach.
4. Get into a position that is as comfortable and natural as possible.
5. Wash your penis with warm water and soap. If soap and water are not available, use a moist disposable towelette.
6. If you are not circumcised, pull back the foreskin and keep it back during the catheterization.
7. Squeeze some of the water-soluble lubricant onto a paper towel.
8. Lubricate the catheter tip and 2 inches up from the tip by gently rolling the catheter in the lubricant on the paper towel.
9. Position the draining end of the catheter so that the urine can flow into the toilet or the collection container.
10. Hold your penis erect or at a right angle to your body.

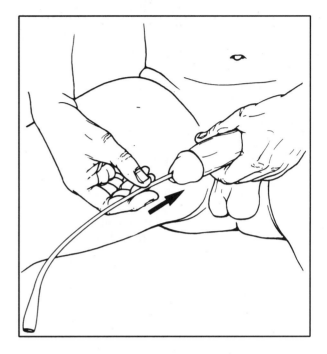

11. Slowly insert the catheter.
12. When urine begins to flow, insert the catheter about 2 more inches. This is to make sure the catheter is in your bladder.
13. When the urine stops flowing, change your position or press (strain) your stomach muscles. This helps to empty your bladder completely.
14. Withdraw the catheter slowly. Keep the catheter tip pointed up to avoid dribbling urine.
15. If you are not circumcised, pull your foreskin forward again.
16. Wash your hands and get dressed.
17. Complete your *Self-Catheterization Log.*
18. Follow the steps for catheter care.

Catheter Care

1. Wash the dirty catheter with warm water and soap. (If there is no soap and water, wipe it with a moist disposable towelette and put it into the bag or jar. Complete total catheter care when soap and water are available.)
2. Rinse the catheter (inside and out) with clear clean water.
3. Dry the catheter completely with a clean towel.
4. Put the catheter in a plastic bag or glass jar.

5. When all of the catheters are used (or once a week), boil them for 20 minutes in water.
6. Store the boiled catheters in clean towels, clean glass jars, or fresh plastic bags. KEEP BOILED CATHETERS IN A SEPARATE LOCATION FROM USED CATHETERS.
7. Use each catheter only once after it has been boiled.
8. Buy new catheters to replace ones that crack or become hard.

IMPORTANT POINTS

1. Follow your catheterization schedule at all times.
2. Take your medications as prescribed.
3. Take liquid refreshments at evenly spaced times between the time you get up and 2 hours before you go to bed. Do not drink large amounts in short periods of time.
4. Avoid caffeine (coffee, tea, cocoa, cola, and chocolate).
5. Limit the calcium-rich foods in your diet (milk, milk products, eggs, green leafy vegetables, broccoli, legumes, nuts, and whole grains).

6. Limit the phosphorus-rich foods in your diet (milk, milk products, lean meats, processed foods, and soft drinks).
7. Be accurate when recording information on your *Self-Catheterization Log.*
8. Keep extra supplies for catheterization at home and at work.
9. If you are incontinent (have uncontrolled urination) between catheterizations,
    a. Wash the wet skin with soap and water,
    b. Dry the skin completely,
    c. Expose the skin to the air for as long as possible,
    d. Use powder or cornstarch sparingly,
    e. Change into dry underwear and clothes,
    f. Consider the use of an external urine collection device.
10. Ask the nurse or doctor anything you are unsure of or have questions about.
11. Urine is usually a light yellow color with little odor. Dark urine with a strong odor may be a sign of not drinking enough fluids or of a urinary tract infection. Some foods and drugs (medications) can cause a urine odor. Call your nurse or doctor if you notice dark, strong-smelling urine.

OTHER INSTRUCTIONS

Self-Catheterization Log

Date	Time	Amount of Urine Returned	Changes in Urine		
			COLOR	ODOR	CLARITY

Intermittent self-catheterization (male).

Urinary Catheter Care (Female)

GENERAL INFORMATION

A urinary catheter drains urine continuously from the bladder, through a clear plastic tube, and into a collection bag. It is held inside the bladder by a small balloon filled with sterile saline.

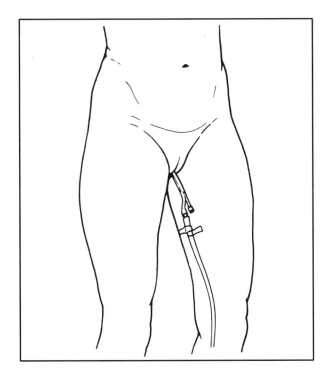

Urinary catheters come in different sizes.

- Your catheter size is _____.
- Your balloon size is _____.

GUIDELINES

The following suggestions will help you take care of your urinary catheter.

1. Wash your hands with soap and water (or a moist disposable towelette) before and after handling your catheter, tube, and collection bag.
2. Do not tug on or pull the catheter.
3. Check the tube for kinks and for loops to make sure that the urine has a clear and easy pathway to the collection bag.
4. Do not lie or sit on the catheter tube or collection bag.
5. Make sure the collection bag is below the level of your bladder at all times.

6. Empty the collection bag as often as necessary, but at least every 8 hours. A leg bag should be emptied at least every 3 hours.
7. Clean the drain of the collection bag with alcohol or a povidone-iodine solution before and after emptying the bag.
8. Drink at least eight to ten 8-ounce glasses of fluid each day. Water and fresh cranberry juice are especially good.
9. Keep a record of your daily fluid intake and your daily urine output. The nurse can teach you how to do this.
10. Wash the area around your catheter with soap and warm water every day. Move the catheter around as little as possible.
11. Do not use powders or lotions around the catheter.
12. Change the tube and collection bag
    a. Every 3 days if you are reusing the equipment,
    b. At least every 2 weeks if you are not reusing the equipment.
13. If you use a leg bag or want to reuse plastic collection bags,
    a. Clean the bag with soapy water,
    b. Rinse the bag well with clean tap water,
    c. Soak the bag for 30 minutes in a solution of one part vinegar to three parts water,
    d. Empty the bag,
    e. Air dry the bag,
    f. Put a cap that has been disinfected with alcohol on the connecting tip,
    g. Store the bag in a clean glass jar or plastic bag.
14. Replace tubes and catheter bags that are cracked, hardened, or difficult to see into.
15. Notify the nurse or doctor if you have
    a. Cloudy urine,
    b. Urine with a foul (bad) smell,
    c. Urine with gritty or crusty deposits,
    d. Urine with blood,
    e. Urine with mucus,
    f. Burning at the urinary opening,
    g. Pain or discomfort around the catheter,
    h. Stomach pain,
    i. A fever,
    j. Chills,
    k. Leaking around the catheter,
    l. Constipation.
16. Notify the nurse or doctor if the urinary catheter is accidentally pulled out of the bladder.

OTHER INSTRUCTIONS

Urinary Catheter Care (Male)

GENERAL INFORMATION

A urinary catheter drains urine continuously from the bladder, through a clear plastic tube, and into a collection bag. It is held inside the bladder by a small balloon filled with sterile saline.

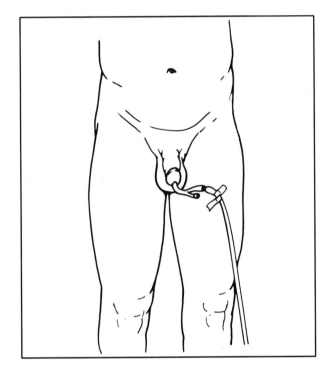

Urinary catheters come in different sizes.

- Your catheter size is _____.
- Your balloon size is _____.

GUIDELINES

The following suggestions will help you take care of your urinary catheter.

1. Wash your hands with soap and water (or a moist disposable towelette) before and after handling your catheter, tube, and collection bag.
2. Do not tug on or pull the catheter.
3. Check the tube for kinks and for loops to make sure that the urine has a clear and easy pathway to the collection bag.
4. Do not lie or sit on the catheter tube or collection bag.
5. Make sure the collection bag is below the level of your bladder at all times.
6. Empty the collection bag as often as necessary, but at least every 8 hours. A leg bag should be emptied at least every 3 hours.
7. Clean the drain of the collection bag with alcohol or a povidone-iodine solution before and after emptying the bag.
8. Drink at least eight to ten 8-ounce glasses of fluid each day. Water and fresh cranberry juice are especially good.
9. Keep a record of your daily fluid intake and your daily urine output. The nurse can teach you how to do this.
10. Wash the area around your catheter with soap and warm water every day. Move the catheter around as little as possible.
11. Do not use powders and lotions on your penis.
12. Change the tube and collection bag
    a. Every 3 days if you are reusing the equipment,
    b. At least every 2 weeks if you are not reusing equipment.
13. If you use a leg bag or want to reuse plastic collection bags,
    a. Clean the bag with soapy water,
    b. Rinse the bag well with clean tap water,
    c. Soak the bag for 30 minutes in a solution of one part vinegar to three parts water,
    d. Empty the bag,
    e. Air dry the bag,
    f. Put a cap that has been disinfected with alcohol on the connecting tip,
    g. Store the bag in a clean glass jar or plastic bag.
14. Replace tubes and catheter bags that are cracked, hardened, or difficult to see into.
15. Notify the nurse or doctor if you have
    a. Cloudy urine,
    b. Urine with a foul (bad) smell,
    c. Urine with gritty or crusty deposits,
    d. Urine with blood,
    e. Urine with mucus,
    f. Burning at the urinary opening,
    g. Pain or discomfort around the catheter,
    h. Stomach pain,
    i. A fever,
    j. Chills,
    k. Leaking around the catheter,
    l. Constipation.
16. Notify the nurse or doctor if the urinary catheter is accidentally pulled out of the bladder.

OTHER INSTRUCTIONS

Urostomy Care

GENERAL INFORMATION

An ostomy is a created opening into the body. The new opening is called a stoma. A urostomy is formed as a passageway for urine to the outside.

Guidelines

These guidelines will help you in caring for your urostomy.

1. Gather all supplies.
2. Roll or fold up one paper towel into the shape of a small "tootsie-roll candy." These are called "wicks," and you will need to prepare about 10 of these. Some patients use a tampon as a wick.
3. Gently remove the soiled pouching system. Use one hand to press down against the skin. Use the other hand to peel away the system.

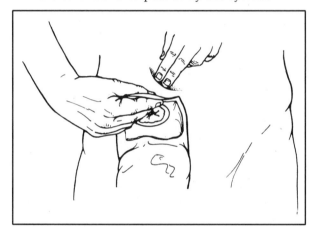

4. Measure your stoma with a measuring guide. Compare the measured stoma size with the size of the pouching system you are using. The size of the pouch opening should be no more than ⅛ inch larger than the stoma.

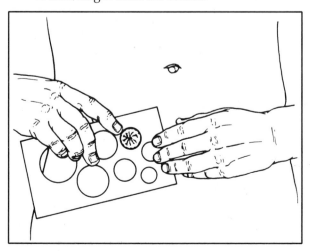

5. Use one paper towel wick or tampon to cover the stoma as you wash and prepare your skin. Replace it when it is soaked; this is to prevent urine from dripping onto your washed, dried skin.

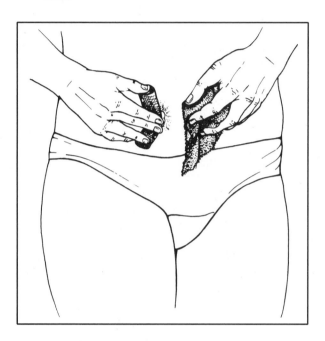

6. Clean the skin around the stoma with warm water and a paper towel or soft white washcloth. Do not use toilet paper, since it breaks apart when wet. There is no need to scrub the skin.

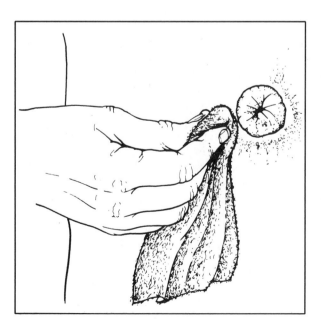

7. Using soap is not necessary. Soap can leave a residue and lead to skin irritation and poor pouch bonding. If soap is used, be sure it is nonalkaline and nondrying (such as Dove, Basis, Purpose, or a castile soap).

8. Rinse well with warm water. Pat the skin dry. Never rub your skin, as it may become irritated. Dry skin helps pouch bonding.

9. Look for any redness or rash on the skin around the stoma. For irritated skin, follow the skin care directions given by your nurse or doctor.

10. Apply your pouching system by following the instructions for your pouching system (see *Pouching System Instructions*).

11. Close the drainage spout at the bottom of the pouch. Using an antireflux pouch prevents backflow of urine.

12. Urostomy pouches should be emptied every 2 hours or so. Stand or sit near the toilet, release the spout, empty the contents, and reclose the spout tightly. Use a large, straight bedside drainage bag at night or while you are in bed. This will reduce stagnation of urine in the pouch, odor, and backflow of urine onto the stoma.

13. If you are using a removable, reusable pouch, you should remove the pouch *only* every morning and replace it with a clean one. It is easier to change the pouch after limiting fluids for 2 to 3 hours, such as before breakfast. Pouches should be washed with liquid dish soap and warm water and hung up to dry.

14. The entire system is changed at designated intervals. Each person's wearing time is different and should average 5 to 7 days. It is advisable to change the system at least every 7 days.

15. For odor control,
    a. Squeeze 8 to 10 drops of commercially available ostomy deodorizer directly into the pouch or onto a cotton ball and drop it into the pouch once a day.
    b. Eating asparagus increases urine odor.
    c. Frequent cleansing of the urinary pouch and thorough cleaning of the skin around the stoma will help reduce odor.
    d. Using one part vinegar to two to three parts water to rinse and soak pouches reduces odor.

16. If mucus control is necessary, a mucus dispersant is commercially available. Check with your ostomy supplier.

Pouching System Instructions
One-Piece Precut Pouching System

1. Remove any protective papers or backing from the pouch adhesive.

2. Carefully center the pouch opening over the stoma.

3. Press the adhesive gently but firmly onto the skin.

Two-Piece Snap-On Pouching System

1. Use a pencil to trace the stoma outline onto the backing of the adhesive wafer.

2. Using small scissors, cut out the pattern as evenly and smoothly as you can. By placing some of your fingers inside the bag once a small hole is made, you can keep the bag open to prevent cutting a hole through it.

3. Peel paper backing off the adhesive wafer.

4. Place the adhesive side toward your skin. Center the opening over the stoma.

5. Press the adhesive gently but firmly onto the skin.

6. Center the pouch over the wafer. Align the snap seals.

7. Firmly press in a circular motion until the pouch is completely snapped on.

Two-Piece System with an Adhesive Wafer and Adhesive-Backed Pouch

1. Remove the backing paper from the adhesive pouch. Lay the pouch flat, with the adhesive side up.

2. Leave the backing paper on the wafer. Hold the wafer with the paper side up. Center the wafer over the adhesive area of the pouch. Press into place, aligning the edges of each as best you can.

3. Use a pencil to trace the stoma outline onto the backing paper of the adhesive wafer.

4. Cut out the pattern as evenly and smoothly as you can. Use small scissors.

5. Peel the paper backing off the adhesive wafer.

6. Place the adhesive side toward your skin. Center the opening over the stoma.

7. Press the adhesive gently but firmly onto the skin.

Faceplated System with Three or More Pieces (Reusable Faceplate and/or Gasket, Wafer, Pouch)

1. Use a pencil to trace the stoma outline onto the backing of the adhesive wafer.

2. Using small scissors, cut out the pattern as evenly and smoothly as possible.

3. Peel the paper backing off the adhesive wafer.

4. Place the adhesive side toward your skin. Center the opening over the stoma.

5. Press the adhesive gently but firmly onto the skin.

6. Peel off one side of the paper backing of the double-sided adhesive gasket.
7. Place the back of the reusable faceplate onto the adhesive gasket. Be very careful to fit the faceplate to the gasket to avoid wrinkles. Wrinkles may cause leakage.
8. Peel off the remaining paper backing from the gasket. Center the faceplate over the stoma.
9. Press the faceplate onto the wafer already on your skin.
10. Attach the pouch to the faceplate. Depending on the brand, you may need to stretch the pouch collar over the faceplate or use an adhesive ring.
11. Place the belt onto the faceplate (if desired). You should be able to slip two fingers between your skin and the belt. A belt supports the pouch and prevents loosening of the seal.

IMPORTANT POINTS

1. Keeping your skin healthy is most important.
   a. Always remove a leaking pouch system as soon as possible. This prevents skin irritation.
   b. If the skin around the stoma has a rash or sore or is red and weepy, call your nurse or doctor immediately.

   c. Be sure your pouch system is the right size. Your size may change, especially in the first 12 weeks after the operation. If you have questions before you buy a system of a different size, call your nurse or doctor. Leakage and skin irritation may occur if the size is not right.
2. Eat a well-balanced diet.
3. Drink 2 to 3 quarts of fluid each day.
4. You should be able to return to your usual activities. Check with your nurse or doctor for any special instructions.
5. Call your nurse or doctor if
   a. Your ostomy stops working.
   b. You have fever, cloudy or foul-smelling urine, pink or red urine, or flank pain (pain in your side). These are the symptoms of urinary tract infection.
6. You can obtain free information from your ostomy supply company and from

   United Ostomy Association (UOA)
   36 Executive Park, Suite 120
   Irvine, California 92714-6744.

   Other Resources
   American Cancer Society
   1599 Clifton Road NE
   Atlanta, Georgia 30329.

OTHER INSTRUCTIONS

Digestive Alterations

Measuring Liquid Intake and Output

GENERAL INFORMATION

A written record of liquid intake and output gives a reliable picture of whether or not an individual's body is getting and holding onto enough necessary fluid. Ideally, a person's liquid intake during a 24-hour period is about two times greater than the liquid output. To keep a written record of liquid intake and output, you need,

- A urine collection device (bedpan, urinal, clean jar, commode, or bucket),
- A calibrated container (if the urine collection device is not calibrated),
- Measuring cup,
- *Intake and Output Record,*
- A pen or pencil,
- Bathroom scale.

GUIDELINES

1. Measure all liquids in the measuring cup before the patient drinks them. Liquids include anything liquid at room temperature like ice cream or gelatin.
2. Write on the intake side of the *Intake and Output Record* what time the patient drinks (*Time*), what the patient drinks (*Type*), and how much liquid he or she drinks (*Amount*). Be as accurate as possible.
3. Write on the output side of the *Intake and Output Record* what time the patient urinates (*Time*) and how much the patient urinates (*Urine Output Amount*). Be as accurate as possible.
4. Wash the urine collection device or measuring container after each use. Rinse it with bleach to prevent odors.
5. If the patient wears diapers or uses absorbent pads, weigh the wet diaper or pad. A dietary or infant scale is needed. Subtract the weight of a dry diaper or pad from the weight of the wet diaper or pad. Write this number (*Urine Output Amount*) and the time (*Time*) of urination on the output side of the *Intake and Output Record.*
6. If the patient is incontinent (unable to control the bladder), put a check in the *Incontinent Episode* column of the *Intake and Output Record,* and write the time (*Time*) the patient urinated. Under the *Urine Output Amount* column, write your best estimate of whether it is a small, moderate, or large amount of urine.
7. If the patient vomits, has diarrhea, or perspires heavily, write the time (*Time*) on the *Intake and Output Record.*
8. Daily weights are the most accurate measurement for incontinence. Daily weights taken at the same time each day also help in monitoring body fluid. It is best to do this when the patient wakes and while he or she is wearing the same clothing.

WASH YOUR HANDS WITH SOAP AND WARM WATER AFTER MEASURING THE URINE AND CLEANING THE EQUIPMENT.

Measuring Liquid Intake and Output

INTAKE AND OUTPUT RECORD

Date _____

Time	INTAKE Type	Amount	Time	OUTPUT Urine Output Amount	Incontinent Episode
24-hour total			24-hour total			

Daily Weight

Vomiting   Time

Heavy Perspiration   Time

Diarrhea   Time

OTHER INSTRUCTIONS

Nutrition and Diet Measures

Calorie-Restricted Diets

Calorie-Restricted Diet for Diabetes Management

DESCRIPTION

Proper nutrition is vital in the treatment of persons with diabetes. Making appropriate food choices and behavior changes can

- Keep blood glucose as near to normal as possible,
- Keep blood lipid levels at optimal levels,
- Provide adequate calories to achieve reasonable weight for adults and normal growth for children,
- Treat or prevent complications of hypoglycemia or hyperglycemia,
- Delay or prevent long-term complications of diabetes.

ADEQUACY

Accurate and effective nutrition education is based on many factors, such as the type of diabetes, weight status, and how long the person has known that he or she has diabetes. Education will address the following areas:

- Weight status
- Lifestyle
- Exercise
- Food choices and spacing of meals
- Insulin needs, if appropriate

Standardized meal plans can be useful initially until a dietitian can develop an individualized plan. Meal plans use lists of food that categorize foods according to nutrient and calorie content. These lists are called exchange lists because any food within the lists can be exchanged for another food within the list. Following are some standardized meal plans for common caloric levels and the "Exchange Lists for Meal Planning" with which they should be used. Caloric levels of 1200 calories or more can meet the recommended dietary allowances.

Standardized Meal Plans

Calories	Total	Breakfast	Lunch	Dinner	Night Snack
1000					
Starch	5	1	1	2	1
Fruit	2	1	1	—	—
Milk	1	½	—	—	½
Vegetable	2	—	1	1	—
Meat	4	1	2	1	—
Fat	1	—	1	—	—
1200					
Starch	6	2	1	2	1
Fruit	2	1	1	—	—
Milk	2	½	½	½	½
Vegetable	2	—	1	1	—
Meat	4	1	2	1	—
Fat	2	1	—	1	—

Table continued on following page

Standardized Meal Plans *Continued*

Calories	Total	Breakfast	Lunch	Dinner	Night Snack
1400					
Starch	7	2	2	2	1
Fruit	3	1	1	1	—
Milk	2	½	½	½	½
Vegetable	2	—	1	1	—
Meat	5	1	2	2	—
Fat	2	1	—	1	—
1500					
Starch	7	2	2	2	1
Fruit	3	1	1	1	—
Milk	2	½	½	½	½
Vegetable	3	—	1	2	—
Meat	5	1	2	2	—
Fat	3	1	1	1	—
1600					
Starch	8	3	2	2	1
Fruit	3	1	1	1	—
Milk	2	1	½	—	½
Vegetable	2	—	1	1	—
Meat	6	1	2	2	1
Fat	3	1	1	1	—
1800					
Starch	9	3	2	3	1
Fruit	4	1	1	1	1
Milk	2	1	½	½	—
Vegetable	3	—	1	2	—
Meat	6	1	2	2	1
Fat	3	1	1	1	—
2000					
Starch	10	3	3	3	1
Fruit	4	1	1	1	1
Milk	2	1	½	½	—
Vegetable	4	—	2	2	—
Meat	7	1	3	2	1
Fat	4	1	1	1	1
2200					
Starch	11	3	3	3	2
Fruit	4	1	1	1	1
Milk	2	1	1	—	—
Vegetable	4	—	2	2	—
Meat	9	1	3	3	2
Fat	4	1	1	1	1
2400					
Starch	11	3	3	3	2
Fruit	5	1	1	2	1
Milk	2	1	1	—	—
Vegetable	4	—	2	2	—
Meat	10	1	4	3	2
Fat	5	1	1	2	1

From Chilton Memorial Hospital, Pompton Plains, NJ.

Exchange Lists for Meal Planning

Starch List

Cereals, grains, pasta, breads, crackers, snacks, starchy vegetables, and cooked beans, peas, and lentils are starches. In general, one starch is equivalent to:

- ½ cup of cereal, grain, pasta, or starchy vegetable
- 1 oz of a bread product, such as 1 slice of bread
- ¾ to 1 oz of most snack foods (Some snack foods may also have added fat.)

Selection Notes

1. Starchy vegetables prepared with fat count as one starch and one fat.
2. Bagels or muffins can be 2 oz, 3 oz, or 4 oz in size, and can, therefore, count as two, three, or four starch choices.
3. Beans, peas, and lentils are also found on the Meat and Meat Substitutes list.
4. Regular potato chips and tortilla chips are found on the Other Carbohydrates list.
5. Most of the serving sizes are measured after cooking.

One Starch Exchange Equals 15 g Carbohydrate, 3 g Protein, 0–1 g Fat, and 80 Calories.

BREAD

Bagel	½ (1 oz)	Pita, 6 in. across	½
Bread, reduced-calorie	2 slices (1½ oz)	Raisin bread, unfrosted	1 slice (1 oz)
Bread, white, whole wheat,	1 slice (1 oz)	Roll, plain, small	1 (1 oz)
pumpernickel, rye		Tortilla, corn, 6 in. across	1
Bread sticks, crisp, 4 in. long × ½ in.	2 (⅔ oz)	Tortilla, flour, 7–8 in. across	1
English muffin	½	Waffle, 4½ in. square, reduced-fat	1
Hot dog or hamburger bun	½ (1 oz)		

CEREALS AND GRAINS

Bran cereals	½ cup	Millet	¼ cup
Bulgur	½ cup	Muesli	¼ cup
Cereals	½ cup	Oats	½ cup
Cereals, unsweetened, ready-to-eat	¾ cup	Pasta	½ cup
Cornmeal (dry)	3 tbsp	Puffed cereal	1½ cups
Couscous	⅓ cup	Rice milk	½ cup
Flour (dry)	3 tbsp	Rice, white or brown	⅓ cup
Granola, low-fat	¼ cup	Shredded Wheat	½ cup
Grape Nuts	¼ cup	Sugar-frosted cereal	½ cup
Grits	½ cup	Wheat germ	3 tbsp
Kasha	½ cup		

STARCHY VEGETABLES

Baked beans	⅓ cup	Plantain	½ cup
Corn	½ cup	Potato, baked or boiled	1 small (3 oz)
Corn on cob, medium	1 (5 oz)	Potato, mashed	½ cup
Mixed vegetables with corn, peas, or	1 cup	Squash, winter (acorn, butternut)	1 cup
pasta	½ cup	Yam, sweet potato, plain	½ cup
Peas, green			

CRACKERS AND SNACKS

Animal crackers	8	Pretzels	¾ oz
Graham crackers, 2½ in. square	3	Rice cakes, 4 in. across	2
Matzoh	¾ oz	Saltine-type crackers	6
Melba toast	4 slices	Snack chips, fat-free (tortilla, potato)	15–20 (¾ oz)
Oyster crackers	24	Whole wheat crackers, no fat added	2–5 (¾ oz)
Popcorn (popped, no fat added or low-fat microwave)	3 cups		

BEANS, PEAS, AND LENTILS
(COUNT AS 1 STARCH EXCHANGE, PLUS 1 VERY LEAN MEAT EXCHANGE.)

Beans and peas (garbanzo, pinto, kidney, white, split, black-eyed)	½ cup	Lima beans	⅔ cup
		Lentils	½ cup
		Miso*	3 tbsp

Table continued on following page

Starch List *Continued*

STARCHY FOODS PREPARED WITH FAT
(COUNT AS 1 STARCH EXCHANGE, PLUS 1 FAT EXCHANGE.)

Biscuit, 2½ in. across	1	Pancake, 4 in. across	2
Chow mein noodles	½ cup	Popcorn, microwave	3 cups
Corn bread, 2 in. cube	1 (2 oz)	Sandwich crackers, cheese or	3
Crackers, round butter type	6	peanut butter filling	
Croutons	1 cup	Stuffing, bread (prepared)	⅓ cup
French-fried potatoes	16–25 (3 oz)	Taco shell, 6 in. across	2
Granola	¼ cup	Waffle, 4½ in. square	1
Muffin, small	1 (1½ oz)	Whole wheat crackers, fat added	4–6 (1 oz)

* 400 mg or more sodium per exchange.

From the American Dietetic Association and the American Diabetes Association. (1995) Exchange Lists for Meal Planning. Copyright © 1995 by the American Diabetes Association and the American Dietetic Association.

The Exchange Lists are the basis of a meal planning system designed by a Committee of the American Diabetes Association and the American Dietetic Association. While designed primarily for people with diabetes and others who must follow special diets, the Exchange Lists are based on the principles of good nutrition that apply to everyone.

Fruit List

Fresh, frozen, canned, and dried fruits and fruit juices are on this list. In general, one fruit exchange is equivalent to:

- 1 small to medium fresh fruit
- ½ cup of canned or fresh fruit or fruit juice
- ¼ cup of dried fruit

Selection Notes

1. Count ½ cup cranberries or rhubarb sweetened with sugar substitutes as free foods.
2. Encourage clients to read the Nutrition Facts on the food label. If one serving has more than 15 g of carbohydrate, the size of the serving will need to be adjusted.
3. Fresh, frozen, and dried fruits have about 2 g of fiber per choice.
4. Portion sizes for canned fruits are for the fruit and a small amount of juice.
5. Whole fruit is more filling than fruit juice and may be a better choice.
6. Food labels for fruits may contain the words "no sugar added" or "unsweetened." This means that no sucrose (table sugar) has been added.
7. Generally, fruit canned in extra light syrup has the same amount of carbohydrate per serving as the "no sugar added" or the juice pack. All canned fruits on the fruit list are based on one of these three types of pack.

One Fruit Exchange Equals 15 g Carbohydrate and 60 Calories.
The Weight Includes Skin, Core, Seeds, and Rind.

FRUIT

Apple, unpeeled, small	1 (4 oz)	Grapefruit sections, canned	¾ cup
Applesauce, unsweetened	½ cup	Grapes, small	17 (3 oz)
Apples, dried	4 rings	Honeydew melon	1 slice (10 oz) or 1 cup cubes
Apricots, fresh	4 whole (5½ oz)	Kiwi	1 (3½ oz)
Apricots, dried	8 halves	Mandarin oranges, canned	¾ cup
Apricots, canned	½ cup	Mango, small	½ fruit (5½ oz) or ½ cup
Banana, small	1 (4 oz)	Nectarine, small	1 (5 oz)
Blackberries	¾ cup	Orange, small	1 (6½ oz)
Blueberries	¾ cup	Papaya	½ fruit (8 oz) or 1 cup cubes
Cantaloupe, small	⅓ melon (11 oz) or 1 cup cubes	Peach, medium, fresh	1 (6 oz)
Cherries, sweet, fresh	12 (3 oz)	Peaches, canned	½ cup
Cherries, sweet, canned	½ cup	Pear, large, fresh	½ (4 oz)
Dates	3	Pears, canned	½ cup
Figs, fresh	1½ large or 2 medium (3½ oz)	Pineapple, fresh	¾ cup
Figs, dried	1½	Pineapple, canned	½ cup
Fruit cocktail	½ cup	Plums, small	2 (5 oz)
Grapefruit, large	½ (11 oz)		

Table continued on opposite page

Fruit List *Continued*

FRUIT

Plums, canned	½ cup	Strawberries	1¼ cup whole berries
Prunes, dried	3	Tangerines, small	2 (8 oz)
Raisins	2 tbsp	Watermelon	1 slice (13½ oz) or 1¼ cup cubes
Raspberries	1 cup		

FRUIT JUICE

Apple juice/cider	½ cup	Grapefruit juice	½ cup
Cranberry juice cocktail	⅓ cup	Orange juice	½ cup
Cranberry juice cocktail, reduced-calorie	1 cup	Pineapple juice	½ cup
		Prune juice	⅓ cup
Fruit juice blends, 100% juice	⅓ cup		
Grape juice	⅓ cup		

From the American Dietetic Association and the American Diabetes Association. (1995) Exchange Lists for Meal Planning. Copyright © 1995 by the American Diabetes Association and the American Dietetic Association.

The Exchange Lists are the basis of a meal planning system designed by a Committee of the American Diabetes Association. While designed primarily for people with diabetes and others who must follow special diets, the Exchange Lists are based on the principles of good nutrition that apply to everyone.

Milk List

Different types of milk and milk products are on this list. Cheeses are on the Meat list and cream and other dairy fats are on the Fat list. Based on the amount of fat they contain, milks are divided into fat-free/low-fat milk, reduced-fat milk, and whole milk. One choice of these includes:

	Carbohydrate (g)	Protein (g)	Fat (g)	Calories
Fat-free/low-fat	12	8	0–3	90
Reduced-fat	12	8	5	120
Whole	12	8	8	150

Selection Notes

1. One cup equals 8 fl oz or ½ pt.
2. Chocolate milk, frozen yogurt, and ice cream are on the Other Carbohydrates list.
3. Nondairy creamers are on the Free Foods list.
4. Rice milk is on the Starch list.
5. Soy milk is on the Medium-fat Meat list.

One Milk Exchange Equals 12 g Carbohydrate and 8 g Protein.
Fat-Free and Low-fat Milk
(0–3 g Fat per Serving)

Fat-free milk	1 cup	Fat-free dry milk	⅓ cup dry
½% milk	1 cup	Plain yogurt	¾ cup
1% milk	1 cup	Nonfat or low-fat fruit-flavored yogurt sweetened with aspartame or with a non-nutritive sweetener	1 cup
Fat-free or low-fat buttermilk	1 cup		
Evaporated fat-free milk	½ cup		

Reduced-fat Milk
(5 g fat per serving)

2% milk	1 cup
Plain low-fat yogurt	¾ cup
Sweet acidophilus milk	1 cup

Whole Milk
(8 g fat per serving)

Whole milk	1 cup
Evaporated whole milk	½ cup
Goat's milk	1 cup
Kefir	1 cup

From the American Dietetic Association and the American Diabetes Association. (1995) Exchange Lists for Meal Planning. Copyright © 1995 by the American Diabetes Association and the American Dietetic Association.

The Exchange Lists are the basis of a meal planning system designed by a Committee of the American Diabetes Association. While designed primarily for people with diabetes and others who must follow special diets, the Exchange Lists are based on the principles of good nutrition that apply to everyone.

Other Carbohydrates List

Food choices from this list can be substituted for a starch, fruit, or milk choice. However, they do not contain as many important vitamins and minerals as the choices on the Starch, Fruit, or Milk list. Some choices will also count as one or more fat choices.

Selection Notes

1. Because many of these foods are concentrated sources of carbohydrate and fat, the portion sizes are often very small.
2. Many fat-free or reduced-fat products made with fat replacers contain carbohydrate. When eaten in large amounts, they may need to be counted.
3. Fat-free salad dressings can be found in smaller amount on the Free Foods list.

One Exchange Equals 15 g Carbohydrate, or 1 Starch, or 1 Fruit, or 1 Milk.

Food	Serving Size	Exchanges per Serving
Angel food cake, unfrosted	¹⁄₁₂ cake	2 carbohydrates
Brownie, small, unfrosted	2 in. square	1 carbohydrate, 1 fat
Cake, unfrosted	2 in. square	1 carbohydrate, 1 fat
Cake, frosted	2 in. square	2 carbohydrates, 1 fat
Cookie, fat-free	2 small	1 carbohydrate
Cookie or sandwich cookie with creme filling	2 small	1 carbohydrate, 1 fat
Cranberry sauce, jellied	¼ cup	1½ carbohydrates
Cupcake, frosted	1 small	2 carbohydrates, 1 fat
Doughnut, plain cake	1 medium (1½ oz)	1½ carbohydrates, 2 fats
Doughnut, glazed	3¾ in. across (2 oz)	2 carbohydrates, 2 fats
Fruit juice bars, frozen, 100% juice	1 bar (3 oz)	1 carbohydrate
Fruit snacks, chewy (pureed fruit concentrate)	1 roll (¾ oz)	1 carbohydrate
Fruit spreads, 100% fruit	1 tbsp	1 carbohydrate
Gelatin, regular	½ cup	1 carbohydrate
Gingersnaps	3	1 carbohydrate
Granola bar	1 bar	1 carbohydrate, 1 fat
Granola bar, fat-free	1 bar	2 carbohydrates
Honey	1 tbsp	1 carbohydrate
Hummus	⅓ cup	1 carbohydrate, 1 fat
Ice cream	½ cup	1 carbohydrate, 2 fats
Ice cream, light	½ cup	1 carbohydrate, 1 fat
Ice cream, fat-free, no sugar added	½ cup	1 carbohydrate
Jam or jelly, regular	1 tbsp	1 carbohydrate
Milk, chocolate, whole	1 cup	2 carbohydrates, 1 fat
Pie, fruit, 2 crusts	⅙ pie	3 carbohydrates, 2 fats
Pie, pumpkin or custard	⅛ pie	1 carbohydrate, 2 fats
Potato chips	12–18 (1 oz)	1 carbohydrate, 2 fats
Pudding, regular (made with low-fat milk)	½ cup	2 carbohydrates
Pudding, sugar-free (made with low-fat milk)	½ cup	1 carbohydrate
Salad dressing, fat-free*	¼ cup	1 carbohydrate
Sherbet, sorbet	½ cup	2 carbohydrates
Spaghetti or pasta sauce, canned*	½ cup	1 carbohydrate, 1 fat
Sugar	1 tbsp	1 carbohydrate
Sweet roll or Danish	1 (2½ oz)	2½ carbohydrates, 2 fats
Syrup, light	2 tbsp	1 carbohydrate
Syrup, regular	1 tbsp	1 carbohydrate
Syrup, regular	¼ cup	4 carbohydrates
Tortilla chips	6–12 (1 oz)	1 carbohydrate, 2 fats
Vanilla wafers	5	1 carbohydrate, 1 fat
Yogurt, frozen, low-fat, fat-free	⅓ cup	1 carbohydrate, 0–1 fat
Yogurt, frozen, fat-free, no sugar added	½ cup	1 carbohydrate
Yogurt, low-fat with fruit	1 cup	3 carbohydrates, 0–1 fat

* = 400 mg or more sodium per exchange.

From the American Dietetic Association and the American Diabetes Association. (1995) Exchange Lists for Meal Planning. Copyright © 1995 by the American Diabetes Association and the American Dietetic Association.

The Exchange Lists are the basis of a meal planning system designed by a Committee of the American Diabetes Association. While designed primarily for people with diabetes and others who must follow special diets, the Exchange Lists are based on the principles of good nutrition that apply to everyone.

Vegetable List

In general, one vegetable exchange is equivalent to:

- ½ cup of cooked vegetables or vegetable juice
- 1 cup of raw vegetables

Selection Notes

1. One to two vegetable choices at a meal or snack do not have to be counted because they contain only small amounts of calories or carbohydrates.
2. Three cups or more of raw vegetables or 1½ cups of cooked vegetables at one meal count as 1 carbohydrate choice.
3. Starchy vegetables such as corn, peas, winter squash, and potatoes that contain larger amounts of calories and carbohydrates are on the Starch list.
4. Tomato sauce is different from spaghetti sauce, which is on the Other Carbohydrates list.

One Vegetable Exchange Equals 5 g Carbohydrates, 2 g Protein, 0 g Fat, and 25 Calories.

Artichoke	Eggplant	Salad greens (endive, escarole, lettuce, romaine,
Artichoke hearts	Green onions or scallions	spinach)
Asparagus	Greens (collard, kale, mustard, turnip)	Sauerkraut*
Beans (green, wax, Italian)	Kohlrabi	Spinach
Bean sprouts	Leeks	Summer squash
Beets	Mixed vegetables (without corn, peas,	Tomato
Broccoli	or pasta)	Tomatoes, canned
Brussels sprouts	Mushrooms	Tomato sauce*
Cabbage	Okra	Tomato/vegetable juice*
Carrots	Onions	Turnips
Cauliflower	Pea pods	Water chestnuts
Celery	Peppers (all varieties)	Watercress
Cucumber	Radishes	Zucchini

* = 400 mg or more sodium per exchange.

From the American Dietetic Association and the American Diabetes Association. (1995) Exchange Lists for Meal Planning. Copyright © 1995 by the American Diabetes Association and the American Dietetic Association.

The Exchange Lists are the basis of a meal planning system designed by a Committee of the American Diabetes Association. While designed primarily for people with diabetes and others who must follow special diets, the Exchange Lists are based on the principles of good nutrition that apply to everyone.

Meat and Meat Substitutes List

Meat and meat substitutes that contain both protein and fat are on this list. In general, one meat exchange is equivalent to:

- 1 oz meat, fish, poultry, or cheese,
- ½ cup beans, peas, and lentils.

Based on the amount of fat they contain, meats are divided into very lean, lean, medium-fat, and high-fat lists. One ounce (one exchange) of each of these includes:

	Carbohydrate (g)	Protein (g)	Fat (g)	Calories
Very lean	0	7	0–1	35
Lean	0	7	3	55
Medium-fat	0	7	5	75
High-fat	0	7	8	100

Selection Notes

1. Meat should be weighed after cooking and removing bones and fat. Four oz of raw meat is equal to 3 oz of cooked meat. Following are some examples of meat portions:
   1 oz cheese = 1 meat choice and is about the size of a 1-in cube
   2 oz meat = 2 meat choices, such as
              = 1 small chicken leg or thigh
                ½ cup cottage cheese or tuna

Table continued on following page

Meat and Meat Substitutes List *Continued*

3 oz meat = 3 meat choices and is about the size of a deck of cards, such as
1 medium pork chop
1 small hamburger
½ of a whole chicken breast
1 unbreaded fish fillet

2. Limit choices from the high-fat group to three times per week or less.
3. Most grocery stores stock Select and Choice grades of meat. Select grades of meat are the leanest meats. Choice grades contain a moderate amount of fat, and Prime cuts of meat have the highest amount of fat. Restaurants usually serve Prime cuts of meat.
4. "Hamburger" may contain added seasoning and fat, but ground beef does not.
5. Encourage the reading of labels to find products that are low in fat and cholesterol (5 g or less of fat per serving).
6. Beans, peas, and lentils are also found on the Starch list.
7. Peanut butter, in smaller amounts, is also found on the Fat list.
8. Bacon, in smaller amounts, is also found on the Fat list.
9. Some processed meats, seafood, and soy products may contain carbohydrate when consumed in large amounts. If so, these should be counted as a carbohydrate choice as well as a meat choice.

Meal Planning Tips

1. Bake, roast, broil, grill, poach, steam, or boil these foods rather than frying.
2. Place meat on a rack so the fat will drain off during cooking.
3. Use a nonstick spray and a nonstick pan to brown or fry foods.
4. Trim off visible fat before or after cooking.
5. If flour, bread crumbs, coating mixes, fat, or marinades are added when cooking, these may need to be counted in the meal plan.

VERY LEAN MEAT AND SUBSTITUTES LIST
ONE EXCHANGE EQUALS 0 g CARBOHYDRATE, 7 g PROTEIN, 0–1 g FAT, AND 35 CALORIES.

One very lean meat exchange is equal to any one of the following items:

Poultry: Chicken or turkey (white meat, no skin), Cornish hen (no skin)	1 oz
Fish: Fresh or frozen cod, flounder, haddock, halibut, trout; tuna fresh or canned in water	1 oz
Shellfish: Clams, crab, lobster, scallops, shrimp, imitation shellfish	1 oz
Game: Duck or pheasant (no skin), venison, buffalo, ostrich	1 oz
Cheese with 1 g or less fat per ounce:	
Nonfat or low-fat cottage cheese	¼ cup
Fat-free cheese	1 oz
Other: Processed sandwich meats with 1 g or less fat per ounce, such as deli thin, shaved meats, chipped beef,* turkey ham	1 oz
Egg whites	2
Egg substitutes, plain	¼ cup
Hot dogs with 1 g or less fat per ounce*	1 oz
Kidney (high in cholesterol)	1 oz
Sausage with 1 g or less fat per ounce	1 oz

Count as one very lean meat and one starch exchange.

Beans, peas, lentils (cooked)	½ cup

LEAN MEAT AND SUBSTITUTES LIST
ONE EXCHANGE EQUALS 0 g CARBOHYDRATE, 7 g PROTEIN, 3 g FAT, AND 55 CALORIES.

One lean meat exchange is equal to any one of the following items:

Beef: USDA Select or Choice grades of lean beef trimmed of fat, such as round, sirloin, and flank steak; tenderloin; roast (rib, chuck, rump); steak (T-bone, porterhouse, cubed), ground round	1 oz
Pork: Lean pork, such as fresh ham; canned, cured, or boiled ham; Canadian bacon*; tenderloin, center loin chop	1 oz
Lamb: Roast, chop, leg	1 oz
Veal: Lean chop, roast	1 oz
Poultry: Chicken, turkey (dark meat, no skin), chicken (white meat, with skin), domestic duck or goose (well-drained of fat, no skin)	1 oz
Fish:	
Herring (uncreamed or smoked)	1 oz
Oysters	6 medium
Salmon (fresh or canned), catfish	1 oz
Sardines (canned)	2 medium
Tuna (canned in oil, drained)	1 oz
Game: Goose (no skin), rabbit	1 oz

Table continued on opposite page

Meat and Meat Substitutes List *Continued*

Cheese:
4.5%-fat cottage cheese	¼ cup
Grated Parmesan	2 tbsp
Cheeses with 3 g or less fat per ounce	1 oz

Other:
Hot dogs with 3 g or less fat per ounce*	1½ oz
Processed sandwich meat with 3 g or less fat per ounce, such as turkey pastrami or kielbasa	1 oz
Liver, heart (high in cholesterol)	1 oz

MEDIUM-FAT MEAT AND SUBSTITUTES LIST
ONE EXCHANGE EQUALS 0 g CARBOHYDRATE, 7 g PROTEIN, 5 g FAT, AND 75 CALORIES.

One medium-fat meat exchange is equal to any one of the following items:
Beef: Most beef products fall into this category (ground beef, meat loaf, corned beef, short ribs, Prime grades of meat trimmed of fat, such as prime rib)	1 oz
Pork: Top loin, chop, Boston butt, cutlet	1 oz
Lamb: Rib roast, ground	1 oz
Veal: Cutlet (ground or cubed, unbreaded)	1 oz
Poultry: Chicken (dark meat, with skin), ground turkey or ground chicken, fried chicken (with skin)	1 oz
Fish: Any fried fish product	1 oz

Cheese: With 5 g or less fat per ounce
Feta	1 oz
Mozzarella	1 oz
Ricotta	¼ cup (2 oz)

Other:
Egg (high in cholesterol, limit to 3 per week)	1
Sausage with 5 g or less fat per ounce	1 oz
Soy milk	1 cup
Tempeh	¼ cup
Tofu	4 oz or ½ cup

HIGH-FAT MEAT AND SUBSTITUTES LIST
ONE EXCHANGE EQUALS 0 g CARBOHYDRATE, 7 g PROTEIN, 8 g FAT, AND 100 CALORIES.

One high-fat meat exchange is equal to any one of the following items.
Pork: Spareribs, ground pork, pork sausage	1 oz
Cheese: All regular cheeses, such as American,* cheddar, Monterey Jack, Swiss	1 oz
Other: Processed sandwich meats with 8 grams or less fat per ounce, such as bologna, pimento loaf, salami	1 oz
Sausage, such as bratwurst, Italian, knockwurst, Polish, smoked	1 oz
Hot dog (turkey or chicken)*	1 (10/lb)
Bacon	3 slices (20 slices/lb)

Count as one high-fat meat plus one fat exchange.
Hot dog (beef, pork, or combination)*	1 (10/lb)

Count as one high-fat meat plus two fat exchanges.
Peanut butter (contains unsaturated fat)	2 tbsp

* 400 mg or more sodium per exchange.

From the American Dietetic Association and the American Diabetes Association. (1995) Exchange Lists for Meal Planning. Copyright © 1995 by the American Diabetes Association and the American Dietetic Association.

The Exchange Lists are the basis of a meal planning system designed by a Committee of the American Diabetes Association. While designed primarily for people with diabetes and others who must follow special diets, the Exchange Lists are based on the principles of good nutrition that apply to everyone.

Fat List

Fats are divided into three groups, based on the main type of fat they contain: monounsaturated, polyunsaturated, and saturated. Saturated fats are linked with heart disease and cancer. In general, one fat exchange is equivalent to:

- 1 tsp of regular margarine or vegetable oil
- 1 tsp of regular salad dressings

Selection Notes

1. One fat exchange is based on a serving size containing 5 g of fat.
2. Fat-free salad dressings are on the Other Carbohydrates list and the Free Foods list.
3. See the Free Foods list for nondairy coffee creamers, whipped topping, and fat-free products, such as margarines, salad dressings, mayonnaise, sour cream, cream cheese, and nonstick cooking spray.

Monounsaturated Fats List
One Fat Exchange Equals 5 g Fat and 45 Calories.

Avocado, medium	⅛ (1 oz)
Oil (canola, olive, peanut)	1 tsp
Olives: ripe (black)	8 large
green, stuffed*	10 large
Nuts	
almonds, cashews	6 nuts
mixed (50% peanuts)	6 nuts
peanuts	10 nuts
pecans	4 halves
Peanut butter, smooth or crunchy	2 tsp
Sesame seeds	1 tbsp
Tahini paste	2 tsp

Polyunsaturated Fats List
One Fat Exchange Equals 5 g Fat and 45 Calories.

Margarine: stick, tub, or squeeze	1 tsp
lower-fat (30% to 50% vegetable oil)	1 tbsp
Mayonnaise: regular	1 tsp
reduced-fat	1 tbsp
Nuts, walnuts, English	4 halves
Oil (corn, safflower, soybean)	1 tsp
Salad dressing: regular*	1 tbsp
reduced-fat	2 tbsp
Miracle Whip Salad Dressing®: regular	2 tsp
reduced-fat	1 tbsp
Seeds: pumpkin, sunflower	1 tbsp

Saturated Fats List
One Fat Exchange Equals 5 g of Fat and 45 Calories.

Bacon, cooked	1 slice (20 slices/lb)
Bacon, grease	1 tsp
Butter: stick	1 tsp
whipped	2 tsp
reduced-fat	1 tbsp
Chitterlings, boiled	2 tbsp (½ oz)
Coconut, sweetened, shredded	2 tbsp
Cream, half and half	2 tbsp
Cream cheese: regular	1 tbsp (½ oz)
reduced-fat	2 tbsp (1 oz)
Fatback or salt pork†	
Shortening or lard	1 tsp
Sour cream: regular	2 tbsp
reduced-fat	3 tbsp

* = 400 mg or more sodium per exchange.

† Use a piece 1 in. × 1 in. × ¼ in. when eating the fatback cooked with vegetables. Use a piece 2 in. × 1 in. × ½ in. when eating only the vegetables with the fatback removed.

From the American Dietetic Association and the American Diabetes Association. (1995) Exchange Lists for Meal Planning. Copyright © 1995 by the American Diabetes Association and the American Dietetic Association.

The Exchange Lists are the basis of a meal planning system designed by a Committee by the American Diabetes Association. While designed primarily for people with diabetes and others who must follow special diets, the Exchange Lists are based on the principles of good nutrition that apply to everyone.

Free Foods List

A free food is any food or drink that contains less than 20 calories or less than 5 grams of carbohydrate per serving. Foods with a serving size listed should be limited to three servings per day, spread throughout the day. Foods listed without a serving size can be eaten as often as desired.

Fat-Free or Reduced-Fat Foods

Cream cheese, fat-free	1 tbsp
Creamers, nondairy, liquid	1 tbsp
Creamers, nondairy, powdered	2 tsp
Mayonnaise, fat-free	1 tbsp
Mayonnaise, reduced-fat	1 tsp
Margarine, fat-free	4 tbsp
Margarine, reduced-fat	1 tsp
Miracle Whip®, nonfat	1 tbsp
Miracle Whip®, reduced-fat	1 tsp
Nonstick cooking spray	
Salad dressing, fat-free	1 tbsp
Salad dressing, fat-free Italian	2 tbsp
Salsa	¼ cup
Sour cream, fat-free, reduced-fat	1 tbsp
Whipped topping, regular or light	2 tbsp

Sugar-Free or Low-Sugar Foods

Candy, hard, sugar-free	1 candy
Gelatin dessert, sugar-free	
Gelatin, unflavored	
Gum, sugar-free	
Jam or jelly, low-sugar or light	2 tsp
Sugar substitutes	

Sugar substitutes, alternatives, or replacements that are approved by the Food and Drug Administration (FDA) are safe to use. Common brand names include:

Equal (aspartame)
Sprinkle Sweet® (saccharin)
Sweet One (acesulfame K)
Sweet-10® (saccharin)
Sugar Twin® (saccharin)
Sweet 'n Low® (saccharin)

Syrup, sugar-free	2 tbsp

Drinks

Bouillon, broth, consommé*	
Bouillon or broth, low-sodium	
Carbonated or mineral water	
Club soda	
Cocoa powder, unsweetened	1 tbsp
Coffee	
Diet soft drinks, sugar-free	
Drink mixes, sugar-free	
Tea	
Tonic water, sugar-free	

Condiments

Catsup	1 tbsp
Horseradish	
Lemon juice	
Lime juice	
Mustard	
Pickles, dill*	1½ large
Soy sauce, regular or light*	
Taco sauce	1 tbsp
Vinegar	

Seasonings

Some seasonings that contain sodium or are salts, including garlic or celery salt, and lemon pepper
Flavoring extracts
Garlic
Herbs, fresh or dried
Pimento
Spices
Tabasco or hot pepper sauce
Wine, used in cooking
Worcestershire sauce

* 400 mg or more of sodium per exchange.

From the American Dietetic Association and the American Diabetes Association. (1995) Exchange Lists for Meal Planning. Copyright © 1995 by the American Diabetes Association and the American Dietetic Association.

The Exchange Lists are the basis of a meal planning system designed by a Committee of the American Diabetes Association. While designed primarily for people with diabetes and others who must follow special diets, the Exchange Lists are based on the principles of good nutrition that apply to everyone.

Combination Foods List

Combination foods do not fit into any one exchange list. This is a list of exchanges for some typical combination foods.

Food	Serving Size	Exchanges Per Serving
Entrees		
Tuna noodle casserole, lasagna, spaghetti with meatballs, chili with beans, macaroni and cheese*	1 cup (8 oz)	2 carbohydrates, 2 medium-fat meats
Chow mein (without noodles or rice)*	2 cups (16 oz)	1 carbohydrate, 2 lean meats
Pizza, cheese, thin crust†	¼ of 10 in. (5 oz)	2 carbohydrates, 2 medium-fat meats, 1 fat
Pizza, meat topping, thin crust*	¼ of 10 in. (5 oz)	2 carbohydrates, 2 medium-fat meats, 2 fats
Pot pie*	1 (7 oz)	2 carbohydrates, 1 medium-fat meat, 4 fats
Frozen entrees		
Salisbury steak with gravy, mashed potato*	1 (11 oz)	2 carbohydrates, 3 medium-fat meats, 3–4 fats
Turkey with gravy, mashed potato, dressing*	1 (11 oz)	2 carbohydrates, 2 medium-fat meats, 2 fats
Entree with less than 300 calories*	1 (8 oz)	2 carbohydrates, 3 lean meats
Soups		
Bean*	1 cup	1 carbohydrate, 1 very lean meat
Cream (made with water)*	1 cup (8 oz)	1 carbohydrate, 1 fat
Split pea (made with water)*	½ cup (4 oz)	1 carbohydrate
Tomato (made with water)*	1 cup (8 oz)	1 carbohydrate
Vegetable beef, chicken noodle, or other broth-type*	1 cup (8 oz)	1 carbohydrate

Fast Foods

Food	Serving Size	Exchanges Per Serving
Burritos with beef*	2	4 carbohydrates, 2 medium-fat meats, 2 fats
Chicken nuggets*	6	1 carbohydrate, 2 medium-fat meats, 1 fat
Chicken breast and wing, breaded and fried*	1 each	1 carbohydrate, 4 medium-fat meats, 2 fats
Fish sandwich/tartar sauce*	1	3 carbohydrates, 1 medium-fat meat, 3 fats
French fries, thin*	20–25	2 carbohydrates, 2 fats
Hamburger, regular	1	2 carbohydrates, 2 medium-fat meats
Hamburger, large*	1	2 carbohydrates, 3 medium-fat meats, 1 fat
Hot dog with bun*	1	1 carbohydrate, 1 high-fat meat, 1 fat
Individual pan pizza*	1	5 carbohydrates, 3 medium-fat meats, 3 fats
Soft-serve cone	1 medium	2 carbohydrates, 1 fat
Submarine sandwich*	1 sub (6 in.)	3 carbohydrates, 1 vegetable, 2 medium-fat meats, 1 fat
Taco, hard shell*	1 (6 oz)	2 carbohydrates, 2 medium-fat meats, 2 fats
Taco, soft shell*	1 (3 oz)	1 carbohydrate, 1 medium-fat meat, 1 fat

* 400 mg or more sodium per exchange.

From the American Dietetic Association and the American Diabetes Association. (1995) Exchange Lists for Meal Planning. Copyright © 1995 from the American Diabetes Association and the American Dietetic Association.

The Exchange Lists are the basis of a meal planning system designed by a Committee of the American Diabetes Association. While designed primarily for people with diabetes and others who must follow special diets, the Exchange Lists are based on the principles of good nutrition that apply to everyone.

DESCRIPTION

Everyone needs to eat nutritious foods. Good health depends on eating a variety of foods that contain the right amounts of carbohydrate, protein, fat, vitamins, minerals, fiber, and water. The number of calories you need depends on your size, age, and activity level. Eating the right number of calories helps you reach and stay at a reasonable weight. People who are overweight are at risk for developing health problems such as high blood pressure, heart disease, cancer, and diabetes. By following a calorie-restricted balanced nutritious diet along with exercise, you can achieve a reasonable weight.

ADEQUACY

Weight management begins with sound education and individualized counseling provided by a qualified care giver such as a registered dietitian or nurse. Meal planning is essential to staying on a calorie-restricted diet. Use of food exchange lists will make meal planning easier and ensure you are getting adequate nutrients. Standardized meal plans, used with the Exchange Lists for Meal Planning can be used to plan and individualize your calorie-restricted diet. Weight management diets of 1200 calories or more can meet the Recommended Dietary Allowances.

GUIDELINES

1. Eat a variety of food. Choose a variety of foods within the food groups to make sure you are getting all nutrients.

2. Eat healthy carbohydrates, not just those that are high in sugar.

3. Eat less fat. Avoid adding fat during food preparation and let fat drip away from food. Choose mostly lower fat foods within the food exchange lists.

4. Eat more fiber. Try whole grains, fresh fruits, and raw vegetables.

5. Pay attention to portion sizes. Measure food at first to get used to what a portion size looks like.

6. Avoid skipping meals. This can make you extra hungry, moody, and unable to focus.

7. Be physically active. Be active at least 30 minutes on most days. This can be as simple as walking.

8. On a reduction diet an individual may reach a point where weight remains the same for 1, 2, or even 3 weeks. Weight loss will resume, however, if the diet is continued.

9. Usually, fluid or salt restriction is not considered desirable for weight reduction unless it is required for medical reasons.

10. The suggested meal plan may be modified to meet individual desires. For example, if an individual would like a mid-afternoon or evening snack, he or she may reserve some food from the previous meal for that purpose or divide the food for the day into five small meals instead of the suggested three. (This menu plan is to be used with the Exchange Lists for Meal Planning.)

OTHER INSTRUCTIONS

Cardiovascular Diets

Sodium-Controlled Diets

DESCRIPTION

A sodium-controlled diet will help manage high blood pressure (hypertension) in persons who are sodium-sensitive. It will also help prevent water retention. A sodium-controlled diet will allow high blood pressure medication to be more effective.

ADEQUACY

Sodium-controlled meal plans are adequate in all nutrients based on the Recommended Dietary Allowances.

GUIDELINES

Many people need to limit their sodium intake to less than 3000 milligrams (mg) a day. Below are some common levels of sodium restriction and accompanying dietary guidelines.

1. 3000 mg sodium—Eliminate, or eat sparingly, high-sodium processed foods and beverages such as fast foods; salad dressings; smoked, salted, and koshered meats; regular canned foods; pickled vegetables; luncheon meats; and commercially softened water. Allow up to one fourth teaspoon of table salt in cooking or at the table.
2. 2000 mg sodium—Eliminate processed and prepared foods and beverages high in sodium. Limit milk and milk products to 16 ounces daily. Replace regular canned and instant products with low-sodium versions. Do not allow any salt in food preparation or at the table.
3. 1000 mg sodium—Use low-sodium versions of all processed and prepared foods and beverages. Limit regular bread to two servings per day, and limit milk and milk products to 16 ounces per day. Do not allow salt in food preparation or at the table.
4. 500 mg sodium—Omit canned or processed foods containing sodium or salt. Omit vegetables containing high amounts of natural sodium. Limit meat to 5 ounces per day and milk and milk products to 16 ounces per day. Use low-sodium bread in place of regular bread and distilled water for cooking and drinking. Do not use salt in food preparation or at the table.

HELPFUL TIPS

1. Diet education should consider body weight. Persons with hypertension who are over ideal body weight should reduce their weight.
2. Food labels should be read for sodium content. Low sodium foods should have less than 140 mg of sodium per serving. Sodium-free foods should have less than 5 mg of sodium per serving.
3. Many nonprescription medications and other nonfood substances such as chewing tobacco contain sodium. Check labels on medications for sodium content or ask the pharmacist about them.
4. Salt substitutes may contain potassium. If potassium is also restricted in the diet, appropriate salt substitutes should be used.
5. When dining away from home, request food prepared without salt.
6. Limiting alcohol and caffeine can also help manage hypertension.

Following are guidelines for food selection and a sample menu for a 2000 mg sodium diet.

Guidelines for Food Selection for 2000 mg Sodium Diet

Food Category	Allowed	Avoid
Beverages	Milk (limit to 16 oz daily), buttermilk (limit to 1 cup per week); eggnog; all fruit juices; low-sodium, salt-free vegetable juices; low-sodium carbonated beverages	Malted milk, milk shake, chocolate milk; regular vegetable or tomato juices; commercially softened water used for drinking or cooking
Breads and cereals	Enriched white, wheat, rye, and pumpernickel bread, hard rolls, and dinner rolls; muffins, cornbread, pancakes, and waffles; most dry cereals, cooked cereal without added salt; unsalted crackers and breadsticks; low-sodium or homemade bread crumbs	Breads, rolls, and crackers with salted tops; quick breads; instant hot cereals; commercial bread stuffing; self-rising flour and biscuit mixes; regular bread crumbs or cracker crumbs
Desserts and sweets	All; desserts and sweets made with milk should be within allowance	None
Fats	Butter or margarine; vegetable oils; unsalted salad dressings; light, sour, and heavy cream	Regular salad dressings containing bacon fat, bacon bits, and salt pork; snack dips made with instant soup mixes or processed cheese
Fruits	Most fresh, frozen, and canned fruits	Fruits processed with salt or sodium-containing compounds
Meats and meat substitutes	Any fresh or frozen beef, lamb, pork, poultry, fish; some shellfish; canned tuna or salmon, rinsed; eggs and egg substitutes; low-sodium cheese including low-sodium ricotta and cream cheese; low-sodium cottage cheese; regular yogurt; low-sodium peanut butter; dried peas and beans; frozen dinners (<500 mg sodium)	Any smoked, cured, salted, koshered, or canned meat, fish, or poultry including bacon, chipped beef, cold cuts, ham, hot dogs, sausage, sardines, anchovies, marinated herring, and pickled meats; crab, lobster; frozen breaded meats; pickled eggs; regular hard or processed cheese and cheese products, salted nuts
Potatoes and potato substitutes	White or sweet potatoes, squash, enriched rice, barley, noodles, spaghetti, macaroni, and other pastas cooked without salt; homemade bread stuffing	Commercially prepared potato, rice, or pasta mixes; commercial bread stuffing
Soups	Low-sodium commercially canned and dehydrated soups, broths, and bouillons; homemade broth soups without added salt and made with allowed vegetable; cream soups within milk allowance	Regular canned or dehydrated soups, broths or bouillon
Vegetables	Fresh, frozen vegetables and low-sodium canned vegetables	Regular canned vegetables, sauerkraut, pickled vegetables, and others prepared in brine; frozen vegetables in sauces; vegetables seasoned with ham, bacon, or salt pork
Miscellaneous	Salt substitute with physician's approval; pepper, herbs, spices; vinegar, lemon, or lime juice; low-sodium condiments (catsup, chili sauce, mustard); fresh ground horseradish; unsalted tortilla chips, pretzels, potato chips, popcorn	Any seasoning made with salt including garlic salt, celery salt, onion salt, and seasoned salt; sea salt, rock salt, kosher salt; meat tenderizers; monosodium glutamate; regular soy sauce, barbecue sauce, teriyaki sauce, steak sauces, and most flavored vinegars; canned gravy and mixes; regular condiments; salted snack foods

Sample Menu for 2000 mg Sodium Diet

Breakfast	Lunch	Dinner
Orange juice (½ cup)	Low-sodium vegetable soup (1 cup)	Green salad (3½ oz)
Whole grain cereal (¾ cup)	Unsalted crackers (4)	Salt free vinegar and oil dressing
Banana (½)	Lean beef patty (3 oz)	(1 tbsp)
Whole wheat toast (2 slices)	Hamburger bun (1)	Broiled skinless chicken breast (3 oz)
Margarine (2 tsp)	Low-sodium mustard (1 tbsp)	Herbed brown rice (½ cup)
Jelly or jam (1 tbsp)	Low-sodium mayonnaise (1 tbsp)	Steamed broccoli (½ cup)
2% milk (1 cup)	Sliced tomato (2 oz) and lettuce	Whole grain roll (1)
Coffee/tea	Fresh fruit salad (½ cup)	Margarine (2 tsp)
	Graham crackers (4)	Italian fruit ice (½ cup)
	2% milk (1 cup)	Medium apple (1)
	Coffee/tea	Coffee/tea

From Chilton Memorial Hospital, Pompton Plains, NJ.

Seasonings for Sodium-Restricted Diets (1000 mg or Above)

Allowed

Allspice	Fennel	Pepper, black, red, or white
Almond extract	Garlic, juice or powder	Peppermint extract
Anise seed	Ginger	Pimento
Basil	Horseradish root or horseradish	Poppy seed
Bay leaf	prepared without salt	Poultry seasoning
Bouillon cube, low-sodium dietetic	Hot pepper sauce	Purslane
if less than 5 mg of sodium per	Juniper	Rosemary
cube	Lemon juice or extract	Saccharin
Caraway seed	Lime juice	Saffron
Cardamom	Mace	Sage
Catsup, low sodium	Maple extract	Salt substitutes (if recommended by
Chili powder	Marjoram	the doctor)
Chili sauce, low sodium	Meat extracts, low-sodium dietetic	Savory
Chives	Meat tenderizers, low-sodium dietetic	Sesame seeds
Cinnamon	Mint	Sorrel
Cloves	Mustard, dry	Sugar
Cocoa (1 to 2 tsp)	Mustard, prepared low-sodium	Tarragon
Coconut	Nutmeg	Thyme
Cumin	Onion, fresh, juice, or sliced	Turmeric
Curry	Orange extract	Vanilla extract
Cyclamate, calcium (sugar	Paprika	Vinegar
substitute)	Parsley	Wine, if allowed
Dill	Pepper, fresh green or red	Walnut extract

Avoid

Barbecue sauce	Garlic salt	Relishes
Bouillon cube, regular	Horseradish, prepared with salt	Salt—all types
Catsup, regular	Meat extracts	Salt substitutes unless recommended
Celery leaves, dried or fresh	Meat sauces	by the doctor
Celery salt	Meat tenderizers	Seasoned salt
Celery seed	Monosodium glutamate	Soy sauce, regular and low-sodium
Chili sauce, regular	Mustard, prepared, regular	Steak sauce
Cyclamate, sodium (sugar	Olives	Teriyaki sauce
substitute)	Onion salt	Worcestershire sauce
Flavored vinegars	Pickles	

Note: Read the label on mixed spices to be sure that no sodium compound or nonpermitted seasoning is included.
From Chilton Memorial Hospital, Pompton Plains, NJ.

Cardiac Prevention Diet

DESCRIPTION

The purpose of the Cardiac Prevention Diet is to provide a balanced diet restricted in fat, saturated fat, cholesterol, and sodium. Reduction in these substances should aid in reducing lipids in the blood. This diet is appropriate for people who have elevated serum cholesterol and triglyceride levels, and who are at high risk for heart disease. This diet is intended to be a long-term lifestyle change. It can be used along with medication treatment.

ADEQUACY

This diet provides all essential nutrients and adequate calories based on Recommended Dietary Allowances.

GUIDELINES

1. Adjust calorie intake to achieve and maintain ideal body weight.
2. Increase consumption of fruits, vegetables, whole grains, and high fiber foods.
3. Decrease consumption of refined sugars, and processed and packaged foods (usually high in saturated fats, cholesterol, and sodium). Use simple foods, not convenience or processed items. Vegetables should be fresh, frozen, or "no salt" canned. Prepare all foods without butter, cream, or high-fat sauces.
4. Reduce consumption of foods high in cholesterol and saturated fats. Saturated fats are found in animal products and some plant products (for example, coconut, palm, and palm kernel oil). Most saturated fats are high in cholesterol (for example, cheese, butter, eggs, cream, whole milk, fatty beef, pork, lamb, and poultry skin), which can form fat deposits within the arteries and eventually block them.
5. Increase consumption of polyunsaturated and monounsaturated fats derived largely from vegetables and plant sources (for example, safflower oil and olive oil).
6. Limit total fat to less than 30 percent of total calories.
7. Limit the sodium content of the diet. Avoid seasoning your food with salt. Eliminate processed and convenience foods, all food items with visible salt on them, and those foods preserved in salt.

HELPFUL TIPS FOR EATING IN RESTAURANTS

1. Order broiled, baked, or poached foods with sauces on the side.
2. Ask how a dish is prepared. Knowing all the ingredients lets you control your fat intake.
3. Look for restaurants that have low fat options on the menu.
4. Ask for substitutions, even if the menu says "no substitutes." Most restaurants will bring skim milk instead of cream for coffee, unbuttered toast, and so on.
5. Try fresh fruit or sorbet for dessert.

Cardiac Prevention Diet

	Allowed	Avoid
Beverages (limit to 16 oz milk daily)	Fat-free and low-fat fluid, evaporated, or powdered milk, coffee, tea, decaffeinated coffee	Whole milk, whole milk products, evaporated whole milk, 2% milk, sweetened condensed milk, chocolate and malted milk
Breads, cereals, potatoes, crackers (6–11 servings daily)	Most commercial loaf breads; English muffins; plain bagels; unsalted saltines; matzos; graham crackers; melba toast; unsalted pretzels, cooked and most commercial dry cereals; potatoes; rice; noodles; spaghetti; macaroni	High-fat dinner rolls; egg or cheese bread or bagels; bakery and packaged mixes of doughnuts, biscuits, muffins, sweet rolls, pancakes, waffles, French toast; potato chips; french fries; high-fat party crackers; any breads, rolls, and crackers with visible salt toppings; commercial granola cereals, granola bars; egg noodles
Desserts (allowed within calorie restriction)	Frozen low-fat yogurt; fruit ices; sherbet; angel food cake; gelatin; cakes, pies, or cookies made with allowed margarine, fat-free milk and egg whites or substitute	Commercially prepared pies, cakes, cookies, or pastries; ice cream; whole milk puddings; custards; desserts made with chocolate or coconut; nondairy whipped topping
Eggs	Limit 3 to 4 egg yolks per week (including those used in cooking); cholesterol-free egg substitute	Fried eggs
Fats and oils (limit to 3 servings daily)	Oils: olive, canola, peanut, safflower, sunflower, corn, soybean, cottonseed; (margarines with liquid oil listed as first ingredient on the label; the fats you buy should contain more polyunsaturated than saturated fatty acids); mayonnaise; salad dressings: French, Italian, Thousand Island, or mayonnaise-type (Look for reduced calorie, low-sodium salad dressings.) Nuts: unsalted walnuts, pecans, almonds	Butter; cocoa butter; coconut oil; palm oil; palm kernel oil; meat drippings; gravies containing animal fat; solid vegetable shortening; lard; salt pork; cream (heavy, sweet, sour, or whipped); half and half; nondairy creamers made with coconut oil; cream cheese; salad dressing containing cheese and other restricted ingredients; olives
Fruit (four servings)	All unsweetened canned fruits and fruit juices; fresh fruit as tolerated; avocado in small amounts	Sweetened fruits and juices
Meat, fish, poultry, cheese (limit to 4–6 oz per day)	Fresh and frozen fish; crab; lobster; scallops; clams; oysters; low-sodium water packed tuna or salmon; poultry (without skin); lean cuts of veal, beef, and pork (trimmed of visible fat), (no more than 15% fat); unsalted fresh ground peanut butter (2 tbsp = 1 oz meat); low-fat cottage cheese; part skim milk cheeses (eg, mozzarella and ricotta cheese); low-fat, low-sodium cheese (6 grams fat, 30 mg sodium or less/oz); dry, grated cheese (eg, Parmesan—limit 2 tsp); tofu	Processed and cured meats (luncheon meat, frankfurters, sausage, ham, corned beef and bacon); "Prime" grade, heavily marbled and fatty meats; organ meats; fried fish, chicken, or meat; duck, goose, or capon; meats canned in gravy or sauce; canned pork and beans; processed cheese; cheese spreads; cream cheese and all other regular cheeses; caviar; sardines; herring; anchovies; Kosher prepared meats; shrimp and crayfish are moderately high in cholesterol—can be eaten occasionally

Table continued on following page

Cardiac Prevention Diet *Continued*

	Allowed	Avoid
Soups	Homemade (fat skimmed) soups made with allowed foods; low-sodium broth; cream soups made with allowed ingredients	Commercial soups; cream-based soups made with whole milk, cream, or eggs; bouillon cubes; canned bouillon; dry soup mixes
Sugar (allowed within calorie restriction)	Sugar, hard candy, gum drops, honey, jam, jelly, syrup, chewing gum, marshmallows, cocoa powder, molasses	Candies made with butter, cream, coconut, coconut or palm oil, chocolate, whole milk, cocoa butter
Vegetables (4 servings per day)	Fresh, frozen, or low-sodium canned vegetables as tolerated; low sodium tomato juice and vegetable juice cocktail; gas-forming vegetables as tolerated	Fried vegetables, sauerkraut, and pickled vegetables
Miscellaneous	All herbs, spices, dry cocoa, carob powder, pepper, Mrs. Dash. Salt substitute (if ordered by physician) Limit catsup, mustard, or Worcestershire sauce to 1 tbsp	Salt, seasoned salts, BBQ sauce, pickles, relish, olives, soy sauce, chili sauce, MSG (monosodium glutamate), gravies made with animal fat, cream sauce made from butter and cream, coconut, chocolate

Sample Menu for Cardiac Prevention Diet

Breakfast	Lunch	Dinner
Orange juice (½ cup)	Homemade vegetable soup (1 cup)	Green salad (3½ oz)
Whole-grain cereal (¾ cup)	Crackers (4)	Vinegar and oil dressing (1 tbsp)
Banana (½)	Lean beef patty (3 oz)	Broiled skinless chicken breast (3 oz)
Whole-wheat toast (2 slices)	Hamburger bun (1)	Herbed brown rice (½ cup)
Reduced-fat margarine (2 tsp)	Mustard (1 tbsp)	Steamed broccoli (½ cup)
Jelly or jam (1 tbsp)	Low-fat mayonnaise (2 tsp)	Whole-grain roll (1)
Fat-free or low-fat milk (1 cup)	Sliced tomato (2 oz) and lettuce	Reduced fat margarine (2 tsp)
Decaf. coffee/Decaf. tea	Fresh fruit salad (½ cup)	Low-fat frozen yogurt (½ cup)
	Graham crackers (4)	Medium apple (1)
	Fat-free or low-fat milk (1 cup)	Decaf. coffee/Decaf. tea
	Decaf. coffee/Decaf. tea	

From Chilton Memorial Hospital, Pompton Plains, NJ.

Gastrointestinal Diets

Bland Diet*

DESCRIPTION

This diet is based on regular eating habits restricted by individual tolerance with elimination of particular items that cause gastric irritation. The diet is supplemental to the primary therapy of medication.

GUIDELINES

1. Eat a well-balanced diet. There is little rationale for completely eliminating a particular food unless it causes repeated discomfort.
2. Foods in general that may cause discomfort include red and black pepper, chili powder, caffeine, cocoa, chocolate, and alcohol. Use of vinegar, pickles, and mustard is cautioned.

*From Chilton Memorial Hospital, Pompton Plains, NJ.

3. Highly seasoned foods, decaffeinated beverages, citrus juice, and tomatoes may be consumed according to individual tolerance.
4. Beverages that stimulate gastric secretion, such as decaffeinated and caffeinated beverages, should not be ingested on an empty stomach or before bedtime.
5. Eat meals at regular intervals. Add frequent snacks *only* if relief is gained with food.
6. Do not use milk in excessive amounts (stimulates gastric acid).
7. Chew food well, especially raw fruits and vegetables.
8. Take small, frequent (4 to 6) feedings throughout the day.
9. Caution should be used in introducing gas-producing foods into the diet. Introduce only one food at a time and then in a small amount.

OTHER INSTRUCTIONS

Fiber- and Residue-Restricted Diet

DESCRIPTION

A fiber-restricted diet uses limited amounts of well-cooked or canned vegetables and canned, cooked, or very ripe fruits. Whole-grain breads and cereals are replaced with refined foods. Legumes, nuts, and seeds are omitted.

GUIDELINES

Following the diet guidelines results in a diet that contains less than 20 grams of fiber daily.

Guidelines for Food Selection for Fiber- and Residue-Restricted Diet

Food Group	Allowed	Avoid
Beverages	Coffee, tea, carbonated beverages, strained fruit drinks, milk as tolerated*	Any containing fruit or vegetable pulp; prune juice†
Breads	Refined breads, rolls, biscuits, muffins, crackers; pancakes or waffles; plain pastries	Any made with whole-grain flour, bran, seeds, nuts, coconut, or raw or dried fruits; cornbread, graham crackers
Cereals	Refined cooked cereals including grits and farina; refined cereals including puffed rice and puffed wheat	Oatmeal; any whole grain, bran or granola cereal; any containing seeds, nuts, coconut, or dried fruit
Desserts and sweets	Plain cakes and cookies; pie made with allowed fruits; plain sherbet, fruit ice, frozen pops, yogurt, gelatin, and custard; jelly; plain hard candy; marshmallows; ice cream as tolerated*	Any made with whole-grain flour, bran, seeds, nuts, coconut, or dried fruit
Fats	Margarine, butter, salad oils and dressings, mayonnaise; bacon; plain gravies	Any containing whole-grain flour, bran, seeds, nuts, coconut, or dried fruit
Fruits	Most canned or cooked fruits,† applesauce,† fruit cocktail,† ripe banana†	Dried fruit; all berries; most raw fruit
Meats and meat substitutes	Ground or well-cooked, tender beef, lamb, ham, veal, pork, poultry, fish, organ meats; eggs and cheese	Tough, fibrous meats with gristle†; any made with whole-grain ingredients, seeds, or nuts; dried beans, peas, lentils, legumes; peanut butter
Potato and potato substitutes	Cooked white and sweet potatoes without skin; white rice; refined pasta	All others
Soups	Bouillon, broth, or cream soups made with allowed vegetables, noodles, rice, or flour	All others
Vegetables	Most well-cooked and canned vegetables without seeds† except those excluded; lettuce if tolerated; strained vegetable juice	Sauerkraut, winter squash, peas, and corn; most raw vegetables and vegetables with seeds
Miscellaneous	Salt, pepper, sugar, spices, herbs, vinegar, ketchup, mustard	Nuts, coconut, seeds, and popcorn

Sample Menu for Fiber- and Residue-Restricted Diet

Breakfast	Lunch	Dinner
Strained orange juice (½ cup)	Broth (1 cup)	Strained tomato juice (½ cup)
Corn flakes (¾ cup)	Saltine crackers (4)	Broiled lean hamburger (3 oz)
Applesauce (½ cup)	Tuna salad (no vegetables) on white bread	Baked potato without skin
Plain English muffin	Ripe banana (½ cup)	Cooked spinach (½ cup)
Margarine (2 tsp)	Vanilla wafer cookies (2)	White roll (1)
Jelly (tbsp)	Low-fat milk (1 cup)	Margarine (2 tsp)
Low-fat milk (1 cup)	Coffee/tea	Low-fat ice cream (½ cup)
Coffee/tea		Coffee/tea

* Mixed consensus exists regarding the inclusion of milk on a low-residue diet. It has been suggested that because milk is not considered a high-residue food, it should not be eliminated from the low-residue diet unless an individual has lactase deficiency. Some practitioners continue to limit milk and products containing milk to 2 cups per day, as suggested in previous literature.

† These foods are not necessarily high in fiber but may increase colonic residue; assess patient food tolerance and limit as needed. Residue may be further reduced by excluding all fruits and vegetables with the exception of strained juices and white potatoes without skin.

Guidelines © 1996, The American Dietetic Association. *Manual of Clinical Dietetics.* Used by permission. Menu from Chilton Memorial Hospital, Pompton Plains, NJ.

OTHER INSTRUCTIONS

High-Fiber Diet

DESCRIPTION

The high-fiber diet is a general diet with an emphasis on fiber-rich food sources including fruits, legumes, vegetables, whole-grain breads, and cereals. The diet may be used in several bowel conditions such as constipation and diverticulosis. The National Cancer Institute recommends a diet with 25 to 30 grams of fiber daily. A high-fiber diet can be achieved by making changes in the *type* of foods one normally eats.

TERMS

The term *dietary fiber* refers to the part of plant food that cannot be digested in the intestinal tract. There are two main types of dietary fiber, water-insoluble and water-soluble. Examples of water-insoluble fiber are cellulose, hemicellulose, and lignin. This fiber is unchanged during digestion. Insoluble fiber may help prevent and treat constipation and diverticular disease and may decrease the risk of colon cancer.

Examples of water-soluble fiber are pectin and mucilages. This fiber dissolves in water and is found in oats, barley, and some fruits and vegetables. This type of fiber may improve blood glucose and cholesterol levels.

ADEQUACY

The high-fiber diet is adequate in all nutrients.

GUIDELINES

1. Increased fiber should come from a variety of food sources, rather than from dietary fiber supplements, to ensure the intake of enough vitamins, minerals, and other nutrients.
2. Drink at least eight to ten 8-ounce glasses of water daily.
3. Fiber intake should be increased slowly to minimize bloating, gas, cramps, and diarrhea. These effects usually subside within a few days. If they continue, decrease the fiber content of the diet and call your nurse or doctor.
4. Follow a regular diet pattern with the following guidelines:

High-Fiber Foods		
Food Group	**Allowed**	**Avoid**
Breads, cereals, and starches 6 servings daily	Whole-grain breads, crackers, muffins, pancakes, waffles and biscuits made from whole-wheat flour; whole-grain or bran cereals, dried or cooked; whole-wheat pasta, air-popped popcorn and wheat germ	Refined breads and cereals
Fruits* 4 or more servings daily (½ cup each) one of which is citrus fruit or juice	Fresh, frozen, stewed, canned or dried fruits or juices; eat whole fruits, including their skins, example: raw apples with skin, or orange with white membrane	None
Vegetables* 4–5 servings daily	Fresh, frozen, canned, or dried, served cooked or raw; include 1 or 2 salads daily, emphasizing vegetables such as broccoli, cabbage, carrots, cauliflower, celery, green peppers, tomatoes, and zucchini	None
Beans (servings optional)	Garbanzo beans, kidney beans, lentils, lima beans, split peas, pinto beans, navy beans, and other beans and peas	None
Nuts and seeds (servings optional)	All nuts and seeds including almonds, walnuts, peanuts, peanut butter, sesame seeds, and sunflower seeds	None

* These foods are high in natural fiber and cellullose.

Fiber Content of Common Foods

Food Item	Serving Size	Total Fiber per Serving (g)	Soluble Fiber per Serving (g)	Insoluble Fiber per Serving (g)
CEREALS				
All Bran	⅓ cup	8.6	1.4	7.2
Benefit	¾ cup	5.0	2.8	2.2
Cheerios	1¼ cups	2.5	1.2	1.3
Corn flakes	1 cup	0.5	0.1	0.4
Cream of Wheat, regular, uncooked	2½ tbsp	1.1	0.4	0.7
Fiber One	½ cup	11.9	0.8	11.1
40% Bran Flakes	⅔ cup	4.3	0.4	3.9
Grapenuts	¼ cup	2.8	0.8	2.0
Grits, corn, quick, uncooked	3 tbsp	0.6	0.1	0.5
Heartwise	1 cup	5.7	2.9	2.8
Nutri-Grain wheat	⅔ cup	2.7	0.7	2.0
Oat bran, cooked	¾ cup	4.0	2.2	1.8
Oat bran flakes	½ cup	2.1	0.8	0.3
Oat flakes	⅔ cup	2.1	1.0	1.1
Oatmeal, uncooked	⅓ cup	2.7	1.4	1.3
Product 19	1 cup	1.2	0.3	0.9
Puffed Rice	1 cup	0.2	0.1	0.1
Puffed Wheat	1 cup	1.0	0.5	0.5
Quaker Oat Squares	½ cup	2.2	0.8	1.4
Raisin Bran	¾ cup	5.3	0.9	4.4
Rice Krispies	1 cup	0.3	0.1	0.2
Shredded Wheat	⅔ cup	3.5	0.5	3.0
Shredded Wheat and Bran	⅔ cup	2.5	0.6	1.9
Special K	1 cup	0.9	0.2	0.7
Total, whole wheat	1 cup	2.6	0.6	2.0
Wheat flakes	¾ cup	2.3	0.4	1.9
Wheaties	⅔ cup	2.3	0.7	1.6
GRAINS				
Cornmeal	2½ tbsp	0.4	0.1	0.3
Flour, oat	2½ tbsp	1.8	1.0	0.8
rye	2½ tbsp	2.6	0.8	1.8
white	2½ tbsp	0.6	0.3	0.3
whole wheat	2½ tbsp	2.1	0.3	1.8
Macaroni, white, cooked	½ cup	0.7	0.4	0.3
whole wheat, cooked	½ cup	2.1	0.4	1.7
Noodles, egg, cooked	½ cup	1.4	0.4	1.0
spinach, cooked	½ cup	1.1	0.5	0.6
Popcorn, popped	3 cups	2.0	0.1	1.9
Rice, white, cooked	⅓ cup	0.5	trace	0.5
wild, cooked	⅓ cup	0.4	0.1	0.3
Spaghetti, white, cooked	½ cup	0.9	0.4	0.5
whole wheat, cooked	½ cup	2.7	0.6	2.1
Wheat bran	½ cup	12.3	1.0	11.3
Wheat germ	3 tbsp	3.9	0.7	3.2
BREADS AND CRACKERS				
Bagel, plain	½	0.7	0.3	0.4
Biscuit, baked	1	0.5	0.3	0.2
Bread, bran	1 slice	1.5	0.2	1.3
cornbread	1–2-in cube	1.4	0.3	1.1
cracked wheat	1 slice	1.9	0.3	1.6
French	1 slice	0.9	0.3	0.6
mixed grain	1 slice	1.9	0.3	1.6
oatmeal	½ slice	1.2	0.3	0.9
pita, white	½ pocket	0.5	0.2	0.3
pumpernickel	1 slice	2.7	1.2	1.5
raisin	1 slice	1.2	0.3	0.9
rye	1 slice	1.8	0.8	1.0
sourdough	1 slice	0.8	0.3	0.5
white	1 slice	0.6	0.3	0.3
whole wheat	1 slice	1.5	0.3	1.2

Table continued on following page

Fiber Content of Common Foods *Continued*

Food Item	Serving Size	Total Fiber per Serving (g)	Soluble Fiber per Serving (g)	Insoluble Fiber per Serving (g)
BREADS AND CRACKERS *Continued*				
Bread sticks	2	0.6	0.2	0.4
Bun, hamburger	½	0.7	0.2	0.5
Crackers, matzo	1	1.0	0.5	0.5
saltine	6	0.5	0.3	0.2
saltine, wheat	5	0.5	0.2	0.3
snack, whole wheat	4	2.0	0.3	1.7
wheat	5	0.6	0.2	0.4
English muffin	½	0.8	0.2	0.6
Melba toast, wheat	5 slices	1.8	0.4	1.4
Pretzels, hard	¾ oz	0.8	0.2	0.6
Roll, brown-and-serve	1 roll	0.8	0.3	0.5
Taco shell	2	1.4	0.2	1.2
Tortilla, corn	1	1.4	0.2	1.2
Tortilla, flour	1	0.7	0.3	0.4
Waffle, toasted	1	0.7	0.3	0.4
FRUITS				
Apple, red, fresh w/skin	1 sml	2.8	1.0	1.8
Applesauce, canned, unsweetened	½ cup	2.0	0.7	1.3
Apricots, canned, drained	4 halves	1.2	0.5	0.7
dried	7 halves	2.0	1.1	0.9
fresh w/skin	4	3.5	1.8	1.7
Avocado, fresh, flesh only	⅛	1.2	0.5	0.7
Banana, fresh	½ sml	1.1	0.3	0.8
Blueberries, fresh	¾ cup	1.4	0.3	1.1
Cherries, black, fresh	12 lrg	1.3	0.6	0.7
Cherries, red, canned	½ cup	1.8	0.9	0.9
Currants, dried	2 tbsp	0.4	0.2	0.2
Dates, dried	2½ med	0.9	0.3	0.6
Figs, dried	1½	2.3	1.1	1.2
Fruit cocktail, canned	½ cup	2.0	0.7	1.3
Grapefruit, fresh	½ med	1.6	1.1	0.5
Grapes, red, fresh w/skin	15 sml	0.4	0.2	0.2
Grapes, white, fresh w/skin	15 sml	0.6	0.3	0.3
Kiwifruit, fresh, flesh only	1 lrg	1.7	0.7	1.0
Mango, fresh, flesh only	½ sml	2.9	1.7	1.2
Melon, cantaloupe	1 cup cubed	1.1	0.3	0.8
honeydew	1 cup cubed	0.9	0.3	0.6
watermelon	1¼ cups cubed	0.6	0.4	0.2
Nectarine, fresh	1 sml	1.8	0.8	1.0
Orange, fresh, flesh only	1 sml	2.9	1.8	1.1
Peaches, canned, unsweetened	½ cup	2.0	0.7	1.3
fresh, w/skin	1 med	2.0	1.0	1.0
Pear, canned	½ cup	3.7	0.7	3.0
fresh, w/skin	½ lrg or 1 sml	2.9	1.1	1.8
Pineapple, canned	⅓ cup	1.4	0.2	1.2
fresh	¾ cup	1.4	0.1	1.3
Plum, red, fresh	2 med	2.4	1.1	1.3
Prunes, dried	3 med	1.7	1.0	0.7
stewed, unsweetened, drained	¼ cup	1.6	0.9	0.7
Raisins, dried	2 tbsp	0.4	0.2	0.2
Raspberries, fresh	1 cup	3.3	0.9	2.4
Strawberries, fresh	1¼ cups	2.8	1.1	1.7

Table continued on opposite page

Fiber Content of Common Foods *Continued*

Food Item	Serving Size	Total Fiber per Serving (g)	Soluble Fiber per Serving (g)	Insoluble Fiber per Serving (g)
VEGETABLES				
Asparagus, cooked	½ cup	1.8	1.7	1.1
Bean sprouts, fresh	1 cup	1.6	0.6	1.0
Beets, flesh only, cooked	½ cup	1.8	0.8	1.0
Broccoli, cooked	½ cup	2.4	1.2	1.2
Brussels sprouts, cooked	½ cup	3.8	2.0	1.8
Cabbage, fresh	1 cup	1.5	0.6	0.9
red, cooked	½ cup	2.6	1.1	1.5
Carrots, canned	½ cup	1.5	0.7	0.8
fresh	1 7½-in long	2.3	1.1	1.2
sliced, cooked	½ cup	2.0	1.1	0.9
Cauliflower, cooked	½ cup	1.0	0.4	0.6
Celery, fresh	1 cup chopped	1.7	0.7	1.0
Corn, whole kernel, canned	½ cup	1.6	0.2	1.4
Cucumber, fresh	1 cup	0.5	0.2	0.3
Green beans, canned	½ cup	2.0	0.5	1.5
French style, cooked	½ cup	2.8	1.1	1.7
Kale, chopped, frozen	½ cup	2.5	0.7	1.8
Lettuce, iceberg	1 cup	0.5	0.1	0.4
Mushrooms, fresh	1 cup pieces	0.8	0.1	0.7
Okra, frozen, cooked	½ cup	4.1	1.0	3.1
Olives, canned	10 sml	1.0	0.1	0.9
Onion, cooked	½ cup chopped	2.0	1.1	0.9
fresh	½ cup chopped	1.7	0.9	0.8
Peas, green, canned	½ cup	3.2	0.4	2.8
green, frozen, cooked	½ cup	4.3	1.3	3.0
Pepper, green, fresh	1 cup chopped	1.7	0.7	1.0
Potato, sweet, canned	⅓ cup	0.8	0.3	0.5
sweet, flesh only, cooked	⅓ cup	2.7	1.2	1.5
Pumpkin, fresh, cooked	1 cup	1.2	0.4	0.8
Snow peas, fresh, cooked	½ cup	1.4	0.6	0.8
Spinach, cooked	½ cup	1.6	0.5	1.1
Squash, yellow, crookneck, frozen	½ cup	0.7	0.3	0.4
Tomato, canned	½ cup	1.3	0.5	0.8
fresh	1 med	1.0	0.1	0.9
sauce	⅓ cup	1.1	0.5	0.6
Turnip, cooked	½ cup	4.8	1.7	3.1
V-8 juice	½ cup	0.7	0.2	0.5
Zucchini, sliced, cooked	½ cup	1.2	0.5	0.7
LEGUMES				
Black beans, cooked	½ cup	6.1	2.4	3.7
Black-eyed peas, canned	½ cup	4.7	0.5	4.2
Broad beans, no pods, cooked	½ cup	5.1	1.0	4.1
Butter beans, dried, cooked	½ cup	6.9	2.7	4.2
Chick peas, dried, cooked	½ cup	4.3	1.3	3.0
Garbanzo beans, canned	⅓ cup	2.8	0.3	2.5
Kidney beans, dark red, dried, cooked,	½ cup	6.9	2.8	4.1
light red, canned	½ cup	7.9	2.0	5.9
Lentils, dried, cooked	½ cup	5.2	0.6	4.6
Lima beans, canned	½ cup	4.3	1.1	3.2
Mung beans, dried, cooked	½ cup	3.3	0.7	2.6
Navy beans, dried, cooked	½ cup	6.5	2.2	4.3
Pinto beans, canned	½ cup	6.1	1.4	4.7
dried, cooked	½ cup	5.9	1.9	4.0
Split peas, dried, cooked	½ cup	3.1	1.1	2.0
White beans, Great Northern, canned	½ cup	7.2	2.2	5.0
dried, cooked	½ cup	5.0	1.4	3.6

Table continued on following page

Fiber Content of Common Foods *Continued*

Food Item	Serving Size	Total Fiber per Serving (g)	Soluble Fiber per Serving (g)	Insoluble Fiber per Serving (g)
NUTS AND SEEDS				
Almonds	6 whole	0.6	0.1	0.5
Brazil nuts	1 tbsp	0.5	0.1	0.4
Coconut, dried	1½ tbsp	1.5	0.1	1.4
fresh	2 tbsp	1.1	0.1	1.0
Hazelnuts (filberts)	1 tbsp	0.5	0.2	0.3
Peanut butter, smooth	1 tbsp	1.0	0.3	0.7
Peanuts, roasted	10 lrg	0.6	0.2	0.4
Sesame seeds	1 tbsp	0.8	0.2	0.6
Sunflower seeds	1 tbsp	0.5	0.2	0.3
Walnuts	2 whole	0.3	0.1	0.2

High-Fiber Diet Suggested Menu

Breakfast	Lunch	Dinner
Orange (4 oz)	Chicken (2 oz)	Vegetable soup (1 cup)
Whole wheat cereal (¾ cup)	Baked potato	Roast beef (3 oz)
Whole wheat toast (2)	Spinach (½ cup)	Brown rice (½ cup)
Butter or margarine (1 tsp)	Tossed salad (1 cup)	String beans (½ cup)
Low-fat milk (8 oz)	Whole wheat bread (1)	Celery and carrot salad (½ cup)
Coffee or tea	Butter or margarine (1 tsp)	Whole wheat roll (1)
	Apricots (½ cup)	Butter or margarine (1 tsp)
	Coffee or tea	Fresh apple (1)
	Low-fat milk (8 oz)	Coffee or tea

High-Fiber Foods and menu from Chilton Memorial Hospital, Pompton Plains, NJ.

Fiber Content of Common Foods © 1996 The American Dietetic Association. *Manual of Clinical Dietetics.* Used by permission.

OTHER INSTRUCTIONS

Lactose-Controlled Diet

DESCRIPTION

This diet is used in cases of lactose intolerance.

ADEQUACY

This diet is adequate in all nutrients, except calcium.

Lactose-Controlled Diet

You need a lactose-controlled diet if you are unable to digest the milk sugar lactose. This diet will help prevent uncomfortable side effects such as bloating, cramping, or diarrhea that may occur when you consume milk or milk products. Side effects should stop 3 to 5 days after following this diet. Because there are varying degrees of lactose intolerance, you will need to experiment with foods to determine your individual tolerance.

Food Categories	Foods Recommended	Foods That May Cause Distress	Tips
▲ **BREADS, CEREALS, RICE, AND PASTA 6–11 SERVINGS EACH DAY**			
Serving size = 1 slice bread, 1 cup ready-to-eat cereal, ½ cup cooked cereal, rice, or pasta, ½ bun, bagel, or English muffin	Whole-grain or enriched breads, cereals, rice, barley, and pastas made with milk-free ingredients	Any prepared with milk, milk products, or mixes containing lactose	Try lactose-reduced milk on ready-to-eat cereals, or choose hot cereals such as oatmeal that can be prepared with water.
▲ **VEGETABLES 3–5 SERVINGS EACH DAY**			
Serving size = 1 cup raw leafy, ½ cup cooked, ¾ cup juice	All	Vegetables prepared with milk or milk products	Select salad bar items or a chef salad without cheese or other milk products.
▲ **FRUITS 2–4 SERVINGS EACH DAY**			
Serving size = 1 medium size, ½ cup canned, ¾ cup juice, ¼ cup dried	All fruits and fruit juices	None	
▲ **MILK, YOGURT, AND CHEESE 2–3 SERVINGS EACH DAY**			
Serving size = 1 cup, 1½ oz natural cheese, 2 oz processed cheese	Soy milk, lactose-reduced milk, and lactose-free supplements Hard, aged, and processed cheese, if tolerated Yogurt, if tolerated	Milk, milk products, goat's milk, and acidophilus milk	Experiment with lactose-reduced or lactose-free milk or cheese available in most supermarkets. Small amounts of milk (½ cup or less) may be tolerated *with* meals.
▲ **MEATS, POULTRY, FISH, DRY BEANS AND PEAS, EGGS, AND NUTS 2–3 SERVINGS OR TOTAL OF 6 OZ DAILY**			
Serving size = 2–3 oz cooked; count 1 egg, ½ cup cooked beans, 2 tbsp peanut butter, or ⅓ cup nuts as 1 oz of meat	All meats, poultry, fish, and eggs Dry peas and beans Nuts and peanut butter	Cold cuts and frankfurters that contain lactose filler	Avoid meat, poultry, or fish that is creamed, breaded, or topped with a cheese- or milk-containing sauce.

Table continued on following page

Lactose-Controlled Diet *Continued*

Food Categories	Foods Recommended	Foods That May Cause Distress	Tips
▲ Fats, Snacks, Sweets, Condiments, and Beverages			
	Butter or margarine, nondairy creamer, and oil-based salad dressings Cakes, cookies, pies, flavored gelatin desserts, and fruit ices made with milk-free ingredients Sugar, corn and pure maple syrup, honey, jellies, jams, and pure sugar candies All milk-free beverages	Salad dressings containing milk or cheese Cream soups Any dessert prepared with milk or milk products such as sherbet, ice cream, pudding, and some cakes, cookies, and pies Chocolate or caramels or any candies made with milk or milk products Instant drink mixes	In place of milk, use a non-dairy creamer or lactose-reduced milk in baked products; use broth for sauces and gravies. Heated milk products such as soup, custard, or pudding may be better tolerated than cold milk products.

Important Points to Keep in Mind

- Scan all product ingredient lists and check to see if they contain milk. Terms like milk solids, whey, curds, skim milk powder, and skim milk solids mean that lactose is present.
- Look for cookbooks with recipes adapted for a lactose-controlled diet.
- Try to include plenty of other sources of calcium in your diet. Some good sources include dark green vegetables, canned fish with fine bones (sardines and salmon), and dry beans
- Talk to your doctor, registered dietitian, or pharmacist about lactase enzymes in tablet or droplet form for use with products containing milk.

Sample Menu for a Lactose-Controlled Diet

Breakfast	Lunch	Dinner
Orange juice (¾ cup)	Vegetable barley soup (1 cup)	Apple-raisin salad (1 cup)
Oat-bran cereal (1 cup)	Crackers (4)	Broiled skinless chicken breast (3 oz)
Banana (1 medium)	Lean beef patty (3 oz)	Baked potato (1 medium)
Whole-wheat toast (2 slices)	Hamburger bun (1)	Whole-grain roll (1)
Margarine (2 tsp)	Tossed salad (1 cup)	Margarine (1 tsp)
Jelly or jam (1 tbsp)	Sliced tomato (2 oz)	Lemon ice (½ cup)
Lactose-reduced milk* (1 cup)	Vinegar and oil dressing (1 tbsp)	Coffee or tea
Coffee or tea	Orange (1 medium)	
	Lactose-reduced milk* (1 cup)	
	Coffee or tea	

* If lactose-reduced milk is not tolerated, substitute ½ cup nondairy creamer at breakfast and fruit juice at lunch. A calcium supplement should also be provided if this substitution is made.

© 1996 The American Dietetic Association. *Manual of Clinical Dietetics.* Used with permission.

OTHER INSTRUCTIONS

Fat-Controlled Diet (50 grams)

DESCRIPTION

This diet is designed for people who have trouble digesting or absorbing fat.

ADEQUACY

This diet meets the Recommended Dietary Allowances.

GUIDELINES

1. All foods should be prepared without added butter, cream, or other fats and oils, unless as part of the fat allowance.
2. Individual food tolerances may vary greatly. If patients experience no discomfort from strongly flavored vegetables such as broccoli, brussels sprouts, cabbage, cauliflower, cucumber, onion, dried peas, beans and lentils, peppers, radish, turnips, as well as raw apples, avocado, berries, and melon, they may be included.

OTHER INSTRUCTIONS

Fat-Controlled Diet

You need a fat-controlled diet if you have trouble digesting or absorbing fat. This diet will help prevent uncomfortable side effects such as diarrhea, bloating, and cramping that may occur when you consume high-fat foods. In addition, eating too much fat may interfere with the absorption of other important nutrients in your diet.

Food Categories	Foods Recommended	Foods That May Cause Distress	Tips
▲ BREADS, CEREALS, RICE, AND PASTA 6–11 SERVINGS EACH DAY			
Serving size = 1 slice bread, 1 cup ready-to-eat cereal, ½ cup cooked cereal, rice, or pasta, ½ bun, bagel, or English muffin	Whole-grain or enriched breads, cereals, rice, barley, and pastas Low-fat and fat-free crackers	Breads prepared with eggs or cheese Granola-type cereals Biscuits, pancakes, croissants, muffins, or doughnuts High-fat snack crackers	Choose a tomato-based sauce instead of cream sauce for pastas. Use fruit spreads on breads in place of butter or margarine.
▲ VEGETABLES 3–5 SERVINGS EACH DAY			
Serving size = 1 cup raw leafy, ½ cup cooked, ¾ cup juice	Fresh, frozen, or canned vegetables	Vegetables prepared with added fat, cream sauces, or cheese sauces	Cook vegetables in broth or sprinkle with herbs and spices to add flavor.
▲ FRUITS 2–4 SERVINGS EACH DAY			
Serving size = 1 medium, ½ cup canned, ¾ cup juice, ¼ cup dried	All fresh, frozen, canned, or dried fruit Fruit juices	Avocado	Snack on fresh or dried fruits instead of chips or cookies.
▲ MILK, YOGURT, AND CHEESE 2–3 SERVINGS EACH DAY			
Serving size = 1 cup milk or yogurt, 1½ oz natural cheese, 2 oz processed cheese	Fat-free milk, and fat-free milk and fat-free cheeses Reduced-fat or nonfat yogurt and cottage cheese	1%, 2%, and whole milk, buttermilk, chocolate milk, and cream Regular and processed cheese	In recipes, substitute fat-free or evaporated fat-free milk, or reduced-fat yogurt for whole milk and cream.
▲ MEATS, POULTRY, FISH, DRY BEANS AND PEAS, EGGS, AND NUTS 2–3 SERVINGS OR UP TO 6 OZ DAILY			
Serving size = 2–3 oz cooked*; count 1 egg and ½ cup cooked beans as 1 oz of meat	Lean beef such as sirloin, round, chuck; veal Lean pork such as tenderloin, ham, Canadian bacon Lean lamb such as chops or leg Poultry without the skin All fresh, frozen, or canned fish packed in water Luncheon meats (95% fat-free) Legumes cooked without added fat Egg whites	All fried, fatty, or heavily marbled meat, poultry, or fish such as: ground beef, pork, or lamb; ribs; corned beef; sausage, duck, goose Canned fish packed in oil Most luncheon meats including bologna, salami, and pimento loaf; frankfurters Dry peas and beans prepared with fat or high-fat meat Nuts and peanut butter Egg yolks	Broil, roast, grill, or boil meats, poultry, and fish instead of frying. Trim all visible fat before cooking. Select or prepare meats in their natural juice instead of with sauces and gravies.

*3 oz of cooked meat is about the size of a deck of cards.

▲ FATS LIMIT TO 3–5 SERVINGS DAILY

One serving equals:
1 tsp of margarine, butter, regular mayonnaise, oil, shortening, and bacon fat
1 tbsp of diet margarine, reduced-calorie mayonnaise, reduced-calorie creamy salad dressing, regular oil-based salad dressing, cream cheese, and whipping cream
2 tbsp of reduced-calorie salad dressing (oil-based), shredded coconut, liquid coffee whitener, and sour cream

▲ SNACKS, SWEETS, CONDIMENTS, AND BEVERAGES

Fat-free broth or soups	Cream or cheese sauces and gravies
Sherbet, fruit ice, gelatin, angel food cake, graham crackers, and nonfat frozen desserts	Cakes, cookies, pies, and ice cream
	Coconut, chocolate, and creamed candy
Honey, jams, jellies, syrups, and hard candy	High-fat snacks such as chips and buttered popcorn
Coffee, tea, soda, and other nondairy drinks	
	Try lemon juice, vinegar, or garlic or onion powder on cooked foods in place of butter or margarine.

Important Points to Keep in Mind

• Scan cookbooks for low-fat cooking tips and low-fat recipes.
• Convenience foods such as frozen and canned dinners are usually high in fat. Read food labels carefully and look for high-fat ingredients such as cheese, oil, shortening, and butter or margarine. Look for "light" frozen dinners with less than 300 calories and less than 10 g of fat.
• Use fat-free items sparingly. Some contain very small amounts of fat. Contact the manufacturer for the specific fat content.
• When dining out, ask for sauces or salad dressings on the side and use sparingly.

Sample Menu for a Fat-Controlled Diet
(50 g of fat)

BREAKFAST	LUNCH	SNACK	DINNER
Orange juice (¾ cup)	Fat-free vegetable soup (1 cup)	Graham crackers (4)	Tossed green salad (1 cup)
Whole-grain cereal (½ cup)	Saltine crackers (4)	Fat-free milk (1 cup)	Fat-free salad dressing (1 tbsp)
Banana (1 medium)	Lean roast beef (3 oz)		Broiled boneless skinless chicken breast (3 oz)
Whole-wheat toast (2 slices)	Whole-wheat bread (2 slices)		Herbed brown rice (½ cup)
Diet margarine (1 tbsp)	Mustard (1 tbsp)		Whole-grain roll (1)
Jelly or jam (1 tbsp)	Reduced-calorie mayonnaise (1 tbsp)		Diet margarine (1 tbsp)
Fat-free milk (1 cup)	Sliced tomato and lettuce		Fruit ice (½ cup)
Coffee or tea	Orange (1 medium)		Apple (1 medium)
	Coffee or tea		Coffee or tea

© 1996 The American Dietetic Association. *Manual of Clinical Dietetics*. Used with permission.

Gluten-Restricted, Gliadin-Free Diet

DESCRIPTION

This diet is designed for people who are unable to digest gliadin, one of the proteins that make up gluten.

ADEQUACY

This diet meets the Recommended Dietary Allowances.

OTHER INSTRUCTIONS

Gluten-Restricted, Gliadin-Free Diet

You need a gluten-restricted, gliadin-free diet if you are unable to digest gliadin, one of the proteins that make up gluten. This diet will help prevent uncomfortable side effects such as diarrhea, abdominal bloating, weight loss, and fatigue. Once you have removed gliadin from your diet, symptoms should gradually disappear. The gliadin-free diet should be continued for life.

Food Categories	Foods Recommended	Foods To Omit	Tips
▲ **BREADS, CEREALS, RICE, AND PASTA 6–11 SERVINGS EACH DAY**			
Serving size = 1 slice bread, 1 cup ready-to-eat cereal, ½ cup cooked cereal, rice, or pasta, ½ bun, bagel, or English muffin	Breads or bread products made from tapioca, arrowroot, corn, or potato starch; corn, potato, rice, or soy flour, or gluten-free bread mix Corn or rice cereals containing malt flavoring derived from corn, puffed rice, cream of rice, cornmeal, hominy, and grits Enriched brown and wild rice; rice noodles, and pastas made with allowed flours	Any bread or bread product made from wheat, rye, kasha, barley, buckwheat, durum, graham, wheat starch, or low-gluten flour Commercial mixes for biscuits, cornbread, muffins, pancakes, or waffles Wheat germ, bran, bulgur, millet, and triticale Cereals containing malt flavoring or malt derived from grains listed above Most crackers	Toast or warm gluten-free bread products for added flavor. Experiment with gluten-free products to add variety and nutrients to your diet. Some of these products may be purchased from your supermarket, health food store, or direct from the manufacturer.
▲ **VEGETABLES 3–5 SERVINGS EACH DAY**			
Serving size = 1 cup raw leafy, ½ cup cooked or chopped, ¾ cup juice	All plain, fresh, frozen, or canned vegetables made with allowed ingredients	Any creamed or breaded vegetables (unless allowed ingredients are used), canned baked beans	Buy plain, frozen, or canned vegetables and season with herbs, spices, or sauces made with allowed ingredients.
▲ **FRUITS 2–4 SERVINGS EACH DAY**			
Serving size = 1 medium size, ½ cup canned, ¾ cup juice, ¼ cup dried	All fruits and fruit juices	Any thickened fruit sauces and some commercial fruit pie fillings	
▲ **MILK, YOGURT, AND CHEESE 2–3 SERVINGS EACH DAY**			
Serving size = 1 cup milk or yogurt, 1½ oz natural cheese, 2 oz processed cheese	All milk and milk products except those made with gluten additives Aged cheese	Chocolate milk, malted milk, and instant milk drinks Any cheese or cheese spread containing oat gum	Contact the food manufacturer for product information if the ingredient list is not on the label.
▲ **MEATS, POULTRY, FISH, DRY BEANS AND PEAS, EGGS, AND NUTS 2–3 SERVINGS OR TOTAL OF 6 OZ DAILY**			
Serving size = 2–3 oz cooked; count 1 egg, ½ cup cooked beans, 2 tbsp peanut butter, or ⅓ cup nuts as 1 oz of meat	All meat, poultry, fish, and shellfish; eggs Dry peas and beans, nuts, peanut butter, soybean Cold cuts, frankfurters, or sausage without fillers	Any prepared with wheat, rye, oats, barley, gluten stabilizers, or fillers including some frankfurters, cold cuts, sandwich spreads, sausages, and canned meats Self-basting turkey	When dining out select meat, poultry, or fish made without breading, gravies, or sauces.

Table continued on following page

Gluten-Restricted, Gliadin-Free Diet *Continued*

Food Categories	Foods Recommended	Foods To Omit	Tips
▲ FATS, SNACKS, SWEETS, CONDIMENTS, AND BEVERAGES	Butter, margarine, salad dressings, sauces, soups, and desserts made with allowed ingredients Sugar, honey, jelly, jam, hard candy, plain chocolate, coconut, molasses, marshmallows, meringues Pure instant or ground coffee, tea, carbonated drinks, wine (made in United States), rum Most seasonings and flavorings	Commercial salad dressings, prepared soups, condiments, and seasonings prepared with ingredients listed above Hot cocoa mixes, nondairy cream substitutes, flavored instant coffee, alcohol distilled from cereals such as gin, vodka, whiskey, and beer	Store all gluten-free products in your refrigerator or freezer because they do not contain preservatives.

Important Points to Keep in Mind

- Read all food labels carefully! Avoid all products that contain wheat, rye, barley, oats, gluten stabilizers, and hydrolyzed or texturized vegetable protein.
- Look for specialty cookbooks adapted for a gluten-restricted, gliadin-free diet.
- Check with your doctor or pharmacist before taking any medications because some may contain gluten.
- When in doubt about any commercial product, do not use it until you consult a registered dietitian or obtain information from the manufacturer.

Sample Menu for a Gluten-Restricted Gliadin-Free Diet

Breakfast	Lunch	Snack	Dinner
Orange juice (¾ cup) Cream of rice cereal (½ cup) Banana (½) Gluten-free toast (2 slices) Margarine (2 tsp) Jelly (1 tbsp) Milk (1 cup)	Tomato juice (¾ cup) Lean beef patty (3 oz) Gluten-free bread (2 slices) Pure mayonnaise (1 tbsp) Tomato and lettuce Milk (1 cup) Coffee or tea	Rice cakes (2) Fruit juice (¾ cup)	Tossed salad (1 cup) Pure oil and vinegar dressing (1 tbsp) Broiled chicken breast (3 oz) Herbed brown rice (½ cup) Steamed broccoli (½ cup) Gluten-free bread (1 slice) Margarine (2 tsp) Orange sherbet (½ cup) Coffee or tea

© 1996 The American Dietetic Association. *Manual of Clinical Dietetics*. Used with permission.

Nutritional Management of Gastroesophageal Reflux Disease (GERD)

DESCRIPTION

The diet is designed to decrease symptoms associated with the reflux of gastric fluid into the esophagus.

ADEQUACY

The diet is adequate in all essential nutrients depending on individual food tolerance. If citrus fruits and juices are not tolerated, other sources of foods high in vitamin C or a vitamin supplement should be included.

GUIDELINES

1. Eat a well-balanced, low-fat diet.
2. Avoid known irritants such as chocolate, alcohol, mint, carbonated beverages, citrus juice, tomato products, and coffee (with or without caffeine) depending on individual tolerance.
3. If weight loss is needed, ask your nurse or doctor about a calorie-restricted diet.
4. Eat smaller, more frequent meals.
5. Avoid eating within 3 hours before bedtime.
6. Maintain an upright position during and after eating for at least 30 minutes.
7. Avoid tight clothing in the waist area.
8. Elevate the head of the bed when sleeping.
9. Stop smoking.

Guidelines for Food Selection for Gastroesophageal Reflux Disease Diet

Food Groups	Allowed	Eliminated
Beverages	Fat-free milk, 1% and 2% low-fat buttermilk; juices (any except citrus); decaffeinated, non-mint tea	Whole milk, chocolate milk, chocolate shakes or drinks; citrus drinks/juices; carbonated beverages; tomato juice, vegetable juice; mint tea; coffee (regular or decaffeinated); alcoholic beverages
Breads and cereals	Plain (with or without whole-grain flour) bread, cereals, rolls, biscuits, crackers; pancakes, waffles, French toast; muffins made with low-fat ingredients; bagels; corn tortillas	Breads and cereals prepared with high-fat ingredients such as croissants, doughnuts, sweet rolls, muffins
Desserts	Angel food cake, sponge cake, low-fat cookies; gelatin; fruit-based desserts; sherbet; fruit ice, low-fat yogurt, reduced-fat ice cream; pudding or custard made with 1% or 2% low-fat milk	All other pies, cookies, and cakes; ice cream; any desserts containing chocolate
Fats	Nonfat or low-fat dressings and mayonnaise; nonfat liquid or powdered cream substitutes, nonfat sour cream	Gravies; bacon; meat drippings; butter, margarine, vegetable oils, heavy cream, sour cream
Fruits	Fresh, frozen, and canned fruits as tolerated	Orange, lemon, tangerine, pineapple, grapefruit, citrus juices
Meats and meat substitutes	Lean meat; poultry (without skin); lean pork; fish (fresh or water-packed), shellfish; nonfat/low-fat yogurt; low-fat cheeses; tofu; dried beans (includes fat-free refried beans) and peas; eggs (limit to 3–4 egg yolks per week)	Fried meat, poultry, fish, or eggs; regular luncheon meats, hot dogs, sausages, refried beans

Table continued on following page

Guidelines for Food Selection for Gastroesophageal Reflux Disease Diet *Continued*

Food Groups	Allowed	Eliminated
Potatoes and potato substitutes	Baked, boiled, and mashed potatoes without added fat; enriched pasta (noodles, spaghetti, macaroni); rice	French fries, potato chips; pastas served with cream sauces
Soups	Fat-free broths, homemade soups prepared with one or all of the following: lean meat, vegetables, pasta, peas, and low-fat ingredients (eg, fat-free milk, egg whites)	Regular cream and tomato-based soups
Sweets	Sugar; honey; jam; jelly; molasses; maple syrup; hard candy; marshmallows	Butter, coconut, chocolate, and cream candies
Vegetables	Plain fresh, frozen, and canned vegetables prepared without added fat	Fried or creamy style vegetables; tomatoes and tomato products
Miscellaneous	Salt, garlic, oregano, sage, pepper; other spices and herbs	Spices and herbs in tomato-based sauces; spearmint, peppermint; chili and jalapeño peppers; vinegar

Sample Menu for Gastroesophageal Reflux Disease Diet

Breakfast	Lunch	Midday Snack	Dinner
Cranberry juice (½ cup) Bran flakes (¾ cup) Banana (½) English muffin Margarine (1 tsp) Jelly or jam (2 tbsp) Fat-free milk (1 cup) Coffee (if tolerated) or tea	Vegetable soup (1 cup) Saltine crackers (4) Tuna salad (3 oz) on whole-wheat bread (2 slices) Lettuce Coffee (if tolerated) or tea	¼ cantaloupe, ripe Vanilla wafers (6) Fat-free milk (1 cup)	Tossed vegetable salad (with 1 tbsp dressing) Broiled skinless chicken breast (3 oz) Rice pilaf (½ cup) Steamed spinach (½ cup) Whole-grain roll (1) Margarine (1 tsp) Low-fat ice cream (½ cup) Fresh strawberries (¾ cup) Coffee (if tolerated) or tea

Guidelines © the American Dietetic Association. *Manual of Clinical Dietetics.* Used by permission.
Menu from Chilton Memorial Hospital, Pompton Plains, NJ.

OTHER INSTRUCTIONS

Diet After Ostomy Placement

Diet After Ostomy Placement

The following suggestions are provided to prevent or limit unpleasant odor, gas, and blockage after your ostomy placement. It is important that you follow an ostomy diet for 6 to 8 weeks after placement. After 6 to 8 weeks, add new foods one at a time to make certain you can tolerate them.

Food Categories	Foods Recommended	Tips
▲ **BREADS, CEREALS, RICE, AND PASTA 6–11 SERVINGS EACH DAY**		
Serving size = 1 slice bread 1 cup ready-to-eat cereal ½ cup cooked cereal, rice, or pasta ½ bun, bagel, or English muffin	White bread, rolls, crackers Refined cereal (cream of wheat, cream of rice, oatmeal) White rice	During the first 6 to 8 weeks after surgery, limit foods containing insoluble fiber such as wheat, bran, corn, and nuts. Then, add these foods gradually to see if you can handle them.
▲ **VEGETABLES 3–5 SERVINGS EACH DAY**		
Serving size = ½ cup cooked ¾ cup juice	Soft, cooked green beans, carrots, beets, squash, and stewed tomatoes Mashed, boiled, or baked potatoes without the skin Other pureed vegetables	Avoid raw celery, mushrooms, green peppers, raw cabbage, peas, corn, Chinese vegetables, foods with kernels, nuts, and seeds because they may cause stoma obstruction. Remove skins and seeds from fruits and vegetables.
▲ **FRUITS 2–4 SERVINGS EACH DAY**		
Serving size = 1 medium size ½ cup canned or cooked ¾ cup juice	Applesauce, bananas, and canned fruit packed in water or juice Unsweetened citrus juices and lemon juice	Purchase canned fruit packed in water instead of syrup. Include foods that contain soluble fiber such as applesauce, bananas, oatmeal, and rice in your daily menu. Soluble fiber will help prevent loose stools. Eat coconut, pineapple, and raisins in small quantities and chew well to prevent blockage. Avoid dried fruit.
▲ **MILK, YOGURT, AND CHEESE 2–3 SERVINGS EACH DAY**		
Serving size = 1 cup milk or yogurt 1½ oz natural cheese 2 oz processed cheese	Milk and milk products as tolerated All cheeses without seeds	Slowly add milk and milk products to your diet. If these foods cause uncomfortable side effects such as gas and diarrhea, omit from your diet for several days and gradually add them back in small amounts.
▲ **MEATS, POULTRY, FISH, DRY BEANS AND PEAS, EGGS, AND NUTS 2–3 SERVINGS OR TOTAL OF 6 OZ DAILY**		
Serving size = 2–3 oz cooked; count 1 egg, ½ cup cooked beans, or 2 tbsp peanut butter as 1 oz of meat	Lean meat, fish, and poultry Eggs	Broil, roast, grill, or boil meats instead of frying. Select or prepare meats in their natural juice instead of gravies or sauces.

Table continued on following page

Diet After Ostomy Placement *Continued*

Food Categories	Foods Recommended	Tips
▲ FATS, SNACKS, SWEETS, CONDIMENTS, AND BEVERAGES		
	Fat-free broth, bouillon, and cream soups made with fat-free milk and lean meats Low-fat desserts such as angel food cake, vanilla wafers, graham crackers, nonfat frozen dessert, and frozen yogurt Tea and coffee	Choose low-fat snacks such as pretzels instead of potato chips or corn chips. Use fat in moderation including that used in food preparation.

Important Points to Keep in Mind

- Drink at least 8 to 10 cups of liquids each day to prevent dehydration and constipation.
- Gas and odors that occur after you eat some foods can often be controlled with carbon filters or deodorants. Also try to include odor-reducing food in your diet, such as buttermilk, cranberry juice, and yogurt.
- Most ostomy patients do not have to remove these foods from their diet completely. Experiment with small amounts of these foods to determine your individual tolerance.
  Odor-producing foods: Asparagus, eggs, cabbage, alcohol, garlic, onions, cheese, fish, coffee. Cranberry juice, buttermilk, parsley, and yogurt may reduce odor.
  Gas-producing foods: Beer, broccoli, brussels sprouts, carbonated beverages, cabbage, cauliflower, cucumber, dry beans and peas, fatty foods, green pepper, highly spiced foods, melon, milk
- To prevent gas, avoid using straws for beverages and chew slowly with your mouth closed.

Sample Menu Following Ostomy Placement

BREAKFAST	SNACK	SNACK
Orange juice (¾ cup) Oatmeal (½ cup) White toast (2 slices) Jelly (1 tbsp) Margarine (2 tsp) Fat-free milk (1 cup) Coffee or tea	Banana (½) Graham crackers (4) **LUNCH** Pureed vegetable soup (1 cup) Saltine crackers (4) Lean hamburger (3 oz) Hamburger bun (1) Ketchup (1 tbsp) Canned fruit cocktail (½ cup) Iced tea	Applesauce (½ cup) Vanilla wafers (2) Fat-free milk (½ cup) **DINNER** Tomato juice (¾ cup) Boneless skinless chicken breast (3 oz) Herbed white rice (½ cup) Steamed green beans (½ cup) Dinner roll (1) Margarine (2 tsp) Low-fat yogurt (½ cup) Coffee or tea

Note: At first you may find it easier to eat 3 to 4 meals per day. Try not to skip meals. This may cause gas production and watery stools.

© 1996 the American Dietetic Association. *Manual of Clinical Dietetics.* Used with permission.

OTHER INSTRUCTIONS

General Diets

Healthful Eating Plan

Healthful Eating Plan

If you eat more healthfully, you may be able to decrease your risk for common nutrition-related diseases such as diabetes, cardiovascular diseases, osteoporosis, and certain cancers. Eating healthfully doesn't mean giving up your favorite foods. *All* foods have their place in a healthful eating style! The best approach is to learn how to balance your food choices over the course of a day and week and to select more grain-based dishes, vegetables, and fruits.

Food Categories	Choose Most Often	Tips
▲ BREADS, CEREALS, RICE, AND PASTA 6–11 SERVINGS EACH DAY		
Serving size = 1 slice bread 1 oz ready-to-eat cereal ½ cup cooked cereal, rice, or pasta ½ bun, bagel, or English muffin 1 small roll, biscuit, or muffin 3–4 small or 2 large crackers 1 6-inch tortilla	Whole-grain or enriched breads, bagels, tortillas, English muffins, crackers, hamburger/hot dog buns, dinner rolls, and pita bread Whole-grain or enriched ready-to-eat cereals and cooked cereals like oatmeal, grits, and farina Whole-grain or enriched rice, spaghetti, macaroni, or other type of noodles Pancakes, waffles, pretzels, and rice cakes	Build daily menus around breads, cereals, rice, and pasta. Choose whole grains for added fiber. Go easy on biscuits, cakes, cookies, cornbread, croissants, danish, doughnuts, muffins, pie crust, tortilla chips, and fatty sauces or toppings added to foods in this group.
▲ VEGETABLES 3–5 SERVINGS EACH DAY		
Serving size = ½ cup cooked or chopped raw, 1 cup raw leafy, ¾ cup juice	All vegetables like asparagus, broccoli, cabbage, carrots, cauliflower, celery, corn, greens, green beans, onions, peas, peppers, potatoes, snow peas, spinach, squash, sweet potatoes, tomatoes, zucchini	Try adding grated carrots to a salad or pasta sauce, or chopped veggies to an omelette or stir-fry. Go easy on deep-fried vegetables, potato chips, pickled vegetables, and highly salted vegetables or juices.
▲ FRUITS 2–4 SERVINGS EACH DAY		
Serving size = 1 medium size, ¼ melon wedge, ½ cup chopped, cooked, or canned, ¼ cup dried, ¾ cup juice	All fruits and fruit juices like apple, apricot, banana, berries, cherries, dates, figs, grapes, grapefruit, kiwi, mango, melons, orange, papaya, peach, pear, pineapple, prunes, raisins, and tangerine	Fruits contribute vitamins, minerals, and fiber, and they make sweet and tasty snacks and desserts. Citrus fruits such as oranges, grapefruit, or tangerines provide vitamin C.
▲ MILK, YOGURT, AND CHEESE 2–3 SERVINGS EACH DAY		
Serving size = 1 cup milk or yogurt, 1½ oz natural cheese, 2 oz processed cheese	Fat-free and reduced-fat milk and milk products like fat-free or 1% milk, low-fat or nonfat plain yogurt, low-fat cheese and cottage cheese	For added calcium, sprinkle shredded cheese into salads and eggs or add yogurt to dips and salad dressings. Choose nonfat or reduced-fat dairy products to help trim fat.

Table continued on following page

Healthful Eating Plan *Continued*

Food Categories	Choose Most Often	Tips

▲ Meats, Poultry, Fish, Dry Beans and Peas, Eggs, and Nuts 2–3 servings each day

Food Categories	Choose Most Often	Tips
Serving size = 2–3 oz cooked lean meat, poultry, or fish; count 1 egg, ½ cup cooked dried beans, 2 tbsp peanut butter, or ⅓ cup nuts as 1 oz of meat	Lean beef such as sirloin, round, chuck Lean pork such as tenderloin Lean lamb such as chops or leg Veal Light-meat poultry without the skin All fresh, frozen, or canned fish and shellfish packed in water Eggs, dried beans and peas cooked without added fat, tofu	Foods from this group supply protein, iron, and vitamin B12. To minimize fat, select lean cuts of meat and trim surrounding fat, remove skin from poultry, and broil, bake, stir-fry, or grill. Once a weak try going "meatless" for dinner or lunch.

▲ Fats, Snacks, Sweets, Condiments, and Beverages

Food Categories	Choose Most Often	Tips
Use sparingly	Include moderate amounts occasionally: alcoholic beverages, bacon, butter, candy, cream, cream cheese, frosting, fruit drinks, gelatin desserts, honey, jam, jelly, lard, margarine, mayonnaise, molasses, popsicles, salad dressings, shortening, soft drinks, sour cream, sugar, syrup, vegetable oil	Foods in this group add flavor and pleasure to eating but provide mostly calories with few or no nutrients.

Important Points to Keep in Mind

- All foods can be part of a healthful eating style. Use the Food Guide Pyramid to plan your food selections and to help you balance your choices over the course of the day or week.
- Healthful eating and physical activity go hand in hand. Each day participate in activities you like, such as walking, jogging, or swimming. Thirty minutes is recommended, but it need not happen all at once.
- Variety is an important part of eating healthfully. Each week try one new recipe, or when eating out order something you've never tried before.
- When you read food labels, focus on the nutrition information that applies to your eating goals.

Sample Menu for Healthful Eating

BREAKFAST	LUNCH	SNACK	DINNER
Orange juice (¾ cup) Whole-grain cereal (¾ cup) with fresh berries (½ cup) Whole-wheat toast (2 slices) topped with jam (1 tbsp) Reduced-fat milk (1 cup) Coffee or tea	Vegetable soup (1 cup) with crackers (4) Hamburger (3 oz) on a toasted bun (1) with mustard (1 tbsp), ketchup (1 tbsp), sliced tomato (2 oz), and lettuce Fresh fruit salad (½ cup) Coffee or tea	Graham crackers (4) Fresh apple (1 medium) Reduced-fat milk (1 cup)	Tossed salad (1 cup) drizzled with vinegar and oil dressing (1 tbsp) Broiled, savory chicken breast (3 oz)—remove skin before eating Herbed brown rice (½ cup) Steamed broccoli (½ cup) Whole-grain roll (1) topped with margarine (2 tsp) Low-fat frozen strawberry yogurt (½ cup) Coffee or tea

© 1996, The American Dietetic Association. *Manual of Clinical Dietetics.* Used with permission.

OTHER INSTRUCTIONS

Food Guide Pyramid

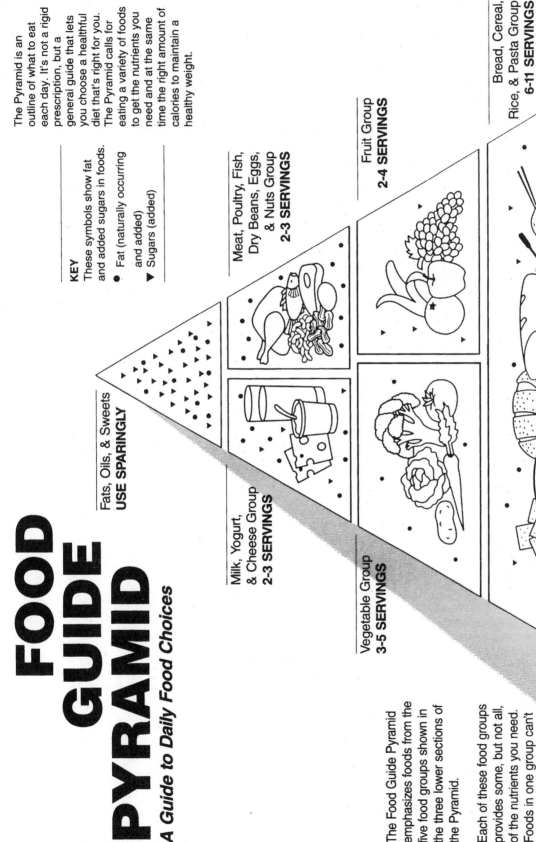

FOOD GUIDE PYRAMID
A Guide to Daily Food Choices

The Pyramid is an outline of what to eat each day. It's not a rigid prescription, but a general guide that lets you choose a healthful diet that's right for you. The Pyramid calls for eating a variety of foods to get the nutrients you need and at the same time the right amount of calories to maintain a healthy weight.

KEY
These symbols show fat and added sugars in foods.
● Fat (naturally occurring and added)
▼ Sugars (added)

Fats, Oils, & Sweets
USE SPARINGLY

Milk, Yogurt, & Cheese Group
2-3 SERVINGS

Meat, Poultry, Fish, Dry Beans, Eggs, & Nuts Group
2-3 SERVINGS

Vegetable Group
3-5 SERVINGS

Fruit Group
2-4 SERVINGS

Bread, Cereal, Rice, & Pasta Group
6-11 SERVINGS

The Food Guide Pyramid emphasizes foods from the five food groups shown in the three lower sections of the Pyramid.

Each of these food groups provides some, but not all, of the nutrients you need. Foods in one group can't replace those in another. No one food group is more important than another — for good health, you need them all.

Source: U.S. DEPARTMENT OF AGRICULTURE and the U.S. DEPARTMENT OF HEALTH AND HUMAN SERVICES.

Provided by: the Education Department of the NATIONAL LIVESTOCK AND MEAT BOARD.

What Counts as 1 Serving?

Bread, Cereal, Rice, & Pasta Group

1 slice of bread

½ cup of cooked rice or pasta

½ cup of cooked cereal

1 ounce of ready-to-eat cereal

Vegetable Group

½ cup of chopped raw or cooked vegetables

1 cup of leafy raw vegetables

Fruit Group

1 piece of fruit or melon wedge

¾ cup of juice

½ cup of canned fruit

¼ cup of dried fruit

Milk, Yogurt, & Cheese Group

1 cup of milk or yogurt

1½ ounces of natural cheese

2 ounces of process cheese

Meat, Poultry, Fish, Dry Beans, Eggs, & Nuts Group

2½ to 3 ounces of cooked lean meat, poultry, or fish

Count ½ cup of cooked beans, or 1 egg, or 2 tablespoons of peanut butter as 1 ounce of lean meat

Fats, Oils, & Sweets

LIMIT CALORIES FROM THESE especially if you need to lose weight

▲ The amount you eat may be more than one serving. For example, a dinner portion of spaghetti would count as 2 or 3 servings.

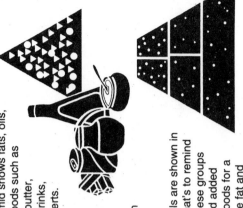

A Closer Look at Fat and Added Sugars

The small tip of the Pyramid shows fats, oils, and sweets. These are foods such as salad dressings, cream, butter, margarine, sugars, soft drinks, candies, and sweet desserts.

Alcoholic beverages are also part of this group. These foods provide calories but few vitamins and minerals. Most people should go easy on foods from this group.

Some fat or sugar symbols are shown in the other food groups. That's to remind you that some foods in these groups can also be high in fat and added sugars. When choosing foods for a healthful diet, consider the fat and added sugars in your choices from all the food groups, not just fats, oils, and sweets from the Pyramid tip.

	Women & some older adults	Children, teen girls, active women, most men	Teen boys & active men
Calorie level*	about 1,600	about 2,200	about 2,800
Bread group	6	9	11
Vegetable group	3	4	5
Fruit group	2	3	4
Milk group	2-3**	2-3**	2-3**
Meat group	2 for a total of 5 ounces	2 for a total of 6 ounces	3 for a total of 7 ounces

*These are the calorie levels if you choose lowfat, lean foods from the 5 major food groups and use foods from the fats, oils, and sweets group sparingly.

**Women who are pregnant or breastfeeding, teenagers, and young adults to age 24 need 3 servings.

Source: U.S. DEPARTMENT OF AGRICULTURE and the U.S. DEPARTMENT OF HEALTH AND HUMAN SERVICES.

Provided by: the Education Department of the NATIONAL LIVESTOCK AND MEAT BOARD.

Guidelines for Pediatric Nutrition

DESCRIPTION

Nutrition during the first years of life provides for the future health, growth, and development of the infant. The following guidelines are for full-term healthy babies up to 24 months. Feeding guidelines for preschool- and school-aged children are also included.

ADEQUACY

The provision of adequate amounts of breast milk, formula, and solid food can meet the Recommended Dietary Allowances for the infant.

GUIDELINES FOR BREAST-FEEDING (see Unit 15 for specific instructions for breast-feeding)

GUIDELINES FOR FORMULA-FEEDING

1. Bottle-feeding should be on demand. Formula can be at body temperature, room temperature, or at a cool temperature. Newborns need at least 6 to 8 feedings a day with 2–5 oz at each feeding. As the baby gets older, *decrease* the number of feedings, but increase the amount to 6–8 oz at each feeding.

2. Any infant foods heated in a microwave oven should be thoroughly mixed and checked for temperature to avoid burns. It is better to warm the bottle in a pan of hot tap water.

3. Adding cereal, sugar honey, or corn syrup to formula *is not* recommended. Honey and corn syrup may contain botulism, which can harm the infant.

4. Six wet diapers a day is a good sign that feeding is going well.

5. Never prop or put your baby to bed with a bottle. The baby could choke.

GUIDELINES FOR INTRODUCING SOLID FOODS

1. The diet for the child up to 1 year of age should be individualized according to the pediatrician's recommendations and the child's tolerance of foods.

2. Consistency of food should be governed by the age and development of the child. Progress toward whole foods should be made as rapidly as possible.

3. Size or portion varies with age, growth periods, and activity. Appetite is greater during the first 12 months than it is in the second year because growth is not as rapid during this period.

How to Feed Your Baby Step-By-Step

Every baby is very special. Don't worry if your baby eats a little more or less than this guide suggests. In fact, this is perfectly normal. The suggested serving sizes are only guidelines to help you get started.

Age	Food Group	Foods	Daily Servings	Suggested Serving Size	Feeding Tips
0–4 Months	Milk	Breast milk *or* Formula* 0–1 month 1–2 months 2–3 months 3–4 months	On demand (about 8–12) 6–8 5–7 4–7 4–6	 2–5 oz 3–6 oz 4–7 oz 6–8 oz	• Nurse baby at least 5–10 minutes on each breast. • Six wet diapers a day is a good sign. • There's no need to force baby to finish a bottle. • Putting baby to bed with a bottle could cause choking! • Heating formula in the microwave is not recommended. *Table continued on following page*

Table continued on following page

How to Feed Your Baby Step-By-Step *Continued*

Age	Food Group	Foods	Daily Servings	Suggested Serving Size	Feeding Tips
4–6 Months	Milk	Breast milk *or* Formula*	4–6 4–6	6–8 oz	• May need to start baby cereal (iron-fortified). • Feed only one new cereal each week. • There's no need to add salt or sugar to cereal. • Offer baby extra water. • Use the microwave with caution.
	Grain	Baby cereal (iron-fortified)	2	1–2 tbsp	
6–8 Months	Milk	Breast milk *or* Formula*	3–5 3–5	6–8 oz	• Add strained fruits and vegetables at first. Add mashed or finely chopped fruits and cooked vegetables later on. • Feed only one new fruit or vegetable each week. • Take out of the jar the amount of food for one feeding. Refrigerate the remaining food. • Try giving baby fruit juice in a cup.
	Grain	Baby cereal (iron-fortified)	2	2–4 tbsp	
		Bread, Crackers	Offer	½ 2 crackers	
	Fruit	Fruit	2	2–3 tbsp	
		Fruit juice	1	3 oz (from cup)	
	Vegetable	Vegetables	2	2–3 tbsp	
8–12 Months	Milk	Breast milk *or* Formula*	3–4 3–4	6–8 oz	• Add strained or finely chopped meats now. • Feed only one new meat a week. • Wait until baby's first birthday to feed egg whites. Some babies are sensitive to the egg white. It's okay to give baby the yolks. • Be patient. Babies make a mess when they feed themselves. • Always taste heated foods before serving them to baby.
		Cheese	4	½ oz	
		Plain yogurt	Offer	½ cup	
		Cottage cheese		¼ cup	
	Grain	Baby cereal (iron-fortified)	2–3	2–4 tbsp	
		Bread *or* Crackers	2–3	½ slice 2 crackers	
	Fruit	Fruit	2	3–4 tbsp	
		Fruit juice	1	3 oz (from cup)	
	Vegetable	Vegetables	2–3	3–4 tbsp	
	Meat	Chicken, beef, pork Cooked, dried beans *or* Egg yolks	2	3–4 tbsp	
12–24 Months	Milk	Whole milk, yogurt	4	½ cup	• Add whole milk now. • Offer small portions and never force your toddler to eat. • "Food jags" are common now. Don't make a big deal out of them. • Respect your toddler's likes and dislikes. Offer rejected foods again. • Make meals fun and interesting. Serve colorful foods that are crunchy, smooth, or warm. • Toddlers need meals *and* snacks. • Feed your toddler at least 3 snacks every day.
		Cheese		½ oz	
		Cottage cheese		¼ cup	
	Grain	Cereal, pasta or rice	6	¼ cup	
		Bread, muffins, rolls Crackers		½ 2 crackers	
	Fruit	Cooked or juice Whole	2	3 oz ½ medium	
	Vegetable	Cooked or juice Whole	3	3 oz ½ medium	
	Meat	Fish, chicken, turkey, beef, pork	2	1 oz	
		Cooked, dried beans *or* peas		¼ cup	
		Egg		1	

*If you are bottle feeding, most doctors recommend iron-fortified formula. Ask your doctor which formula is best for your baby.

Courtesy of the NATIONAL DAIRY COUNCIL®.

GUIDELINES FOR PRESCHOOL- AND SCHOOL-AGED CHILDREN

1. A child should not be forced to eat. Short periods of rebellion against specific foods are best ignored.

2. When new foods are introduced, the child must become accustomed to the taste and texture. Give a small amount first at the beginning of the meal when the child is hungry. Only one new food should be introduced at a time. Do not introduce it if a child is not feeling well. If a new food is turned down, do not force the child to eat. Try again in several days.

3. Very young or very active children may need between-meal feedings. These should be nutritious snacks rather than sweet cookies or candy snacks. Offer such nutritious snacks as cheese or yogurt, saltine or graham crackers, fruit, a bagel or bread, whole milk or fruit juice, unsweetened cereals (such as Cheerios), pudding, steamed vegetables, frozen juice pops, milkshake, pretzels.

4. Sweets such as candy, cookies, and cake should be given only at the end of a meal. Sweets depress appetite and may take the place of other foods the body needs. Sugar-coated cereals are not recommended. Sweets should not be used as a bribe—this will make them more appealing.

5. Clear broth has little nutritive value and should not be given in place of more nutritious food.

6. Sweetened, carbonated drinks should not be given. Water should be given to the child between meals to prevent dehydration.

7. Vitamins and other food supplements should be given only as directed by the doctor.

8. For the hospitalized child, eating at a table with other children should be encouraged, since this improves appetite and acceptance of unfamiliar foods.

9. Some foods are hard for children to chew without a full set of teeth. Watch your child closely to be sure the child can chew and swallow well when giving these foods. To prevent choking, never leave your child alone when eating.

   - Apple chunks and slices,
   - Grapes,
   - Hot dogs,
   - Sausage,
   - Peanut butter,
   - Popcorn,
   - Peanuts—all nuts and seeds,
   - Round candies,
   - Hard chunks of uncooked vegetables such as carrots.

Serving Guidelines for All Ages

Food Group	Servings					Foods	Serving Size
		Children			Adults		
	1–3	4–5	6–8*	9–18*	19+		
Milk group	3†	3‡	3	4	3–4	• milk • yogurt • cheese • cottage cheese • pudding • ice cream, frozen yogurt	1 cup 1 cup 1½–2 oz ½ cup ½ cup ½ cup
Meat group	2†	2	2	2	2–3	• cooked lean meat, fish or poultry • egg • peanut butter • cooked dried peas • cooked dried beans • nuts, seeds	2–3 oz 1 2 tbsp ½ cup ½ cup ⅓ cup
Vegetable group	3†	3	3	3	3–5	• cooked vegetables • chopped, raw vegetables • raw, leafy vegetables • vegetable juice	½ cup ½ cup 1 cup ¾ cup
Fruit group	2†	2	2	2	2–4	• apple, banana, orange, pear • grapefruit • cantaloupe • raw, canned, or cooked fruit • raisins, dried fruit • fruit juice	1 medium ½ ¼ ½ cup ¼ cup ¾ cup
Grain group	6†	6‡	6	6	6–11	• bread • tortilla, roll, muffin • bagel, English muffin, hamburger bun • rice, pasta, cooked cereal, grits • ready-to-eat cereal	1 slice 1 ½ ½ cup 1 oz
"Others" category	Eat in moderation					• fats, oils, and spreads • candy • cookies • chips and other salty snacks • soft drinks	1 tsp/1 tbsp 1 oz 2 small 1 oz 12 oz

*These represent the *minimum* number of servings recommended each day for children and teens ages 6–18.

†For children 1–3, serving sizes are about two-thirds of typical serving sizes.

‡For children 4–5, serving sizes depend on the appetite of the child. If you offer smaller-sized servings, you should increase the number of servings so that children 4–5 eat the equivalent of 3 cups of milk, 4 oz of meat, 6 slices of bread, etc. daily.

Courtesy of the NATIONAL DAIRY COUNCIL®.

Colic in Infants*

BASIC INFORMATION

Colic is repeated episodes of excessive crying that cannot be explained. Crying ranges from fussiness to agonized screaming. Colic is not contagious and occurs more often in boys. Colic affects infants up to 5 months old and is most common in a first child.

Frequent signs and symptoms of colic are excessive crying with the following characteristics:

- Crying bouts usually occur in late afternoon or evening.
- Crying bouts usually begin at 2 to 4 weeks and last through 3 or 4 months.
- The infant's abdomen may rumble, and the child may draw up the legs as if in pain.
- No specific disease, such as an ear infection, hernia, allergy, or urinary infection, can be discovered.

The cause of colic is unknown. It may be related to physical pain or emotional upset. Some likely possibilities include hunger, insufficient sleep, milk that is too hot, overfeeding, food allergy, reactions to tension in the home, loneliness, or tiredness.

There are no known risk factors or specific preventive measures for colic. Remove any causes that can be identified.

All babies cry, and many have fussy periods. Crying is an important activity and a means of communication. Colic is a distressing, but not dangerous, condition. The symptoms can sometimes be relieved. Colic will usually disappear after the third to fourth month.

TREATMENT

General Measures

- Be patient and tolerant. Since colic is normal and not the parents' fault, do not blame yourself.

---

*Modified from Moore, S. (1998). Griffith's Instructions for Patients. 6th edition. Philadelphia: WB Saunders.

- Don't feed the baby every time he or she cries. Look for a reason, such as a gas bubble, cramped position, too much heat or cold, soiled diaper, open diaper pin, or a desire to be cuddled.
- When the baby has an attack of gas, hold the baby securely, and gently massage the lower abdomen. Rocking may be soothing.
- Offer the baby a pacifier.
- Playing music may help.
- Allow the baby to cry if you are certain everything is all right (not hungry, not soiled, no fever, no open pins) and you have done all you can. Colic is distressing, but not harmful.
- Ask someone to take care of the baby to relieve you as often as possible.
- Notify your health care provider if the baby's rectal temperature rises to 101°F (38.3°C) or higher or if the baby is taking a prescription drug, and new, unexplained symptoms develop. The drug may produce side effects.

Medications

Medications are usually not helpful for colic. Simethicone (for gas) may be prescribed.

Activity

There are no restrictions.

Diet

- Interrupt bottle feedings after every ounce and burp the baby. Interrupt breast feedings every 5 minutes.
- Allow at least 20 minutes to feed the baby. Don't prop the baby for feedings.
- Nipple holes should not be too large. A vigorous baby may require blind nipples in which you can make small, homemade nipple holes.
- A short trial of milk substitute is useful to determine if an intolerance to milk is the problem.

OTHER INSTRUCTIONS

Guidelines for Older Adults

DESCRIPTION

Recommended Dietary Allowances for the older person do not differ much from those for middle-aged persons, except for the amount of calories, which are lower. The older person needs the same basic foods every day to provide the recommended amounts of protein, minerals, and vitamins (see Food Guide Pyramid). Excess fat may decrease the appetite. Use low-fat gravies and avoid frequent use of pastries and fried foods. There should be no more than 15 hours between dinner and breakfast. Special attention may need to be given to the texture of food for the very old and for those with poor teeth or ill-fitting dentures. Age-related physical changes may require special dietary changes.

The table lists potential problems and possible solutions.

Dietary Suggestions for Older Adults

Problem	Comment
Decreased sense of smell, taste, and sight	Provide adequate lighting, serve colorful, attractive, flavorful food. Try different textures and seasonings.
Less efficient digestion	Serve small, frequent meals. Allow sufficient time for eating.
Missing teeth or poor-fitting dentures	Adjust texture of food. For example, meat may need to be chopped, ground, or pureed. Meat should be moist and well seasoned. Fruits and vegetables may be served either cooked or raw and, as with meat, may be chopped or strained if the person has difficulty chewing.
Constipation	Encourage consumption of fruits, vegetables, whole-grain breads, and cereals. Provide adequate liquids.
Dehydration	Encourage drinking liquids.
Lactose intolerance; osteoporosis	Many people can tolerate a small amount of milk at a time. Try buttermilk, yogurt, and cheese or cooked milk products such as pudding, custard, or cream soups.
	Encourage use of dark-green leafy vegetables, or calcium-fortified beverages to reduce risk of osteoporosis.
Decreased fat tolerance	Use added fat and fatty foods in moderation.
	Choose lean meats, low-fat, or fat-free milk and milk products. Avoid fried foods.
Iron deficiency	Encourage nutritionally balanced meals, including good sources of protein-lean meat, chicken, and fish.
	Iron-rich foods can be eaten with vitamin C foods. For example, orange juice improves iron absorption.
Arthritis	Provide easy-to-open containers.
	Finger foods may be more easily managed.
	Encourage healthy eating for weight control.

Sample Menu for Older Adults

BREAKFAST	LUNCH	AFTERNOON SNACK	DINNER
Grapefruit juice (½ cup)	Vegetable soup (1 cup)	Vanilla wafer cookies (6)	Tossed green salad (1 cup)
Cornflakes (¾ cup)	Saltine crackers (4)	1% milk (1 cup)	Salad dressing (1 tbsp)
Banana (½)	Lean beef patty (3 oz)		Baked turkey breast (3 oz)
Whole-wheat toast (2 slices)	Hamburger bun (1)		Mashed potatoes (½ cup)
Margarine (2 tsp)	Mustard or ketchup (1 tbsp)		Carrots (½ cup)
Jelly or jam (1 tsp)	Sliced tomato (2 oz) and lettuce		Stuffing (⅓ cup)
1% milk (1 cup)	Canned fruit salad (½ cup)		Margarine (2 tsp)
Coffee/tea			Low-fat ice cream (½ cup)
			Canned peaches (½ cup)
			Decaffeinated coffee/tea

From Chilton Memorial Hospital, Pompton Plains, NJ.

Modified Consistency Diets

Clear Liquid Diet

DESCRIPTION

The clear liquid diet is used to supply fluid and calories in a form that requires little digestion. It is used in preparation for bowel surgery or a colonoscopy, immediately after abdominal surgery, and in acute stages of gastrointestinal problems or other illnesses. The diet is intended for short-term use only—24 to 72 hours. A low-residue or clear liquid oral supplement may be needed if the diet is being used more than 3 days. Solid foods should be started as soon as possible.

ADEQUACY

This diet is not adequate in calories or most nutrients except for vitamin C. It is typically used only for very brief periods (24 to 48 hours).

A protein supplement is given if the diet is continued for more than 3 days, at the discretion of the doctor and dietitian.

Note: A commercially prepared "chemically defined diet" may be useful if a clear liquid diet is necessary for more than a few days or if the patient is seriously undernourished.

Clear Liquid Diet Foods

Food Group	Allowed	Avoid
Beverages	Clear fruit juices (e.g., apple, cranberry, or grape); strained juices (e.g., orange, lemonade, or grapefruit) Clear coffee or tea with lemon and carbonated beverages as allowed and tolerated	All others/beverages including nectars, milk, cream, juices with pulp, cocoa
Soups	Clear broths or bouillon	All others
Sweets and desserts	Clear fruit-flavored or unflavored gelatin; fruit ice made from clear fruit juice or fruit drink; plain hard candy; sugar; honey; sugar substitutes; frozen pops	All others and any not tolerated or contraindicated by medical condition
Miscellaneous	Clear liquid commercially prepared low-residue nutritional supplements, such as protein increased broth or gelatin Consult with health care provider before using	All others

Sample Menu for Clear Liquid Diet

Breakfast	Midmorning Snack	Lunch	Midafternoon Snack	Dinner	Evening Snack
Strained orange juice (4 oz) Gelatin dessert (½ cup) Tea/coffee Sugar (1 tsp)	Gelatin dessert (½ cup)	Apple juice (4 oz) Broth (6 oz) Fruit flavored ice (½ cup) Tea/coffee	Carbonated soda (6 oz)	Cranberry juice (4 oz) Broth (6 oz) Gelatin dessert (½ cup) Carbonated soda (6 oz) Tea/coffee	Fruit flavored ice (½ cup)

From Chilton Memorial Hospital, Pompton Plains, NJ.

Blenderized Liquid Diet

DESCRIPTION

The blenderized liquid diet can be used by people who are unable to chew, swallow, or digest solid foods. This diet consists of fluids and foods blenderized to a liquid form with a consistency ranging from that of fruit juice to cream soup. All liquids can be used to blenderize foods.

ADEQUACY

The diet can be adequate in all nutrients.

GUIDELINES

1. Small, frequent feedings (6 to 8 per day) may help provide adequate calories and protein.

2. Food may blenderize more readily when cut into small pieces before placing it in the blender or food processor.
3. Most foods can be liquefied by mixing equal parts of solids and liquids. Some foods, such as fruits and vegetables, do not need equal amounts of liquid added due to their high fluid content.
4. Blenderized foods should be used immediately but can be refrigerated up to 48 hours or frozen immediately after blenderizing to prevent growth of harmful bacteria.
5. Use of gravy, vegetable juices, cream soups, cheese and tomato sauces, milk, and fruit juices is recommended, rather than water, to increase nutritional value, color, and flavor.

Blenderized Liquid Diet Foods

Food Groups	Allowed	Avoid
Beverages	Milk; thin milk shakes; all beverages	Thickened milk products; alcohol
Breads and cereals	Soft breads and crackers can be blenderized; cereals thinned with milk	All others
Desserts	Thinned custards and puddings; blenderized and thinned cake, pie; milk shakes; sherbet shakes; gelatin	All others
Fats	Butter or fortified margarine; cream and cream substitutes; cooking fats and oils; gravy; whipped topping	All others
Fruits	Fruit juices; strained, thinned nectars; blenderized fruits	All others
Meats and meat substitutes	Blenderized, thinned meats, poultry, fish; beans; smooth peanut butter; eggs; cheese sauce	All others
Potatoes and potato substitutes	Thinned, mashed, creamed potatoes; blenderized, thinned rice and noodles	All others
Soups	Strained or blenderized soups, broth, or bouillon; strained or blenderized cream soups	All others
Sweets	Jelly; honey; sugar; sugar substitute; chocolate syrup, maple syrup	All others
Vegetables	Vegetable juices; blenderized, cooked, and thinned vegetables (no seeds—very fibrous vegetables may be difficult to blenderize)	All others
Miscellaneous	Seasonings and spices as desired	Nuts, coconut, and foods with seeds may not blenderize well

Sample Menu for Blenderized Liquid Diet

BREAKFAST	LUNCH	DINNER
Orange juice, strained (½ cup) Farina (1 cup), thinned with milk (¼ cup) 2% milk (1 cup) Coffee/tea	Cream of chicken soup (1 cup), blenderized with saltine crackers (4) Pureed lean beef patty (3 oz) thinned with beef broth (1 tbsp) Hamburger bun (1) Ketchup (2 tbsp) Pureed green beans (½ cup) thinned with chicken broth (2 tbsp) Coffee/tea	Beef broth soup (1 cup), blenderized with saltine crackers (4) Pureed chicken (3 oz), thinned with chicken broth (2 tbsp) Mashed potatoes (½ cup), thinned with milk Tomato juice (6 oz) Coffee/tea
MIDMORNING SNACK	MIDAFTERNOON SNACK	EVENING SNACK
Thin milk shake made with 2% milk (1 cup), blenderized with a banana and flavored syrup (2 tbsp)	Pureed apricots, thinned with liquid 2% milk (1 cup)	Blenderized fruit (½ cup), thinned with orange juice (2 tbsp) Low fat chocolate milk (1 cup)

© 1996, The American Dietetic Association. *Manual of Clinical Dietetics.* Used by permission.

OTHER INSTRUCTIONS

Mechanically Soft Diet

DESCRIPTION

A mechanically soft diet is designed for people who have difficulty chewing food. The foods recommended on this diet are blended, chopped, ground, or pureed and prepared with added liquids to make them easier to eat.

ADEQUACY

Based on individual food choices, the diet is adequate in all nutrients.

GUIDELINES

1. Avoid any foods containing raw fruit and vegetables or seeds, nuts, dried beans, coconut, and dried fruits.
2. Soften waffles, pancakes, and other bread products in syrups or gelatin or commercial thickener slurry.
3. Moisten ground meats or poultry with gravy, broth, or sauces.
4. For added flavor, add cooked ground meats and soft vegetables to soups, casseroles, or a thick puree base.
5. For food safety reasons, cook eggs until yolks and whites are set. Do not add raw eggs to milk shakes or drinks.
6. Season vegetables with butter or margarine and ground spices.
7. Soften vegetables in soups and sauces.
8. To boost calories, add sauces to vegetables, noodles, and rice.
9. Soften desserts such as cakes or soft cookies with fruit juice or pureed fruit.
10. Blend fruit in milk shakes or yogurt.

Mechanically Altered Foods

Food Category	Allowed	Avoid
Beverages	Milk and other dairy beverages; coffee, tea; carbonated beverages; hot cocoa	Beverages containing raw eggs
Breads	All breads and baked goods made without nuts, seeds, dried fruits and hard to chew crusts. Plain crackers and breads may be softened in liquid.	Dry, crisp, hard breads, crackers and snacks; breads containing seeds, nuts and dried fruit
Cereals	Plain dry or cooked cereals without added fruit or nuts; dry cereals should be softened in liquid.	Those containing seeds, nuts and dried fruit; those remaining hard in liquid. Nuts; shredded wheat, granola, Grape Nuts, or cereal that remains crunchy in milk
Desserts	Plain puddings, custards, gelatins and frozen desserts; fruit whips; yogurt; Soft cakes and cookies without nuts and fruits	Those containing seeds, nuts, or whole or dried fruits; any hard, tough, or chewy desserts
Fats and oils	All except those to avoid	Nuts, seeds, bacon
Fruits	Fruit juices and cooked, canned or mashed ripe fruits without seeds or skins	Those containing tough or fibrous membranes or skins, seeds, or dried fruits
Meats and meat substitutes	Ground, pureed, or chopped meat and poultry—broth, gravy, or sauces may be added to moisten; soft, flaked fish without bones; casseroles made of ground meat; beanless chili or chili with mashed beans; meat loaf; smooth peanut butter; cottage cheese, soft cheeses, cheese sauces; soft, cooked eggs and egg substitutes	Whole pieces of meat or poultry, fried fish, crunchy peanut butter
Potatoes and starches	Mashed, baked, (skinless) boiled potatoes; skinless sweet potatoes; rice or noodles; soft pastas	Fried potatoes and those with skins
Soups	All except those to avoid	Any with chunks of meats and crunchy vegetables

Table continued on opposite page

Mechanically Altered Foods *Continued*

Food Category	Allowed	Avoid
Sweets	Clear jelly; honey; sugar; sugar substitutes; syrup	All candies, dried fruits
Vegetables	Well-cooked, soft, mashed or pureed vegetables without skin or seeds; vegetable juices	All others
Seasonings and condiments	Seasonings (for example, salt and pepper), ground spices, smooth condiments	Nuts, coconuts, seeds, olives

Sample Menu for Mechanically Soft Diet

Breakfast	Lunch	Snack	Dinner
Prune juice (½ cup)	Pea soup (1 cup)	Vanilla wafers (6)	Tomato juice (½ cup)
Oatmeal (¾ cup)	Saltine crackers, softened in soup (4)	Applesauce (½ cup)	Meatloaf
Corn muffin (small)	Egg salad on soft bread		Noodles
Margarine (2 tsp)	Canned peaches (½ cup)		Steamed carrots (½ cup)
1% milk (1 cup)	2% milk (1 cup)		Soft dinner roll (1)
Coffee/tea	Coffee/tea		Margarine (2 tsp)
			Low-fat ice cream (½ cup)
			Coffee/tea

From Chilton Memorial Hospital, Pompton Plains, NJ.

OTHER INSTRUCTIONS

Soft Diet

DESCRIPTION

The soft diet can be used for people who are not able to digest all foods on a general diet.

ADEQUACY

This diet is adequate in the Recommended Dietary Allowances if foods from each of the basic food groups are eaten daily.

Soft Diet Foods

Food Groups	Allowed	Avoid
Beverages	Milk and milk products; all other beverages	Alcoholic beverages
Breads and cereals	All breads, soft rolls, and crackers; cooked or ready-to-eat cereals except those to avoid	Coarse cereals (e.g., bran); whole-grain breads, crackers, bread products with nuts, seeds, or dried fruits
Desserts	Cakes, cookies, pies, pudding, custard, frozen desserts, and gelatin made with allowed foods	Those containing nuts, seeds, coconut, or dried fruits, fried pastries (e.g., doughnuts)
Fats and oils	All except those to avoid	Highly seasoned salad dressings
Fruits	All fruit juices; cooked or canned fruit without seeds	Other fresh and dried fruits
Meats and meat substitutes	All lean, tender meats, poultry, fish and shellfish; eggs; mild-flavored cheeses; creamy peanut butter; soybean and other meat substitutes; plain or flavored yogurt	Connective tissue of meat and poultry, strong-smelling or highly seasoned meats, cheeses, or fish (e.g., luncheon meats; frankfurters, sausage); yogurt with nuts or dried fruits
Potatoes and other starches	Potatoes; white and sweet, enriched rice, barley, spaghetti, macaroni, and other pasta	Fried, highly seasoned potatoes and other starches
Vegetables	All vegetable juices; cooked vegetables except those not allowed, and lettuce as tolerated; salads made from allowed foods	Raw and fried vegetables; whole kernel corn; gas-producing vegetables (e.g., broccoli, brussels sprouts, cabbage, onions, leeks, cauliflower, cucumber, green pepper, rutabagas, turnips, sauerkraut, dried peas, dried beans)
Soups	Soups made with allowed foods	Highly seasoned soups and soups made with gas-producing vegetables
Sweets	Sugar, syrup, honey, jelly and seedless jam, hard candies, plain chocolate candies, molasses, marshmallows	Any with nuts or coconut
Miscellaneous	Iodized salt; flavorings; mildly flavored gravies and sauces; pepper, herbs, spices, ketchup, mustard, vinegar in moderation	Strongly flavored seasonings and condiments (e.g., garlic, chili sauce, chili pepper, horseradish), pickles, popcorn, nuts and coconut

Sample Menu for Soft Diet

Breakfast	Lunch	Dinner
Orange juice (½ cup)	Vegetable soup (1 cup)	Tomato juice (6 oz)
Oatmeal (¾ cup)	Saltine crackers (4)	Broiled, skinless chicken breast (3 oz)
Banana slices (½ cup)	Tuna salad (3 oz) on white bread	Mashed potatoes
Plain English muffin (2 slices)	Lettuce leaf	Steamed carrots (½ cup)
Margarine (2 tbsp)	Canned peaches (½ cup)	Soft dinner roll (1)
Jelly (1 tbsp)	Vanilla wafers (2)	Margarine (2 tsp)
1% milk (1 cup)	1% milk (1 cup)	Low-fat ice cream (½ cup)
Coffee/tea	Coffee/tea	Applesauce (½ cup)
		Coffee/tea

From Chilton Memorial Hospital, Pompton Plains, NJ.

Nutrition Management of People With Swallowing Difficulty

DESCRIPTION

Dysphagia is a term used for swallowing problems. No two people are alike. Diets should be individualized based on swallowing ability and food preference. Diet levels are based on an assessment by the doctor. The use of blenders or food processors helps make solid foods an acceptable consistency.

GUIDELINES

In addition to blenderizing food, food thickeners are sometimes necessary. Both commercial and common food thickeners are available.

The following are some common food thickeners:

- Instant cereal,
- Baby strained bananas or banana flakes,
- Potato flakes,
- Finely chopped crackers,
- Flavored plain yogurt,
- Unflavored/flavored gelatin,
- Powdered skim milk,
- Cottage cheese,
- Cream cheese,
- Heavy cream,
- Bread crumbs.

DYSPHAGIA DIET LEVEL I

This diet is designed for people who cannot swallow chewable foods or thin liquids safely.

- Thick, similar textures are emphasized.
- No coarse textures, nuts, raw fruits, or raw vegetables are allowed.
- No water is allowed.
- All liquids are thickened with a commercial thickening agent.

Dysphagia Diet Level I: Recommended Foods

Breads and cereals	Cream of wheat, cream of rice
Eggs	Soft poached
Milk products	Yogurt without fruit; thickened milk
Fruits	Pureed fruits without seeds or skins; thickened juices
Vegetables	Pureed vegetables without seeds or skins; thickened juices
Fats	Gravy; margarine; thickened sauces or broths
Meats and meat substitutes	Pureed, tender meats or casseroles with gravy or broth to moisten
Soups	Pureed, strained soups; thicken as needed
Desserts	Shakes, custard, pudding, ice cream, sherbet; pudding pops, Jello if tolerated
Beverages	All liquids must be cold and thickened with a commercial thickening agent; no water

DYSPHAGIA DIET LEVEL II

This diet is for people who can swallow easily chewed foods but cannot safely swallow thin liquids. This diet has a pureed base with the addition of some texture, flavor, and variety. Small amounts of liquids may be added to get the appropriate consistency for the food.

- Liquids are thickened only as needed with a commercial thickening agent.
- The person may begin to drink very thick juices and milk products without thickeners if tolerated.
- No coarse textures, nuts, raw fruits, or vegetables are allowed.
- No water is allowed.

Dysphagia Diet Level II: Recommended Foods

Breads and cereals	Cream of wheat, cream of rice, thinned oatmeal; pancakes with syrup if tolerated
Eggs	Soft poached, soft scrambled
Milk products	Yogurt; cottage cheese
Fruits	Pureed fruits without seeds or skins; applesauce; ripe, mashed bananas; thickened juices or nectars
Vegetables	Pureed vegetables without seeds or skins; moist mashed potatoes; mashed winter squash; thickened juices
Fats	Gravy; margarine; thickened sauces or broths
Meats and meat substitutes	Pureed, tender meats or casseroles with gravy or broth to moisten; macaroni and cheese if tolerated
Soups	Pureed, or strained creamed soups
Desserts	Shakes, custard, pudding, ice cream, sherbet; pudding pops, Jello if tolerated; avoid hard candies and nuts
Beverages	Very thick juices, nectars, and milk products if tolerated; all other liquids must be cold and thickened with a commercial thickening agent; no water
Miscellaneous	Syrup if tolerated

DYSPHAGIA DIET LEVEL III

This diet is designed for people who have difficulty chewing and swallowing some foods. It consists of soft food items prepared without blenderizing or pureeing. It may be appropriate for persons beginning to chew.

Dysphagia Diet Level III: Recommended Foods

Breads and cereals	Soft breads and graham crackers only; cooked and cold cereals in milk; waffles, pancakes; rice, pasta; avoid Grape Nuts, granola, and whole-grain crackers or crackers with seeds
Eggs	Poached, scrambled; egg salad
Milk products	Yogurt, cottage cheese, American or processed cheese, ricotta, cream cheese
Fruits	Any fresh or canned fruit without seeds, coarse skins, or fibers such as peeled or canned peaches and pears; juices, nectars
Vegetables	Well-cooked or canned vegetables; avoid spinach, lettuce, and peas
Fats	Gravy; sauces, margarine, seasonings as tolerated
Meats and meat substitutes	Small pieces with gravy, meat salads; macaroni and cheese; soft sandwiches; casseroles made with allowed foods; smooth peanut butter if tolerated
Soups	Mixed textures if well cooked with small pieces
Desserts	Soft desserts; avoid nuts and hard candies
Beverages	Juices, nectars, milk products if tolerated; hot liquids and water may be attempted in small amounts (½ tsp); thicken as needed with a commercial thickening agent
Miscellaneous	Syrup; honey

© 1996 The American Dietetic Association. *Manual of Clinical Dietetics.* Used by permission.

- Textures are soft, with no tough skins.
- No nuts or dry, crispy, raw, or stringy foods are allowed.
- Meats should be minced or cut into small pieces.
- Liquids can be used as tolerated.

DYSPHAGIA DIET LEVEL IV

This diet is designed for people who chew soft textures and swallow all liquids safely.

- Soft textures that do not require grinding or chopping are used.
- No nuts or raw, crisp, or deep-fried foods are allowed.

Dysphagia Diet Level IV: Recommended Foods

Breads and cereals	Soft or lightly toasted breads and crackers; cooked or cold cereals in milk; waffles, pancakes; pasta; avoid crunchy or chewy foods such as hard bagels or English muffins, hard breadsticks, unleavened bread, or Melba toast
Eggs	All eggs
Milk products	Any milk and dairy products if tolerated, cheeses
Fruits	Canned, cooked, or overripe fruits; juices, nectars; peeled fresh fruits in small pieces; soft dried fruits if tolerated
Vegetables	Tender, cooked vegetables
Fats	Any as tolerated
Meats and meat substitutes	Fine, moist meats; meat loaf; meat salads; any other soft foods; small amounts of smooth peanut butter if tolerated
Soups	Any soups
Desserts	Soft desserts and candies; avoid chewy desserts such as hard marshmallow or caramel
Beverages	All beverages
Miscellaneous	Any as tolerated; avoid chips, popcorn, chewing gum

© 1996 The American Dietetic Association. *Manual of Clinical Dietetics.* Used by permission.

Nutritional Support

Nasogastric, Orogastric, and Nasointestinal Tube Feedings

Feeding Tubes

There are different types of feeding tubes. Feeding tubes are named according to where they enter the body and where the tip of the tube is located.

Your feeding tube is called a _____ _____ tube. It enters through your _____, and the tip of the tube is in your _____ _____.

GUIDELINES

These guidelines will help you with tube feedings.

PREPARING THE FEEDING

1. Your nurse or doctor will explain the type of feeding you need. Depending on your needs, you may be instructed to use a prepackaged feeding formula or make your own feeding formula.
2. This is your feeding plan:
   a. Feeding type/name: _____
   b. Amount each day: _____
   c. Amount of each feeding or amount each hour: _____
   d. Amount of water each day: _____
   e. Amount of water *after* each feeding:
   _____
3. Make enough feeding formula for 1 day.
4. Label the container with the date and time of mixing.
5. Most mixtures can be kept only 1 to 2 days.
6. Tube feedings may be given by syringe, gravity drip, or pump. Your tube feeding will be given by _____.

PREPARING THE EQUIPMENT

1. Wash your hands.
2. Use a measuring cup to measure the amount of formula needed. Keep unused formula in the refrigerator.

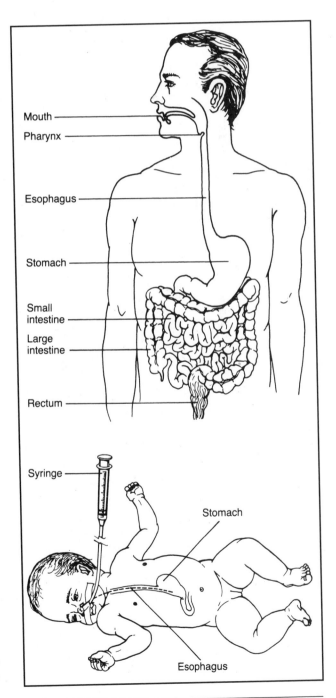

Mouth
Pharynx
Esophagus
Stomach
Small intestine
Large intestine
Rectum

Syringe
Stomach
Esophagus

3. Measure the tap water and pour it into a container.
4. Gather all equipment and follow the directions for your feeding administration set (and pump, if used).
5. If the feeding tube is in your stomach, you must check for correct tube placement *before* giving the feeding.
   a. Draw 10 to 15 milliliters (ml) of air into the syringe for an adult (.5 to 5 ml for a baby).
   b. Insert the tip of the syringe into the end of the feeding tube.
   c. Open the clamp on your feeding tube.
   d. Place the stethoscope over the stomach area, with the ear plugs in your ear.
   e. Inject air into the tube while listening through the stethoscope. You should hear a "whooshing" sound.
   f. If you do not hear the whooshing sound, repeat the above steps.
   g. If you still do not hear the sound, do not give the feeding and call your nurse or doctor.

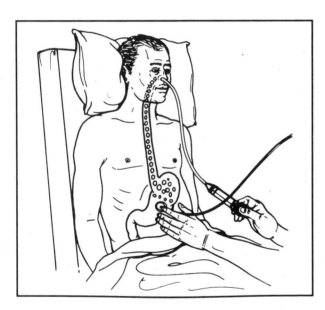

6. If instructed to do so by the nurse or doctor, check the stomach contents.
   a. Attach the syringe to the feeding tube.
   b. Draw back on the syringe's plunger to withdraw the stomach contents (called gastric residual).
   c. Read the amount of gastric residual.

   d. Push the stomach contents back into the stomach with the syringe.
   e. You may be instructed to hold the feeding and to call your doctor or nurse if the gastric residual is greater than _____ ml.

GIVING THE FEEDING

1. For an adult:
   a. Sit upright during the feeding and for 30 to 60 minutes *after* the feeding.
   b. If it is allowed by your doctor, you may stand or walk during your feeding.
   c. Do not lie flat, as this may cause nausea and vomiting.
2. For a child:
   a. If your child is very small and is not being fed continuously, burping may be necessary.
   b. If your child goes to bed after the feeding, place the child on his or her right side. This uses gravity to help the formula flow in the intestinal tract. The head of the bed should also be raised.

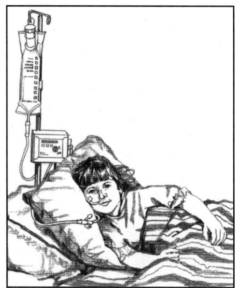

Used with permission of Ross Products Division, Abbott Laboratories, Columbus, OH, from "Tube Feeding Your Child at Home." © 1999 Ross Products Division, Abbott Laboratories.

3. For a baby:
   a. During the feeding, place the baby on his or her back or lying on the right side with the head and chest elevated.

b. If possible, hold the baby during the feeding.
c. Let the baby have a pacifier if it is allowed by your doctor.
d. Burp the baby during the feeding.
e. After the feeding, place the baby on his or her stomach or on the right side for at least 1 hour.
f. Do not lay the baby flat on his or her back, as this may cause nausea and vomiting.
   PICK SYRINGE OR GRAVITY DRIP AND PUMP FOR THE NEXT STEP.

SYRINGE

1. Remove the plunger or bulb from the syringe, then attach the syringe to the feeding tube.
2. Hold the syringe upright and pour in the feeding formula.
3. Open the clamp; the formula should run in.
4. Raising the height of the syringe makes the formula run in more quickly. Lowering the syringe slows the formula. The feeding should last about _____ minutes for an adult (_____ minutes for a baby). Do not force the feeding.

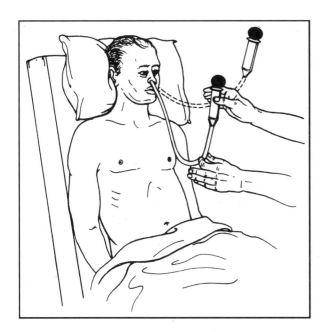

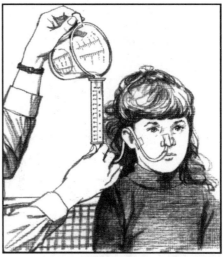

Used with permission of Ross Products Division, Abbott Laboratories, Columbus, OH, from "Tube Feeding Your Child at Home." © 1999 Ross Products Division, Abbott Laboratories.

GRAVITY DRIP AND PUMP

1. Fill the feeding administration set container or bag with feeding formula.

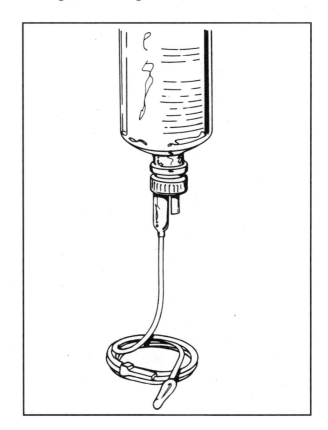

5. Add more formula before the syringe empties. This prevents air from entering the stomach.
6. When all of the formula has been given, pour the premeasured tap water into the syringe.
7. When the water has been flushed through, close the clamp and detach the syringe.
8. See *General Notes*.

2. Hang the feeding set container on an IV pole or a wall hook about 2 feet above your head for an adult or child (6 to 8 inches for a baby).

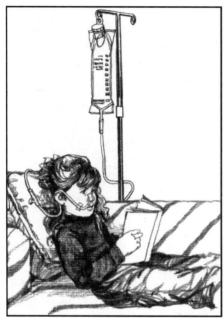

Used with permission of Ross Products Division, Abbott Laboratories, Columbus, OH, from "Tube Feeding Your Child at Home." © 1999 Ross Products Division, Abbott Laboratories.

3. Squeeze the drip chamber until it is about ⅓ to ½ full of formula.
4. Open the flow regulator clamp and fill the tube with formula. Then close the clamp.
5. Attach the tip of the tube to your feeding tube.
6. *For gravity-drip feeding,* open the flow regulator clamp and adjust the flow rate. The formula should run at _____
   _____ .

   For pump feeding, follow the manufacturer's instructions for setting the flow rate. The formula should run at _____
   _____ .

7. When all of the formula has been given, close the flow regulator clamp. Close the clamp before the drip chamber is empty. If you are using a pump, turn off the pump.
8. Pour the premeasured tap water into the container. Open the clamp (remove the tube from the pump if you are using one).
9. When the water has run in, close the clamp.
10. Clamp the feeding tube and detach the administration set's tube from the feeding tube.
11. See *General Notes.*

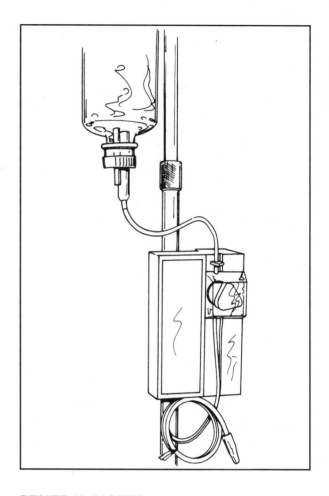

GENERAL NOTES

1. Wash all reusable equipment in warm, soapy water.
2. Keep a daily log of the date, time, and amount of each feeding.
   a. Record the amount of water and any medications given.
   b. Your nurse or doctor will explain any other information that must be recorded.
3. Follow the syringe method for giving medications. Crush and mix the medications as you were instructed.
4. If you have a nasogastric or nasointestinal tube, you may be allowed to chew. Check with your nurse or doctor before chewing anything.
5. Care of the mouth:
   a. Brush the teeth, gums, and tongue at least twice a day.
   b. Use a regular toothbrush and toothpaste.
   c. A lanolin-based moisturizing cream can be used on lips.

6. Care of the nose (nasogastric or nasointestinal):
   a. Clean the edges of both nostrils daily.
   b. You can use a cotton swab moistened with warm water.
   c. A water-soluble lubricant can be used on the nostril edges.
   d. Call your nurse or doctor if you have any signs of redness, bleeding, or numbness in your nose.
7. Taping the tube:
   a. Change the tape holding the tube daily.
   b. Cut the tape before starting.
   c. Hold the tube securely in place before removing the old tape.
   d. Wash the skin with soap and warm water. Rinse well and pat dry.
   e. If you are taping the tube to the cheek, the tube should not pull or rub on the side of the nose or the mouth; do not allow the tube to kink. Change the place on the skin where the tube is taped.

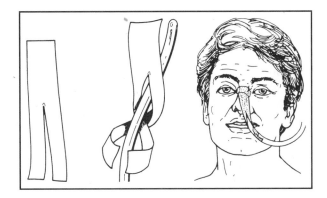

8. If using a tube holder to secure the tube, follow the manufacturer's directions.

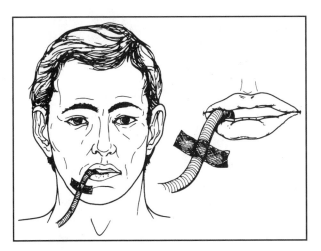

   f. If you are taping the tube to the nose,
      • Cut a piece of tape about 3 inches long,
      • Cut a piece of tape halfway down the center,
      • Place the wide part over the bridge of the nose,
      • Wrap the two thinner pieces around the tube,
      • Be careful that the tube does not rub against the side of the nose.

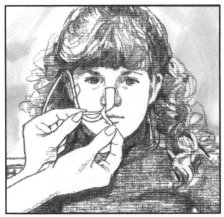

Used with permission of Ross Products Division, Abbott Laboratories, Columbus, OH, from "Tube Feeding Your Child at Home." © 1999 Ross Products Division, Abbott Laboratories.

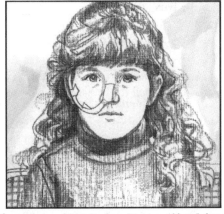

Used with permission of Ross Products Division, Abbott Laboratories, Columbus, OH, from "Tube Feeding Your Child at Home." © 1999 Ross Products Division, Abbott Laboratories.

OTHER INSTRUCTIONS

Ostomy Tube Feedings (Adult)

GUIDELINES

These guidelines will help you with your ostomy tube feeding.

PREPARING THE FEEDING

1. Your nurse or doctor will explain the type of feeding you need. Depending on your needs, you may be instructed to use a prepackaged feeding formula or to make your own feeding formula.
2. This is your feeding plan:
   a. Feeding type/name: _____
   b. Amount each day: _____
   c. Amount of each feeding or amount each hour: _____
   d. Amount of water each day: _____
   e. Amount of water *after* each feeding: _____

   _____
3. Make enough feeding formula for 1 day.
4. Label the container with the date and time of mixing.
5. Most feedings can be kept only 1 to 2 days.
6. Tube feedings may be given by syringe, gravity drip, or pump. Your tube feeding will be given by _____.

PREPARING THE EQUIPMENT

1. Wash your hands.
2. Use a measuring cup to measure the amount of formula needed. Keep unused formula in the refrigerator.
3. Measure the tap water and pour it into a container.
4. Gather all equipment and follow the directions for your feeding administration set (and pump, if used).
5. *If you need to insert the ostomy tube,*
   a. Remove the dressing over the stoma.
   b. Moisten the first 4 inches of the ostomy tube tip with tap water or water-soluble lubricant.
   c. Gently rotate the tube into the stoma about 4 to 6 inches.

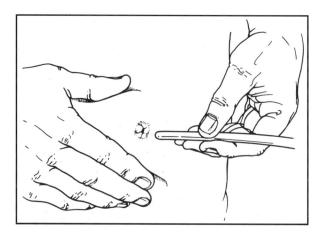

6. *If the ostomy tube, such as a percutaneous endoscopic gastrostomy (PEG) tube, is already in place,* remove the dressing to uncover the tube.

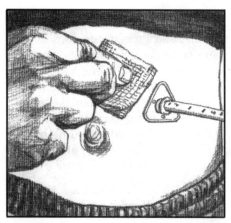

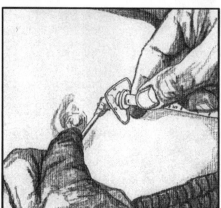

Used with permission of Ross Products Division, Abbott Laboratories, Columbus, OH, from "Tube Feeding Your Child at Home." © 1999 Ross Products Division, Abbott Laboratories.

7. If instructed to do so by the nurse or doctor, check the stomach contents.
   a. Attach the syringe to the ostomy tube (unclamp the ostomy tube if it is clamped).
   b. Draw back on the syringe's plunger to withdraw the stomach contents (called gastric residual).
   c. Read the amount of gastric residual.
   d. Using the syringe, push the stomach contents back into the stomach.
   e. You may be instructed to hold the feeding and to report gastric residual greater than _____ milliliters to your nurse or doctor.

GIVING THE FEEDING

1. Sit upright during the feeding and for 30 to 60 minutes *after* the feeding. If it is allowed by your doctor, you may stand or walk during your feeding.
2. Do not lie flat, as this may cause nausea and vomiting.
   PICK SYRINGE OR GRAVITY DRIP AND PUMP FOR THE NEXT STEP.

SYRINGE

1. Remove the plunger or bulb from the syringe, then attach the syringe to the ostomy tube.
2. Hold the syringe upright and pour in the feeding formula.
3. Open the clamp; the formula should run in.

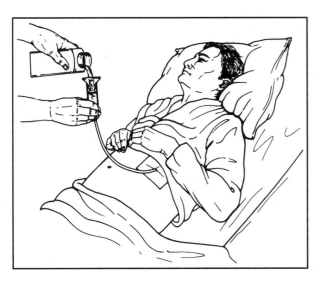

4. Raising the height of the syringe makes the formula run in more quickly. Lowering the syringe slows the formula. The feeding should last about _____ to _____ minutes.

5. Add more formula before the syringe empties. This prevents air from entering the stomach.
6. When all the formula has been given, pour the tap water into the syringe.
7. Close the clamp and detach the syringe.
8. See *General Notes*.

GRAVITY DRIP AND PUMP

1. Fill the feeding administration set container or bag with feeding formula.
2. Hang the feeding set container on an IV pole or a wall hook about 2 feet above your head.
3. Squeeze the drip chamber until it is about ⅓ to ½ full of formula.
4. Open the flow regulator clamp and fill the tube with formula. Then close the clamp.
5. Attach the tip of the tube to your ostomy tube.
6. *For gravity-drip feeding,* open the flow regulator clamp and adjust the flow rate. The formula should run at _____.
   For pump feeding, follow the manufacturer's instructions for setting the flow rate. The formula should run at _____.

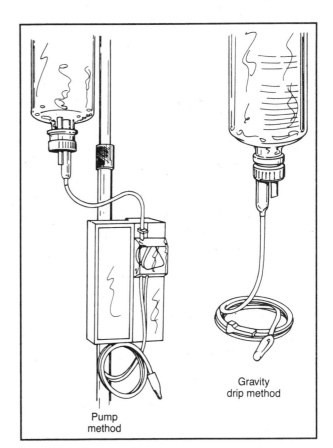

Pump method

Gravity drip method

7. When all of the formula has been given, close the flow regulator clamp. Close the clamp be-

fore the drip chamber is empty. If you are using a pump, turn the pump off.

8. Pour the premeasured tap water into the container. Open the clamp or turn on the pump.
9. When the water has run in, close the clamp or turn off the pump.
10. Clamp the ostomy tube and detach the administration set's tube from the ostomy tube.
11. See *General Notes*.

GENERAL NOTES

1. Wash all reusable equipment in warm soapy water, rinse well, and dry thoroughly. Store equipment in a clean, closed container.
2. Keep a daily log of the date, time, and amount of each feeding.
   a. Record the amount of water and any medications given.

b. Your nurse or doctor will explain any other information that must be recorded.
3. Follow the syringe method for giving medications. Crush and mix the medications as you were instructed to do.
4. Care of the skin around the stoma after a tube feeding:
   a. Wash the skin with warm water and soap.
   b. Rinse the skin well with warm water. Pat the skin dry.
   c. Your doctor may prescribe an ointment to protect the skin.
   d. Call your nurse or doctor if you have any skin redness; bleeding, yellow, or green drainage from the stoma; or a change in the color in the stoma.
   e. Your nurse or doctor will teach you about dressings you may need.

OTHER INSTRUCTIONS

Ostomy Tube Feedings (Infant and Child)

GUIDELINES

These guidelines will help you with your baby's or child's ostomy tube feeding.

PREPARING THE FEEDING

1. Your nurse or doctor will explain the type of feeding you need. Depending on your needs, you may be instructed to use a prepackaged feeding formula or to make your own feeding formula.
2. This is the feeding plan:
   a. Feeding type/name: _____
   b. Amount each day: _____
   c. Amount of each feeding or amount each hour: _____
   d. Amount of water each day: _____
   e. Amount of water *after* each feeding: _____
   _____
3. Make enough feeding formula for 1 day.
4. Label the container with the date and time of mixing.
5. Most feedings can be kept only 1 to 2 days.
6. Tube feedings may be given by syringe, gravity drip, or pump. Your tube feeding will be given by _____.

PREPARING THE EQUIPMENT

1. Wash your hands.
2. Use a measuring cup to measure the amount of formula needed. Keep unused formula in the refrigerator.
3. Measure the tap water and pour it into a container.
4. Gather all equipment and follow the directions for your feeding administration set (and pump, if used).
5. *If you need to change the ostomy tube,*
   a. Before removing the old tube (catheter), test the new catheter:
      • Use the syringe to put 5 milliliters (ml) of water into the shorter tube of the catheter to fill the balloon. Check the balloon for leaks.
      • Use the syringe to remove the water from the balloon.

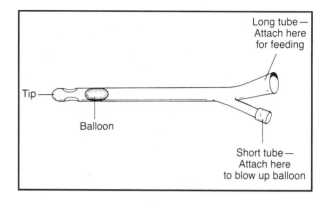

b. Cut three or four small air vents in the wide part of the nipple. Do not cut off the top of the nipple.

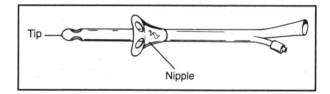

c. Pull the catheter through the top of the nipple with a tweezer.
d. Remove the dressing if there is one.
e. Place the syringe into the shorter tube of the old catheter. Pull back on the syringe plunger to remove the water from the balloon (about 5 ml). This will deflate the balloon.
f. Remove the catheter after deflating balloon.
g. Moisten the tip of the catheter.
h. Gently insert the catheter into the stomach about 2 to 3 inches (depending on the age and size of the child).
i. Fill the syringe with 5 ml of water.

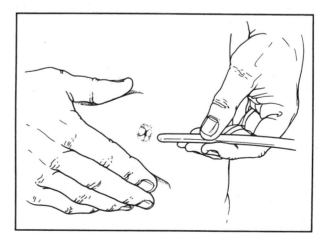

j. Place the syringe into the shorter tube of the catheter. Push the water in to fill the balloon.

k. Gently pull back on the catheter until you feel resistance.

l. Slide the nipple down until it rests against the stomach.

6. If the ostomy tube is already in place, remove the dressing to uncover the tube.

   a. To check gastrostomy or jejunostomy tube placement,

   • Use a nonstretchable tape measure to find the number of inches from the stoma to the end of the tube.

   • Compare this number with previous measurements. If the measurement differs by more than _____ inches, call your nurse or doctor.

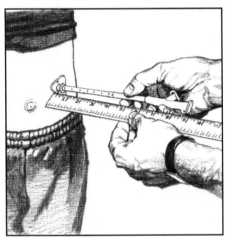

Used with permission of Ross Products Division, Abbott Laboratories, Columbus, OH, from "Tube Feeding Your Child at Home." © 1999 Ross Products Division, Abbott Laboratories.

7. If instructed to do so by the nurse or doctor, check the stomach contents.

   a. Attach the syringe to the ostomy tube (unclamp the ostomy tube if it is clamped).

   b. Draw back on the syringe's plunger to withdraw stomach contents (called gastric residual).

   c. Read the amount of gastric residual.

   d. Using the syringe, push the stomach contents back into the stomach.

   e. You may be instructed to hold the feeding and to report gastric residual greater than _____ ml to your nurse or doctor.

   f. If you cannot obtain stomach contents but your child feels unusually full or nauseated, delay the feeding for 30 to 60 minutes. Check for residual again. If residual is still high, call your nurse or doctor.

g. Residual cannot be obtained when jejunostomy and duodenal tubes are in their proper place.

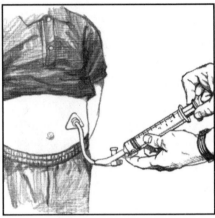

Used with permission of Ross Products Division, Abbott Laboratories, Columbus, OH, from "Tube Feeding Your Child at Home." © 1999 Ross Products Division, Abbott Laboratories.

GIVING THE FEEDING

1. Formula should be at room temperature.
2. Place your child in a highchair, car seat, or other comfortable chair. Be sure that his or her head is raised 45 degrees or more. If possible, hold the baby during the feeding. Let the baby suck on a pacifier if it is permitted by your doctor.
3. After the feeding, keep the baby or child on his or her right side or propped in a sitting position.
4. Do not lay the baby or child flat on his or her back for 1 hour after the feeding, as this may cause nausea and vomiting.

PICK SYRINGE OR GRAVITY DRIP AND PUMP FOR THE NEXT STEP.

SYRINGE

1. Remove the plunger or bulb from the syringe, then attach the syringe to the ostomy tube.
2. Hold the syringe upright and pour in the feeding formula.
3. Open the clamp; the formula should run in.
4. Raising the height of the syringe makes the formula run in more quickly. Lowering the syringe slows the formula. The feeding should last about _____ to _____ minutes.
5. Add more formula before the syringe empties. This prevents air from entering the stomach.
6. When all of the formula has been given, pour the tap water into the syringe.
7. Close the clamp and detach the syringe.
8. See *General Notes.*

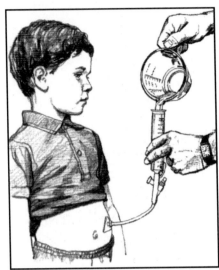

Used with permission of Ross Products Division, Abbott Laboratories, Columbus, OH, from "Tube Feeding Your Child at Home." © 1999 Ross Products Division, Abbott Laboratories.

GRAVITY DRIP AND PUMP

1. Fill the feeding administration set container or bag with feeding formula.
2. Hang the feeding set container on an IV pole or a wall hook. Place your child in a highchair, car seat, or other comfortable chair. Be sure that his or her head is raised 45 degrees or more. For a baby, hang the feeding only about 4 inches above the baby.
3. Squeeze the drip chamber until it is about ⅓ to ½ full of formula.
4. Open the flow regulator clamp and fill the tube with formula. Then close the clamp.
5. Attach the tip of the tube to the ostomy tube.
6. *For gravity-drip feeding,* open the flow regulator clamp and adjust the flow rate.
The formula should run at _____.
For pump feeding, follow the manufacturer's instructions for setting the flow rate. The formula should run at _____.
7. When all of the formula has been given, close the flow regulator clamp. Close the clamp before the drip chamber is empty. If you are using a pump, turn off the pump.
8. Pour the premeasured tap water into the container. Open the clamp or turn on the pump.
9. When the water has run in, close the clamp or turn off the pump.
10. Clamp the ostomy tube and detach the administration set's tube from the ostomy tube.

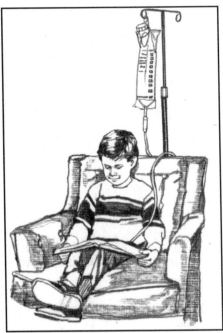

Used with permission of Ross Products Division, Abbott Laboratories, Columbus, OH, from "Tube Feeding Your Child at Home." © 1999 Ross Products Division, Abbott Laboratories.

GENERAL NOTES

1. Wash all reusable equipment in warm soapy water, rinse well, and dry thoroughly. Store equipment in a clean, closed container.
2. Keep a daily log of the date, time, and amount of each feeding.
   a. Record the amount of water given and any medications given.
   b. Your nurse or doctor will explain any other information that must be recorded.
3. Follow the syringe method for giving medications. Crush and mix the medications as you were instructed to do.
4. Care of the skin around the stoma after a tube feeding:
   a. Wash the skin with warm water and soap.
   b. Rinse the skin well with warm water. Pat the skin dry.
   c. Your doctor may prescribe an ointment to protect the skin.
   d. Call your nurse or doctor if you see any skin redness; bleeding, yellow, or green drainage from the stoma; or a change in the color in the stoma.
   e. Your nurse or doctor will teach you about dressings you may need.

Tube Feeding: Special Conditions

Tube feedings can result in some body discomfort. Ways to cope with them are discussed below.

CONDITIONS

Diarrhea

What It Is. Frequent, loose, and watery stools (bowel movements).

What It Feels Like. Frequent, loose, and watery stools; stomach cramping or churning; nausea.

What Causes It. Certain medications, certain types of tube feeding, too much feeding at one time, taking the feeding too fast, and using a tube feeding that is very cold.

What to Do

1. Give feedings slowly and more often, but in smaller amounts.
2. Do not use feedings that have not been refrigerated or feedings that are more than 2 days old.
3. Have the patient relax 30 minutes before and 30 minutes after the feeding. If allowed, a walk after the feeding may help digestion.
4. Be sure all the equipment used for feedings is carefully cleaned and rinsed.
5. Increase the amount of water used after each feeding (about 2 to 4 cups or 500 to 1000 ml a day). Diluting the feeding may also be helpful.
6. *Call your nurse or doctor if diarrhea lasts more than 2 to 3 days.*

Constipation

What It Is. Difficulty in passing stool (bowel movements), infrequent hard stools.

What It Feels Like. Straining to move bowels, loss of appetite, feeling uncomfortably full, headache.

What Causes It. Tube feedings can change bowel movement routines (usually bowel movements occur less often), as can certain medications and changes in diet and activity.

What to Do

1. Establish a routine for bowel movements.
2. Keep a record of bowel movements.
3. Increase amount of water used after feeding.

4. Have one glass of prune juice in warm water at the morning feeding. Rinse the tube with water.
5. *Call your nurse or doctor if constipation lasts more than 5 to 7 days.*

Stomach Upset

What It Is. Stomach discomfort or upset.

What It Feels Like. Nausea, vomiting, feeling of fullness, heartburn, gas pains.

What Causes It. Too much feeding at one time, feedings that are too cold or are too old, intolerance to a certain feeding formula.

What to Do

1. Give feedings slowly and more often, but in smaller amounts. Diluting the feeding may help.
2. Sit upright during feeding and remain upright or walk (if allowed) for at least 30 to 60 minutes after the feeding.
3. Avoid strenuous exercise right after a feeding.
4. If you feel full, wait about an hour before taking the feeding. Do not force a feeding.
5. Do not take a feeding when nauseated or vomiting.
6. *Call your nurse or doctor if you continue to have stomach upset, nausea, or vomiting.*

Dehydration

What It Is. The body is not getting enough fluid or loses too much fluid because of fever, diarrhea, or vomiting.

What It Feels Like. Feeling very thirsty; dry mouth; cracked lips; fever; dry, warm skin; weight loss; weakness; decreasing amount of urine.

What Causes It. Medications; prolonged fever, diarrhea, or vomiting; not taking enough fluid.

What to Do

1. Take the amount of water you have been instructed to take each day.
2. Weigh yourself at least twice a week at the same time of the day.
3. Take extra fluids if you have fever, diarrhea, or symptoms of dehydration.
4. *Call your nurse or doctor if you have symptoms of dehydration or if you lose more than 2 pounds in a week.*
5. Discuss any questions with your nurse or doctor.

Protein-Controlled Diets

Protein-Restricted Diet (40 Grams)

DESCRIPTION

Both animal and vegetable proteins are included in the calculation of protein-restricted diets. In certain stages of some types of liver and kidney disease, protein intake may need to be restricted.

ADEQUACY

Adequacy varies depending on level of protein restriction. Thiamine, riboflavin, niacin, and calcium levels of this diet do not meet the Recommended Daily Allowances.

Protein-Restricted Food Guide	
Food Group	Allowed
Milk (½ cup day)	Milk (fat-free, reduced fat, whole) ½ cup, buttermilk ½ cup, half & half ½ cup, cream cheese 3 tbsp. Ice cream ½ cup, yogurt ½ cup, sherbet 1 cup
Meat (3 oz/day)	Beef, lamb, veal, pork, fish, egg, cheese
Starch choices (4 servings/day)	Spaghetti ½ cup, rice ½ cup, potatoes ½ cup, macaroni ½ cup, noodles ½ cup, bread 1 slice, cereals ¾ cup
Desserts (1 serving/day)	Cake angel food—1 oz, cake 2″ × 2″ square, shortbread cookies 4, vanilla wafers 10, gelatin ½ cup, fruit pie ⅛ pie
Vegetables (2 servings/day)	½ cup serving size
Fruit (4 servings/day)	1 cup juice or ½ cup canned fruit, 1 medium apple, pear, tangerine
Fats (as desired)	1 tsp margarine, butter, mayonnaise, 1 tbsp salad dressing
High-calorie choices (as desired)	Each serving size contains approximately 100 calories and a trace of protein
Carbonated beverages	1 cup
Lemonade	1 cup
Fruit ice	½ cup
Popsicle	1 bar
Sorbet	½ cup
Candy and sweets (as desired)	
Hard candy	4 pieces
Marshmallows	5
Sugar	2 tbsp
Fruit roll-ups	2

From Chilton Memorial Hospital, Pompton Plains, NJ.

High-Calorie, High-Protein Diet

DESCRIPTION

Calories come from all foods and are used by the body for energy. Protein is necessary for growth and repair of body tissues. Calories must be supplied in sufficient amounts to prevent protein from being wasted. If insufficient calories are given, protein would be used for energy instead of important tissue building.

High-Calorie, High-Protein Diet

You may be experiencing problems eating because of loss of appetite or nausea. Or you simply need to gain weight or help your body heal. The following suggestions are provided to help you add more calories and protein to your eating plan.

Food Categories	Foods Recommended	Tips
▲ **BREADS, CEREALS, RICE, AND PASTA 6–11 SERVINGS EACH DAY**		
Serving size = 1 slice bread 1 oz ready-to-eat cereal ½ cup cooked cereal, rice, or pasta ½ bun, bagel, or English muffin 1 small roll, biscuit, or muffin 3–4 small or 2 large crackers 1 6-inch tortilla	All; try whole-grain breads, muffins, croissants, crescent rolls, waffles, pancakes, and granola cereal	Top breads, pancakes, and waffles with extra margarine, jams, cream cheese, dried fruits, nuts, and syrups. Spread peanut butter on crackers, bread, French toast, and waffles. Prepare pasta and rice dishes with cream or cheese sauces.
▲ **VEGETABLES 3–5 SERVINGS EACH DAY**		
Serving size = 1 cup raw leafy, ½ cup cooked or chopped raw, ¾ cup vegetable juice	All Vegetable juices	Add avocado slices or guacamole to salads and sandwiches. Prepare vegetables au gratin, buttered, or creamed. Stuff fruits and vegetables with cottage cheese or ricotta cheese.
▲ **FRUITS 2–4 SERVINGS EACH DAY**		
Serving size = 1 medium size, ½ cup chopped, cooked, or canned, ¾ cup juice, ¼ cup dried	All fresh, dried, or canned in syrup Fruit juices	Blend or whip ice cream or cream with fruit. Select canned fruit with added sugar or canned in syrup. Sweeten fruit with sugar or honey.
▲ **MILK, YOGURT, AND CHEESE 2–3 SERVINGS EACH DAY**		
Serving size = 1 cup milk or yogurt 1½ oz natural cheese 2 oz processed cheese	All; especially whole milk and milk products, full-fat cheeses	Stir powdered milk into soups, sauces, egg dishes, and casseroles. Substitute cream for milk in any recipe. Melt cheese on eggs, fish, hamburgers, and sandwiches.
▲ **MEATS, POULTRY, FISH, DRY BEANS AND PEAS, EGGS, AND NUTS 2–3 SERVINGS EACH DAY**		
Serving size = 2–3 oz cooked lean meat, poultry, or fish; **count** 1 egg, ½ cup cooked dried beans, 2 tbsp peanut butter, ⅓ cup nuts, 3 tbsp textured soy protein, or 2 oz tofu **as 1 oz of meat**	All beef, pork, lamb, veal, poultry, fish Eggs Dried peas and beans Peanut butter Textured soy protein Tofu	Pack more protein into your food by adding extra chopped meat, shredded cheese, textured soy protein, hard-cooked eggs, and egg substitutes to soups, sauces, vegetables, and casseroles. Mix cooked or canned beans into casseroles, rice dishes, pasta, or salad. Add tofu to soups and cheesecake.

Table continued on opposite page

High-Calorie, High-Protein Diet *Continued*

Food Categories	Foods Recommended	Tips
▲ FATS, SNACKS, SWEETS, CONDIMENTS, AND BEVERAGES		
	All kinds of fats; margarine, butter, whipped cream, gravy, cream cheese, salad dressings Jams, jellies, sugar, honey, syrups, candy Cakes, cookies, pies, pudding, custard, ice cream	Add more flavor to your food with herbs and spices, mustard, and lemon. Keep snacks like granola, pudding cups, ice cream, and cookies handy. Boost calories by adding margarine, sour cream, and other fats to food whenever possible.

Important Points to Keep in Mind

- Stock your pantry with your favorite foods.
- Eat smaller meals and snacks every couple of hours.
- Blend instant breakfast into beverages to boost calories and protein.
- Talk to a registered dietitian about commercial supplements that are high in calories and protein.

Sample Menu: High-Calorie, High-Protein Diet

BREAKFAST	SNACK	LUNCH	SNACK	DINNER
Orange juice (¾ cup) Whole-grain cereal with dried fruit (1 cup) Wheat toast (1 slice) with margarine (1 tsp) and jelly (1 tsp) Whole milk* (1 cup)	Peanut butter (2 tbsp) Crackers (4)	Cream soup (1 cup) Hamburger (3 oz) on bun American cheese (1 slice) Mayonnaise (½ tbsp) Fresh fruit salad (1 cup) with yogurt Fruit juice (¾ cup)	Milkshake* with added fruit Chocolate-covered graham crackers (4)	Breaded chicken breast (3 oz) Baked potato (1) with margarine (1 tbsp) and sour cream (4 tbsp) Green beans (½ cup) Chocolate pudding Whole milk* (1 cup)

* Drink double-strength whenever possible. Blend whole milk with dry skim milk powder. Use 1 cup of powder for each quart of milk. Blend well and chill.

© 1996, The American Dietetic Association. *Manual of Clinical Dietetics.* Used with permission.

OTHER INSTRUCTIONS

Nutrition Lists

Guide to Minerals

Guide to Minerals

Mineral	Best Sources	Functions	Deficiency Symptoms
Calcium (1000 mg)	Milk and milk products	Strong bones, teeth, muscle tissue, regulates heart beat, muscle action and nerve function, blood clotting	Soft brittle bones, back and leg pains, heart palpitations, tetany
Chromium (No RDA)	Corn oil, clams, whole-grain cereals, brewer's yeast	Glucose metabolism (energy), increases effectiveness of insulin	Atherosclerosis, glucose intolerance in diabetics
Copper (2 mg)	Oysters, nuts, organ meats, legumes	Formation of red blood cells, bone growth and health, works with vitamin C to form elastin	General weakness, impaired respiration, skin sores
Iodine (150 μg)	Seafood, iodized salt	Component of hormone thyroxine, which controls metabolism	Goiter, dry skin and hair, nervousness, obesity
Iron (18 mg)	Meats and organ meats, fish, leafy green vegetables	Hemoglobin formation, improves blood quality, increases resistance to stress and disease	Anemia (pale skin, fatigue), constipation, breathing difficulties
Magnesium (400 mg)	Nuts, green vegetables, whole grains	Acid/alkaline balance, important in metabolism of carbohydrates, minerals and sugar	Nervousness, tremors, easily aroused anger, disorientation, blood clots
Manganese (No RDA)	Nuts, whole grains, vegetables, fruits	Enzyme activation, carbohydrate and fat production, sex hormone production, skeletal development	Dizziness, poor muscle coordination, ear noises
Phosphorus (1000 mg)	Fish, meat, poultry, eggs, grains	Bone development, important in protein, fat, and carbohydrate use	Poor bones and teeth, arthritis, rickets, appetite loss, irregular breathing
Potassium (No RDA)	Lean meat, vegetables, fruits	Fluid balance, controls activity of heart muscle, nervous system, kidneys	Poor reflexes, irregular heartbeat, dry skin, general weakness
Selenium (50–200 μg provisional RDA)	Seafood, organ meats, lean meats, grains	Protects body tissues against oxidative damage from radiation, pollution and normal metabolic processing	Heart muscle abnormalities
Zinc (15 mg)	Lean meats, liver, eggs, seafood, whole grains	Involved in digestion and metabolism. Important in development of reproductive system, aids in healing	Retarded growth, prolonged wound healing, loss of appetite

Used with permission of the American Institute for Cancer Research, Washington, DC 20069.

Guide to Vitamins

Guide to Vitamins

Vitamin (US RDA)	Best Sources	Functions	Deficiency Symptoms
A (5000 IU)	Liver, eggs, yellow and green fruits and vegetables, milk and dairy products, fish liver oil	Growth and repair of body tissues (resist infection), bone and tooth formation, visual purple production (necessary for night vision)	Night blindness; dry, scaly skin, loss of smell and appetite; susceptibility to infection; frequent fatigue; tooth decay
B_1 Thiamin (1.5 mg)	Wheat germ, yeast, liver, whole grains, nuts, fish, poultry, beans, meat	Carbohydrate metabolism, appetite maintenance, nerve function, growth and muscle tone	Heart irregularity, nerve disorders, fatigue, loss of appetite, forgetfulness
B_2 Riboflavin (1.7 mg)	Whole grains, green leafy vegetables, organ meats	Necessary for fat, carbohydrate, and protein metabolism, cell respiration, formation of antibodies and red blood cells	Eye problems, cracks in corners of mouth, digestive disturbances
B_6 Pyridoxine (2.0 mg)	Fish, poultry, lean meats	Necessary for fat, carbohydrate and protein metabolism, formation of antibodies, maintains sodium/potassium balance (nerves)	Nervousness, dermatitis, blood disorders, muscular weakness, insulin sensitivity, skin cracks, anemia
B_{12} Cobalamin (6 μg)	Organ meats, eggs, milk, fish, cheese	Carbohydrate, fat, protein metabolism, maintains healthy nervous system, blood cell formation	Pernicious anemia, nervousness, neuritis, fatigue, brain degeneration
Biotin (300 μg)	Yeast, organ meats, legumes, eggs	Carbohydrate, fat, and protein metabolism, formation of fatty acids, helps utilize B vitamins	Dry, grayish skin, depression, muscle pain, fatigue, poor appetite
Choline (No RDA)	Organ meats, soybeans, fish, wheat germ, egg yolk	Nerve transmission, metabolism of fats and cholesterol, regulates liver and gallbladder	High blood pressure, bleeding stomach ulcers, liver and kidney problems
Folic Acid Folacin (400 μg)	Green leafy vegetables, organ meats, milk products	Red blood cell formation, protein metabolism, growth and cell division	Anemia, gastrointestinal troubles, poor growth
Niacin (20 mg)	Meat, poultry, fish, milk products, peanuts, brewer's yeast	Fat, carbohydrate and protein metabolism, health of skin, tongue and digestive system, blood circulation	General fatigue, indigestion, irritability, loss of appetite, skin disorders
Pantothenic Acid (10 mg)	Lean meats, whole grains, legumes	Converts nutrients into energy, formation of some fats, vitamin utilization	Vomiting, stomach stress, restlessness, infections, muscle cramps
C Ascorbic Acid (60 mg)	Citrus fruits, vegetables, tomatoes, potatoes	Helps heal wounds, strength to blood vessels, collagen maintenance, resistance to infection	Bleeding gums, slow healing wounds, bruising, aching joints, nosebleeds, poor digestion
D (400 IU)	Fish-liver oils, egg yolks, organ meats, fish, fortified milk	Calcium and phosphorus metabolism (bone formation), heart action, nervous system maintenance	Rickets, poor bone growth, nervous system irritability
E (30 IU)	Vegetable oils, green vegetables, wheat germ, organ meats, eggs	Protects red blood cells, inhibits coagulation of blood, protects fat-soluble vitamins, cellular respiration	Muscular wasting, abnormal fat deposits in muscles, gastrointestinal disease, heart disease
K (No RDA)	Green leafy vegetables, fruit, cereal, dairy products	Important in formation of blood clotting agents	Tendency to hemorrhage

Used with permission from the American Institute for Cancer Research, Washington, DC 20069.

Potassium Content of Common Foods

DESCRIPTION

Potassium plays a role in keeping your heart beat regular and your muscles working properly. It is the job of the kidneys to keep the right amount of potassium in your body. The following are high-potassium foods that you may need to modify in your diet.

High-Potassium Foods—201–350 mg per serving

Fruits	Vegetables	Other Foods
Apricot	Artichokes	Bran/bran products
Avocado	Asparagus	Coffee
Banana	Bamboo shoots	Chocolate
Cantaloupe	Beans, dried	Coconut
Casaba	Beets	Granola
Dates	Broccoli	Ice cream
Dried fruits	Brussels sprouts	Molasses
Figs	Celery	Milk
Honeydew	Escarole	Nuts/seeds
Kiwi	Endive	Salt substitute/lite salt
Mango	Greens (swiss chard, collard, dandelion, mustard, beet)	Snuff/chewing tobacco
Nectarine	Kale	Tea
Orange	Kohlrabi	Yogurt
Papaya	Lentils	
Pear	Legumes	
Plums	Lima beans	
Prunes	Mushrooms	
Raisins	Okra	
Rhubarb	Parsnips	
Juice of these fruits	Pepper-chili	
	Potatoes (french fried, baked, sweet)	
	Pumpkin	
	Rutabagas	
	Spinach	
	Vegetable juice	
	Tomatoes—all products	
	Winter squash	
	Yams	

From Chilton Memorial Hospital, Pompton Plains, NJ.

Hematology and Oncology Alterations

Breast Self-Examination

GENERAL INFORMATION

Breast self-examination should be a routine part of your personal care. It helps you learn how your breasts normally look and feel. Breast self-examination also helps you detect changes in your breasts. Being able to detect changes in your breasts is an important part of finding breast cancer in its early stages. Patients with breast cancers that are found early and treated right away have the best chance of being cured.

GUIDELINES

Use the following guidelines to help you remember how to do breast self-examination.

1. Gather your equipment. You will need
   a. A pillow or folded towel,
   b. A free-standing mirror,
   c. Body lotion.
2. Stand in front of the mirror. Undress to the waist.
3. Relax your arms at your sides.
4. Look at your breasts in the mirror and look for
   a. Changes in shape,
   b. Swelling,
   c. Dimpling of the skin,
   d. Changes in the nipple,
   e. Blue-tinged skin,
   f. Skin that looks like orange peel.
5. Raise your arms up in the air and look again for
   a. Changes in shape,
   b. Swelling,
   c. Dimpling of the skin,
   d. Changes in the nipple,
   e. Blue-tinged skin,
   f. Skin that looks like orange peel.
6. Lower your arms and rest your palms on your hips. Press down firmly on your hips and inspect your breasts. Look at your front, your left side, and your right side.
7. Sweep down your breasts from the collar bone to nipples. Use your palms and fingers. Sometimes, this part of breast self-examination is easier to do when you are in the shower.

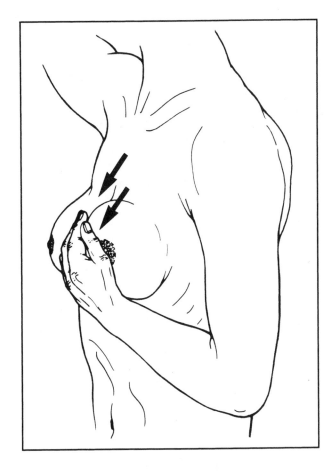

8. Gently grasp the tissue between your underarm and breast, and squeeze gently in a rolling motion. Do this for both sides. You are feeling for lumps.
9. Lie down on your bed. Put the pillow or folded towel under your right shoulder and place your right hand behind your head.
10. Feel your right breast by moving your left hand in a circle (see next page). Your hand should be moving clockwise on your breast (see next page). Start at 12:00 and move on to 1:00, 2:00, etc. Putting body lotion on your fingertips makes this step easier.
11. Inch your fingers toward the nipple and repeat the circle. Continue doing this until you have examined your whole breast. Be alert to any tender areas and any lumps.
12. Squeeze the nipple between your thumb and index finger. Look for any discharge from the nipple.

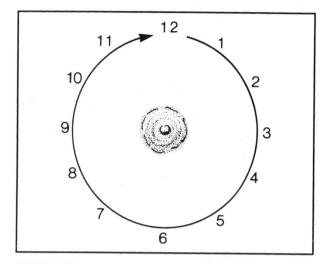

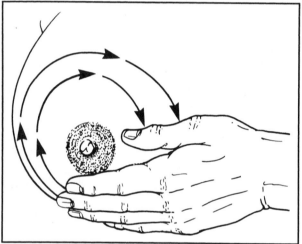

13. Press your nipple with your index and middle fingers, and feel the area underneath the nipple.
14. Put the pillow or folded towel under your left shoulder and place your left hand behind your head. Repeat steps 10 to 13 for the left breast.
15. Do breast self-examination every month. If you are menstruating, examine your breasts 1 week after your period ends. If you are postmenopausal, do it on your birthdate or another easily remembered date of the month.
16. CALL YOUR DOCTOR RIGHT AWAY IF YOU FIND
    - A lump,
    - Discharge from the nipple,
    - Dimpling of the skin,
    - Blue-tinged skin,
    - Swelling,
    - Tenderness,
    - Changes in the shape of your breast,
    - Skin that looks like orange peel.

OTHER INSTRUCTIONS

Hair Loss

GENERAL INFORMATION

Hair loss, or alopecia, usually begins about 2 weeks after chemotherapy treatments have started. It may occur suddenly or slowly. You may lose some of your hair or all of it. The most common site of alopecia is the head. Hair loss may also affect the genital area, the beard, the eyebrows, and the eyelashes.

Alopecia is a temporary side effect. Sometimes your hair regrowth begins while you are still receiving chemotherapy. Usually, though, it begins 2 or 3 months after the chemotherapy treatments have ended. When it does return, your hair may be a slightly different color; it may have a different texture or fullness.

GUIDELINES

The following suggestions will help you deal successfully with alopecia.

Reduce the Hair Loss

1. Make sure your diet is well balanced. The nurse or dietitian can teach you how to do this.
2. Balance your rest and exercise. The nurse can teach you how to conserve your energy by modifying your daily activities.
3. Avoid harsh shampoos; use baby shampoo instead.
4. Blot your hair dry after shampooing. Do not rub it.
5. Do not brush your hair when it is wet. Use a large wide-tooth comb to disentangle and style your hair.
6. When you do brush your hair, use a soft natural-bristle brush.

Disguise the Hair Loss

1. Use a wig. Wigs can be purchased from your hairdresser or from retail stores. The American Cancer Society may also have suitable wigs available. Most wigs have easy instructions for wash and wear. Buy the wig before the alopecia is extreme so you can match it to your own hair color. Practice wearing it so you get used to having it on. Your hairdresser can be very helpful if you want to experiment with wigs of different colors and styles.
2. Wear hats. A milliner can help you choose fashionable hats and headpieces that look good on you.
3. Wear head scarves. Learn how to arrange a scarf in a simple back knot or a more exotic twist. Ask people who routinely wear scarves to teach you. Pretwisted scarves with attached hairpieces are also available through most prostheses shops.
4. Use eyebrow pencil. Select a color slightly lighter than your natural color. Make-up consultants in department stores can assist you. Your eyebrow should start at the point over the inner corner of the eye. The highest arch should be above the outer part of the iris. The end of the brow should not be lower than the beginning. Apply the eyebrow pencil in light tiny lines, using the pencil to fill in gaps between your eyebrow hairs.
5. Use false eyelashes. The cosmetologists in department stores or at your hairdresser's can help you select the best eyelashes for you and can teach you how to apply them.

OTHER INSTRUCTIONS

How to Care for a Dry or Tender Mouth

GENERAL INFORMATION

A dry or tender mouth is a common side effect of many chemotherapeutic agents. The following suggestions can help ease the oral discomfort.

GUIDELINES

1. Rinse with saline, a 1:1 saline/hydrogen peroxide mixture, or a mixture of 1 teaspoon baking soda in 1 cup warm water at least every 2 hours.
2. Do not use commercial mouthwashes.
3. Avoid smoking and alcohol.
4. Avoid extremely hot foods and beverages.
5. Eat soft foods with low acid content.
6. Avoid spices.
7. Use a soft-bristle toothbrush or toothette at least twice a day.
8. Use a topical anesthetic.
9. Suck on popsicles or hard candy.
10. Use a lip balm, water-based lubricant, or petroleum jelly frequently throughout the day.
11. Use artificial saliva.
12. Swish and swallow with a mixture of 1 part orange juice to 3 parts cool water.

OTHER INSTRUCTIONS

How to Cope with Itchy Skin

GENERAL INFORMATION

Itchy skin, or pruritus, is a common side effect of many chemotherapeutic agents. It is also a frequent symptom for people with neoplastic disease. Itchy skin is more than just uncomfortable. It can cause you to scratch enough to open small cuts in your skin, which makes you susceptible to local and body-wide infections.

GUIDELINES

1. Apply a water-based moisturizer frequently throughout the day.
2. Protect skin from temperature extremes.
3. Use cool or lukewarm water for showers and baths.
4. Add cornstarch, baking soda, oatmeal, or soybean powder to bath water.
5. Apply cool wet packs to the skin.
6. Wear lightweight and loose-fitting cotton clothes.
7. Control the itching response by using a vibrator or finger/hand pressure on the itchy area.
8. Control the itching response by using distraction, imagery, or relaxation techniques.

Tell your nurse or doctor if your skin

- Becomes swollen, tender, or very red;
- Develops a rash of any kind;
- Has weeping or oozing blisters.

OTHER INSTRUCTIONS

How to Lessen the Risk of Bleeding

GENERAL INFORMATION

The tendency to bleed is a common side effect of many chemotherapeutic agents. It is also a symptom of many hematologic diseases. The following suggestions can help reduce the risk of bleeding.

GUIDELINES

1. Avoid intramuscular injections when possible.
2. Avoid measuring temperature rectally.
3. Use electric razors.
4. Use soft-bristle toothbrushes.
5. Keep fingernails and toenails short and carefully trimmed.
6. Prevent constipation.
7. Routinely inspect mouth, skin, stool, and urine for blood or signs of bleeding.
8. Avoid strenuous activity and activity that may cause trauma or injury.
9. Avoid the use of aspirin and aspirin-containing substances.
10. Do not walk barefoot.
11. Do not use dental floss.
12. Apply ice and firm pressure to minor cuts of the skin and tongue.

Tell your nurse or doctor *immediately* if you

- Are coughing up blood;
- Have bright red blood in your urine or stool;
- Have bleeding that does not stop.

OTHER INSTRUCTIONS

Postmastectomy Exercises

GENERAL INFORMATION

Postmastectomy exercises are designed to help you increase your ability to move the arm on your operative side. Make these exercises a part of your daily routine in order to get the best results possible. Try to do them in front of a mirror. This will let you see if you are doing the exercises correctly. You may feel some discomfort as you exercise, but the exercises should not cause you pain. If this happens, stop exercising and call the nurse.

EXERCISES

Arm Swings

Stand with your feet 8 inches apart. Bend forward from the waist, allowing your arms to hang toward the floor. Swing both arms up to the sides to reach shoulder level. Swing your arms back to the center, then cross them at the center. Do not bend your elbows.

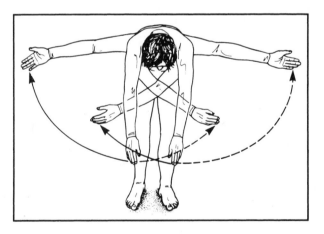

Pulley Motion

Using the arm on the operative side, toss a 6-foot rope over a shower curtain rod (or over the top of a door that has a nail in the top to hold the rope in place for the exercise). Grasp one end of the rope in each hand. Slowly raise the arm on your operative side as far as is comfortable by pulling down on the rope on the opposite side. Keep the raised arm close to your head. Now lower the arm on the operative side in order to raise the other arm. Repeat.

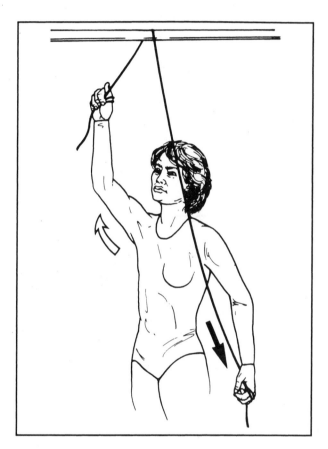

Hand Wall Climbing

Stand facing the wall, with your toes 6 to 12 inches from the wall (see next page). Bend your elbows and place your palms against the wall at shoulder level. Gradually move both hands up the wall, parallel to each other until you feel pulling on your incision or discomfort. Mark that spot on the wall to measure your progress. Work your hands down to shoulder level. Move closer to the wall as your height of reach improves.

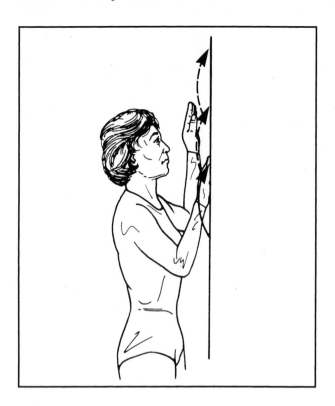

Rope Turning

Tie a rope to a door handle. Hold the rope in the hand of your operative side. Back away from the door until your arm is extended away from your body, parallel to the floor. Swing the rope in as wide a circle as possible. Increase the size of the circle as your mobility returns.

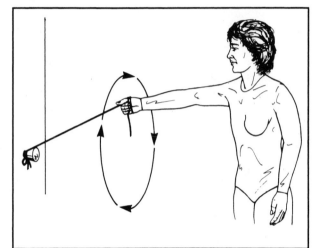

OTHER INSTRUCTIONS

Infusion Therapy

How to Care for a Subcutaneous (SubQ) Infusion

Your physician has ordered a medication that must be given under your skin, or subcutaneously. Usual places for this therapy are in the abdomen or thigh. The amount of medication is more than can be given in a single injection. A subcutaneous or SubQ administration device will be inserted. Once the SubQ set or needle has been inserted just under your skin, _____ milliliters (ml) of solution will be hooked up to a pumping device. The medication will slowly flow, or "infuse," at a rate of _____ ml per hour.

PREVENTING PROBLEMS

This device should be changed anytime it is pulled out of the skin and every 3 days (72 hours). Insertion sites should be rotated from one area (for example, thigh or stomach) to another. Your medication bags must be stored at room temperature or refrigerated (circle one). If the medication must be refrigerated, store it in a clean area away from food. All supplies must be stored in a clean dry place away from children and pets.

You must be careful that an infection does not start where the device enters the skin. Signs of infection include *redness, pain,* and *drainage.* The site must be covered with a dressing and taped so it will not pull out. The clear dressing over the insertion site must be occlusive. This means the dressing sticks tightly to the skin and the SubQ device, with no air pockets, moisture, or peeling edges. Tape may be used outside the dressing to secure the attached tubing for your comfort and help prevent the SubQ device from being accidentally pulled out.

Make sure you have the manufacturer's instructions for your pump. If it is an electronic pump, make sure you always have extra batteries or an alternate power source.

GUIDELINES

Use the following guidelines to help decrease your risk for infection and administer your medication safely.

1. Always wash your hands with antibacterial soap and running water, before handling medication, tubing, or any part of the SubQ device.

2. Keep the dressing clean and dry.

3. Observe for any fluid leaking from under the skin. The device needs to be replaced if it is leaking.

4. Inspect the medication label for correct information:
   - Patient name,
   - Medication name,
   - Correct dose,
   - Expiration date not passed.

   If anything is wrong with the label, *do not use the medication.* Inform your pharmacy provider.

5. Inspect medication container for the following:
   - Cloudy fluid,
   - Particles floating in fluid,
   - Leaking or damage.

   If any of these problems are present, *do not use the medication.* Inform your pharmacy provider.

6. How to administer SubQ medication:
   a. Prepare a work surface by cleaning the selected area with soap/water or alcohol and allowing the area to air-dry.
   b. Wash your hands.
   c. Medication should be at room temperature before infusing.
   d. Gather your equipment
      - Tubing or administration set
      - Alcohol pads
      - Clear dressing or gauze
      - Paper tape
      - Subcutaneous needle set
   e. Prime the medication through the tubing and the SubQ needle set following the pump manufacturer's recommendations.
   f. Select a body site that has enough subcutaneous tissue to accommodate the needle set. Make sure the skin is free of rashes, cuts, or other open areas.
   g. Clean the chosen insertion site with alcohol and allow the skin to air-dry.
   h. Grasp the tissue between thumb and first finger to make a "cushion." Do not pinch hard.

i. Insert the needle swiftly and firmly at a 45-degree angle.

j. Secure the needle in place with clear dressing or gauze and tape.

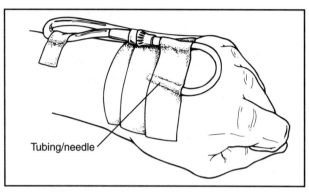

Tubing/needle

k. Discard used materials.

l. Discard used needles in a sturdy container such as a coffee can or laundry detergent bottle with a lid. Dispose of full receptacle according to your town's requirements.

m. Review pump program and re-program as needed.

n. Start infusion.

SPOTTING PROBLEMS

Check your SubQ site for

- Bruising,
- Active bleeding,
- Redness,
- Pain,
- Swelling or hardness.

If any of these signs are noted, stop the infusion. Choose another site and restart administration with a new SubQ set or needle.

OTHER INSTRUCTIONS

How to Care for Your Central Venous Catheter (Cuffed and Noncuffed)

The central venous catheter (central line) is a special intravenous catheter. It is a very flexible tube, generally inserted through the upper chest or neck and into a large vein just outside your heart. There are two general types of central lines. One is cuffed beneath your skin to help secure it; the other is noncuffed and has nothing under your skin to secure it, but may have stitches outside your body to help keep the line in. If your catheter has any external sutures, take care not to loosen or damage the stitches when changing the dressing. Also, the stitches should be examined regularly to ensure they are in place.

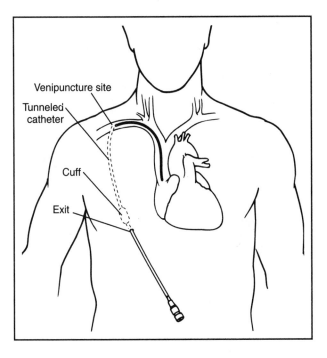

The type of catheter you have is a _____ (brand) and is _____ (cuffed or noncuffed). It has been placed so you can receive intravenous (IV) medications and fluids, and to draw blood for lab work. If properly cared for, this catheter should stay in place until your therapy is complete. The part of the catheter outside the dressing should always have a cap or needleless valve at the end. If a clamp is present, it should be closed when the catheter is not in use. Tape may be used outside the dressing to secure the catheter for your comfort and help prevent it from being accidentally pulled out. Saline and heparin solutions are flushed through the catheter to prevent it from becoming blocked.

PREVENTING PROBLEMS

Because the catheter is in your bloodstream, you must take care that an infection does not enter your body through that opening. An occlusive dressing must always be kept over the insertion site until your doctor gives you other orders. Occlusive means the dressing sticks tightly to the skin, catheter, and insertion site, with no air pockets, moisture, or peeling edges.

This dressing should be changed

- 24 hours after catheter insertion,
- Whenever it becomes wet, soiled, or starts to peel,
- Any time you note the catheter beneath the dressing is pulling out of the vein
- Routinely, every _____ days.

GUIDELINES

Use the following guidelines to help decrease your risk for infection and to keep the catheter in place and working properly.

1. Always wash your hands with antibacterial soap and running water before touching any part of the catheter and prepare a clean work area for supplies before starting any procedure.
2. Keep the dressing dry. With clear occlusive dressings, you should be able to bathe as long as you don't allow water to soak or shower directly on the dressing. Coordinate bathing with your dressing change schedule, so if the dressing starts to loosen, you are prepared to replace it immediately.
3. Make sure the cap or needleless valve stay tightly connected to the catheter and the clamp is closed when the IV line is not in use.
4. Flushing your catheter will keep it from becoming blocked.
   a. Flush with _____ milliliters (ml) of sodium chloride (saline solution) before administration of medications or fluids.
   b. Flush again with the same amount of saline, after the medication or fluid is completed.

c. Finally flush with _____ ml of heparinized solution (heparin lock flush).

d. You may remember this as SASH: *Saline–Administration–Saline–Heparin.*

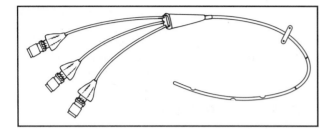

e. If your catheter has more than one lumen or tube, all lumens must be flushed. Lumens not currently being used for medication or fluid administration must be flushed daily. Flush each one with _____ ml of saline and _____ ml of heparin lock flush each day.

5. Prepare the syringe for flushing as follows:

a. Prepare a work surface by cleaning your selected area with soap/water or alcohol, allowing the area to air-dry.

b. Wash your hands.

c. Gather your equipment.
   - 0.9% sodium chloride (saline),
   - Heparinized solution (heparin lock flush) _____ units/ml,
   - Sterile 10-ml syringes with needle attached,
   - Alcohol prep pads.

d. Repeat steps e through j to prepare the saline and heparin syringes needed. Tag the heparin syringe with a label or piece of tape so you know the heparin is the last flush to be given.

e. Pop the cap off the solution bottle, open an alcohol wipe, and use it to clean the rubber top of the bottle.

f. Remove the cap from the needle and pull the plunger back to the _____ ml mark. (*Do not touch the needle or the cleaned bottle top with your fingers. If you accidentally touch the needle, get a fresh one and start again.*)

g. Insert the needle into the rubber top of the bottle.

h. Turn the bottle, needle, and syringe upside down. Inject the air and draw _____ ml of solution.

i. Remove the needle and syringe from the bottle. If air bubbles remain in the syringe, hold the syringe with the needle up. Draw the plunger back slightly and gently tap the barrel of the syringe until the bubbles rise to the top. Push the plunger slightly to get the air out.

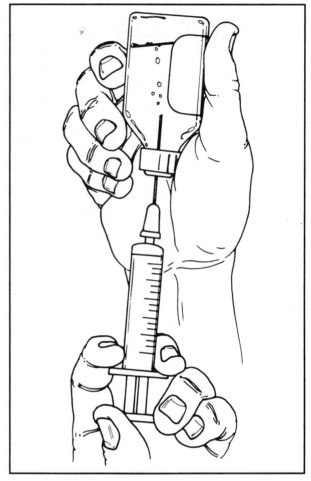

j. Carefully re-cap the needle and lay the syringe down on the cleaned surface.

6. Flush your central venous catheter.

a. Make sure the clamp is open.

b. Clean the cap or needleless valve with alcohol, scrubbing briskly.

c. Allow it to air-dry.

d. While leaving the needle on the syringe, puncture the cap or remove the needle from the syringe for direct connection of the syringe to the needle.

e. Inject fluid by pushing the plunger, until the full amount is used. If resistance is met, *do not force the fluid in. Stop and check for any kinks or pinched off areas of catheter. If none are found, call your home care nurse. Never flush with a syringe smaller than 5 to 10 ml and do not allow a nurse or care giver to do this either. Small syringes create more pressure and could break or damage the catheter.*

f. After flushing, close the catheter clamp.

g. Remove the syringe.

h. Discard all used needles/syringes in a puncture-proof container with a lid. Dispose of full receptacle according to your town's requirements.

7. Change your dressing to prevent infection and keep the catheter in place.

    a. Change your central venous catheter dressing every _____ days and whenever it is wet, loose, or soiled.

    b. Have sterile supplies or dressing change kits available.

    c. Store your supplies in a clean, dry place away from children and pets.

    d. Find a clean, well-lit work area. A mirror may be useful if you change your own dressing.

8. How to change your dressing

    a. Prepare a work surface, by cleaning the selected area with soap/water or alcohol and allowing the area to air-dry.

    b. Wash your hands.
- Remove all jewelry.
- Wash with warm running water and antibacterial liquid soap.
- Scrub fingers, nails, knuckles, back of hands, and 3 inches above the wrist.
- Rinse well.
- Dry your hands with paper towels, and turn the faucet off with those towels. Do not touch the faucet or sink after your hands are clean.
- If caring for someone else's dressing, care givers should put on clean latex gloves after washing and drying their hands.

    c. Gather your supplies
- Prescribed antiseptic cleanser (If alcohol and Betadine are both ordered, use the alcohol first, then the Betadine)
- Sterile dry swabs (large) or prepackaged antiseptic swabs
- Sterile dressing material (gauze or clear occlusive dressing)
  or
- Prepackaged "dressing change kit" with all the above included
- Paper tape
- Bag for waste

    d. Set up your sterile supplies within easy reach.

    e. Remove the old dressing by gently loosening edges. Then remove the dressing over the insertion site by holding the skin and catheter with one hand and stretching the clear dressing out along your skin. Do not pull up and out.

    f. As the dressing is stretched and the adhesive is loosened, gently pull it toward the insertion site. Take care not to pull on the catheter. If sutures are in place, take care not to pull them loose.

    g. Discard the old dressing in the waste bag.

    h. Wash your hands again and change to clean gloves.

    i. *If using alcohol only*: Moisten a dry swab with the antiseptic cleanser or use a premoistened swab to cleanse the insertion site. Move the swab in a circular motion, working out away from the insertion site, about 3 to 6 inches. Include the catheter, as well as the skin and any sutures. Look for signs of infection: redness, swelling, or drainage. If any of these signs are present, finish the procedure and call your nurse.

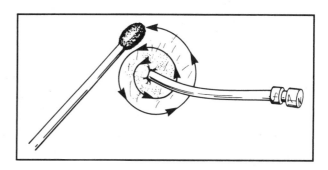

    j. Discard the swab in the waste bag, without touching the dirty end with your hands. Repeat the cleansing with a new antiseptic swab two more times.

    k. Allow the cleaned skin to air-dry.

    l. Gently wipe the catheter with an alcohol wipe from the insertion site to the end cap. DO NOT PULL THE CATHETER.

    m. If using both alcohol and Betadine
- **(1)** Cleanse the insertion site three times as described above with alcohol and allow the area to air-dry;
- **(2)** Cleanse the insertion site three times with Betadine and allow the area to air dry. If too much Betadine is on your skin, causing it to run, blot it with a sterile gauze pad. Do not wipe the Betadine completely off.

    n. Your skin and catheter must be completely dry before replacing the dressing.

    o. If using a clear or transparent dressing
- Remove the paper backing from the clear dressing and apply the sticky side to skin and catheter, so the insertion site is about center.
- Place a piece of tape just outside where the catheter comes out of the dressing to anchor it to the skin.
- If sutures are present, place a small gauze pad over them, under the dressing.

    p. If using gauze and tape
- Place a gauze pad over the insertion site and cover the gauze pad completely with strips of tape.

- Make sure no gauze is exposed.
- Place a piece of tape over the catheter where it comes out of the dressing to anchor it to the skin.

q. Label the dressing with the date it was changed.

r. Dispose of used supplies.

9. How to change the catheter cap

a. The cap or needleless valve must be changed every 7 days to help prevent infection.

b. The best time to change the cap is when you change the dressing.

c. Wash your hands.

d. Gather your supplies
- Sterile cap or valve,
- Syringe filled with saline (as described for flushing the catheter),
- Alcohol pads.

e. IMPORTANT: Make sure the clamp is closed, so that air will not enter your heart.

f. Flush the new sterile cap or valve with saline. Leave it in the packaging so you *do not touch the end that goes to the catheter.*

g. Scrub the old cap with alcohol, especially where the catheter and cap meet.

h. Unscrew and remove the old cap.

i. Use an alcohol pad or gauze to clean the end of the catheter. *Do not allow the end of the opened catheter to touch anywhere. This is a path directly to the bloodstream.*

j. Remove the saline-filled cap from the package and screw it into the catheter. Make sure it fits tightly.

k. Dispose of all used supplies.

SPOTTING PROBLEMS

Call your home health nurse immediately if you experience any of the following:

Signs of Infection

- Swelling, pain, or drainage around insertion site.
- Chills or fever over 101°F.

Signs of Damaged or Blocked Catheter

- Inability to flush the catheter.
- Pain or swelling when you attempt to flush.
- Clear fluid or blood leaking from the insertion site.
- Fluid leaking from any part of catheter during infusion or flushing.

Signs Your Dressing Is No Longer Occlusive

- Air pockets,
- Moisture,
- Loose or peeling edges.

Signs of Serious Complications That May Require Immediate Medical Treatment

If during infusion of medication or flushing of catheter, you have any of these symptoms, it could be an emergency. Activate the Emergency Medical System immediately (call 911).

- Sudden pain in your chest, shoulder, or lower back,
- Cough and shortness of breath,
- Pounding headache,
- Fast, irregular heartbeat,
- Dizziness or fainting.

OTHER INSTRUCTIONS

How to Care for Your Heparin Lock (intravenous catheter less than 1.5 inches)

A heparin lock has been placed in your arm so you can receive intravenous (IV) medications and fluids. Three basic pieces are connected to make up the heparin lock:

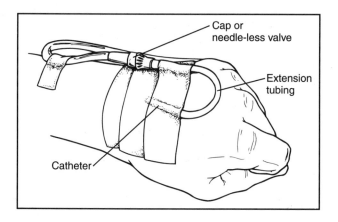

1. The catheter that is in your vein and comes out through the skin is a soft plastic-like material covered by a dressing. You could compare the catheter to a straw. The placement of the catheter will be changed every 2 to 3 days by the nurse.
2. The extension tubing is a length of tubing hooked to the catheter. This piece makes it easier for you or your care giver to use the IV catheter without accidentally pulling it out of the vein. This tubing will have a clamp attached that helps keep the blood from backing up.
3. A cap or needleless valve is attached to the end of the extension. This is where the medication or fluid enters.

PREVENTING PROBLEMS

Because the catheter is in your bloodstream, you must be careful that an infection does not enter your body through that opening. A dressing must be used to keep the catheter insertion site clean and dry. Tape is used outside the dressing to secure the catheter and prevent it from being accidentally pulled out. Saline and heparin solution are flushed through the heparin lock to keep the catheter from becoming blocked.

GUIDELINES

Use the following guidelines to help you decrease your risk for infection and to keep the heparin lock in place and working properly.

1. Always wash your hands with antibacterial soap and running water before touching any part of the heparin lock system.
2. Keep the heparin lock and dressing dry. Cover by wrapping plastic kitchen wrap around your arm, and taping at both ends, before bathing or showering.
3. Make sure all pieces stay connected together tightly and the clamp is in place when the heparin lock is not in use.
4. Check the catheter insertion site frequently before, during, and after use.
   a. Do not remove the clear dressing to check the site. Look through the dressing for signs of redness, swelling, or drainage.
   b. If you have a gauze dressing you cannot see through, gently touch the site to check for swelling or tenderness.
   c. If you have a fever or the site is tender, swollen, or draining, call the nurse immediately.
   d. If the dressing starts to peel off, call the nurse for further instruction. You may have to tape it down until the nurse can arrange a visit.
5. Flushing your catheter will help keep it from becoming blocked.
   a. Flush with _____ milliliters (ml) of sodium chloride (saline solution) before administration of medications or fluids.
   b. Flush again with the same amount of saline, after the medication or fluid is completed.
   c. Finally flush with _____ ml of heparinized solution (heparin lock flush).
   d. You may remember this process as SASH: Saline–Administration–Saline–Heparin.
   e. If medication is given less than every 8 hours, flush with heparin lock flush _____ times a day to prevent blockage.
6. Prepare for syringe flushing as follows:
   a. Prepare a work surface by cleaning the selected area with soap/water or alcohol, and allowing the area to air-dry.

b. Wash your hands.

c. Gather your equipment
  - 0.9% sodium chloride (saline)
  - Heparinized solution (heparin lock flush) _____ units/ml
  - Sterile 10-ml syringes with needle attached
  - Alcohol prep pads

d. Repeat steps e through j to prepare the saline and heparin syringes needed. Tag the heparin syringe with a label or piece of tape so you know the heparin is the last flush to be given.

e. Pop the cap off the solution bottle, open an alcohol wipe, and use it to clean the rubber top of the bottle.

f. Remove the cap from the needle and pull the plunger back to the _____ ml mark. (*Do not touch the needle or the cleaned bottle top with your fingers. If you accidentally touch the needle, get a fresh one and start again.*)

g. Insert the needle into the bottle's rubber top.

h. Turn the bottle, needle, and syringe upside down. Inject the air and withdraw _____ ml of solution.

i. Remove the needle and syringe from the bottle. If air bubbles remain in the syringe, hold the syringe with the needle up. Draw the plunger back slightly and gently tap the barrel of the syringe, until the bubbles rise to the top. Push the plunger slightly to get the air out.

j. Carefully re-cap the needle and lay the syringe down on your clean work surface.

7. Flushing your heparin lock

  a. Make sure the extension clamp is open.

  b. Clean the cap or needleless valve with alcohol, scrubbing briskly. Allow it to air-dry.

  c. Leaving the needle on the syringe, puncture the extension cap or remove the needle from the syringe for direct connection of the syringe to the valve.

  d. Inject fluid by pushing the plunger, until the full amount is used. If resistance is met, DO NOT force the fluid in. Stop and call your home care nurse.

  e. After flushing, close the extension clamp.

  f. Remove the syringe.

  g. Discard all used needles/syringes in a puncture-proof container with a lid. Dispose of full receptacle according to your town's requirements.

OTHER INSTRUCTIONS

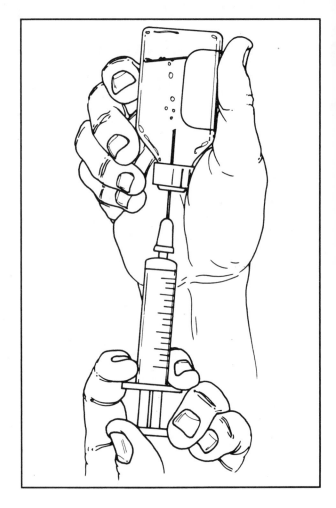

SPOTTING PROBLEMS

Call your home health nurse immediately if you experience any of the following:

Signs of Infection

- Swelling, pain, or drainage around the insertion site.
- Chills or fever over 101°F.

Signs of Dislodged Catheter

- Inability to flush the catheter.
- Pain or swelling when you attempt to flush or during fluid administration.
- Clear fluid or blood leaking from insertion site.

How to Care for Your PICC or Midline Catheter (intravenous catheter greater than 1.5 inches)

The PICC (peripherally inserted central catheter) and midline catheters are special intravenous (IV) catheters. A very soft flexible tube is inserted near the bend of your arm and threaded deeper into the vein. The PICC ends in the vein just outside your heart, and the shorter midline catheter ends near your armpit. The type of catheter you have is a _____ (brand) _____ _____ (PICC or midline). The catheter in your vein is _____ inches long, with _____ inches remaining outside the insertion site beneath the transparent dressing material. It has been placed in your arm so you can receive IV medications and fluids. If properly cared for, this catheter should stay in place until your therapy is complete. The part of the catheter outside the dressing should always have a cap or needleless valve at the end. If a clamp is present, it should be closed when the catheter is not in use. Tape may be used outside the dressing to secure the catheter extension for your comfort and help prevent the catheter from being accidentally pulled out. Saline and heparin solutions are flushed through the IV line to keep the catheter from becoming blocked.

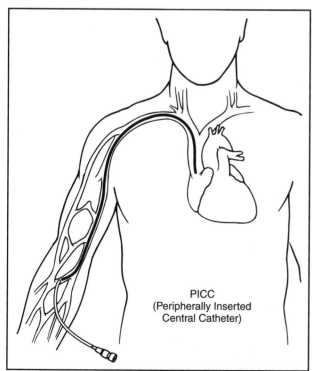

PICC
(Peripherally Inserted
Central Catheter)

PREVENTING PROBLEMS

Because the catheter is in your bloodstream, you must be careful that an infection does not enter your body through that opening. The clear dressing over the insertion site must be occlusive. This means the dressing sticks tightly to the skin, catheter, and insertion site, with no air pockets, moisture, or peeling edges.

This dressing should be changed

- 24 hours after catheter insertion,
- Whenever it becomes wet, soiled, or starts to peel,
- Any time you note the catheter beneath the dressing is pulling out of the vein,
- Every _____ days.

GUIDELINES

Use the following guidelines to help you decrease your risk for infection, and to keep the IV line in place and working properly.

1. Always wash your hands with antibacterial soap and running water before touching any part of the catheter.
2. Keep the dressing dry. Cover it by wrapping plastic kitchen wrap around your arm and taping at both ends before bathing or showering.
3. Make sure the cap, needleless valve, and extensions stay tightly connected and the clamp is closed when the IV line is not in use.
4. Check the catheter insertion site frequently before, during, and after use.
   a. Do not remove the clear dressing without assistance of a nurse or trained care giver.
   b. If you have a fever or the site is tender, swollen, or draining, *call the nurse immediately.*
   c. If the dressing starts to peel off, *call the nurse immediately.*
5. Flushing your catheter will help keep it from becoming blocked.
   a. Flush with _____ milliliters (ml) of sodium chloride (saline solution) before administration of medications or fluids.
   b. Flush again with the same amount of saline, after the medication or fluid is completed.

c. Finally flush with _____ ml of heparinized solution (heparin lock flush).

d. You may remember this as SASH: *Saline–Administration–Saline–Heparin*.

e. If medication is given less than every 8 hours, flush with heparin lock flush _____ times a day to prevent blockage.

6. Prepare the syringe for flushing as follows:

a. Prepare a work surface by cleaning the selected area with soap/water or alcohol and allowing it to air-dry.

b. Wash your hands.

c. Gather your equipment
- 0.9% sodium chloride (saline)
- Heparinized solution (heparin lock flush) _____ units/ml
- Sterile 10-ml syringes with needle attached
- Alcohol prep pads

d. Repeat steps e through j to prepare the saline and heparin syringes needed. Tag the heparin syringe with a label or piece of tape so you know the heparin is the last flush to be given.

e. Pop the cap off the solution bottle, open an alcohol wipe, and use it to clean the rubber top of the bottle.

f. Remove the cap from the needle and pull the plunger back to the _____ ml mark. (*Do not touch the needle or the cleaned bottle top with your fingers. If you accidentally touch the needle, get a fresh one and start again.*)

g. Insert the needle into the rubber top of the bottle.

h. Turn the bottle, needle, and syringe upside down. Inject the air and withdraw _____ ml of solution.

i. Remove the needle and syringe from the bottle. If air bubbles remain in the syringe, hold the syringe with the needle up. Draw the plunger back slightly and gently tap the barrel of the syringe until the bubbles rise to the top. Push the plunger slightly to get the air out.

j. Carefully re-cap the needle and lay the syringe down on the cleaned surface.

7. Flush your PICC or midline catheter.

a. Make sure any clamp on the external catheter is open.

b. Clean the cap or needleless valve with alcohol, scrubbing briskly.

c. Allow it to air-dry.

d. Leaving the needle on the syringe, puncture the cap or remove the needle from the syringe for direct connection of the syringe to the valve.

e. Inject the fluid by pushing the plunger, until the full amount is used. If resistance is met,

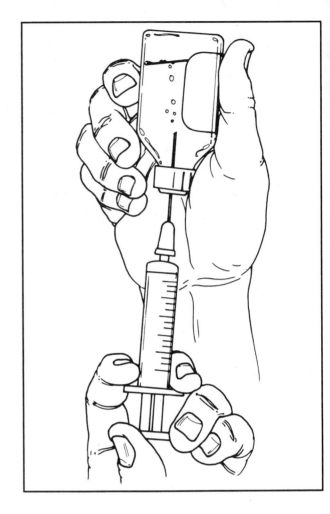

do not force the fluid in. Stop and call your home care nurse. *Never flush with a syringe smaller than 5 to 10 ml and do not allow a nurse or care giver to do this, either. Small syringes exert more pressure that could break the catheter.*

f. After flushing, close the extension clamp.

g. Remove the syringe.

h. Discard all used needles/syringes in a puncture-proof container with a lid. Dispose of full receptacle according to your town's requirements.

SPOTTING PROBLEMS

Call your home health nurse immediately if you experience any of the following:

Signs of Infection

- Swelling, pain, or drainage around insertion site, or in the upper arm.
- Chills or fever over 101°F.

Signs of Damaged or Blocked Catheter

- Inability to flush the catheter.
- Pain or swelling in your arm when you attempt to flush the catheter.
- Clear fluid or blood at the insertion site.
- Fluid leaking from any part of catheter during infusion or flushing.

Signs Your PICC or Midline Dressing Is No Longer Occlusive

- Air pockets,
- Moisture,
- Loose or peeling edges,
- Catheter pulling out of the vein, beneath the dressing.

OTHER INSTRUCTIONS

How to Give Your Intravenous (IV) Medication

Your doctor has ordered a medication that must be given through your bloodstream, using an IV access device. With the support of your home care nursing agency and pharmacy company, you may stay at home and give your own medications. If you are not able, a friend or relative may act as care giver to give your medicine. Under the supervision of a trained home care nurse, this is a safe and convenient way to receive your medication infusion.

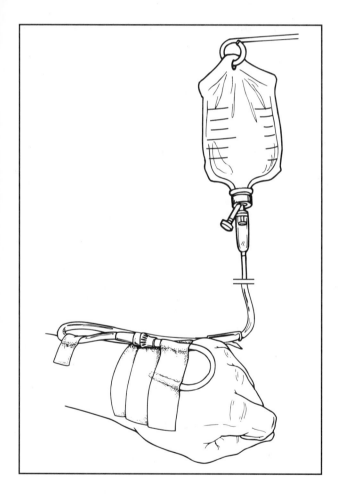

Your medication is _____ . The dose is _____ milligrams (mg) in _____ ml of solution. The schedule is every _____ hours. The medication will flow or "infuse" by gravity drip or will be hooked up to a pumping device. If gravity drip, the rate is _____ drops per minute. If an infusion pump is used the rate is _____ ml per hour.

Your IV tubing may be used for up to _____ hours before it must be replaced.

PREVENTING PROBLEMS

1. Infection is the most preventable problem with IV therapy. Good hand washing is the most important step in preventing infection.
2. All items connected to your IV device must be sterile. If the package is damaged or wet, the item is contaminated (no longer sterile). Discard it.
3. Air should be flushed, or primed, out of any tubing before connecting it to your IV device.
4. If using a pump, make sure you have the manufacturer's instructions. If the pump is electronic, make sure you have extra batteries or an alternate power source.

GUIDELINES

Use the following guidelines to decrease your risk of infection, and take your fluid medication safely.

1. Store all supplies in a clean, dry place, away from children and pets.
2. Store medications per label instructions. If refrigeration is required, place the medication in a section of your refrigerator away from food.
3. Wash hands when you begin, change, or complete an IV infusion:
   - Use antibacterial liquid soap and warm running water.
   - Scrub your hands for about 30 seconds.
   - Dry your hands with paper towels.
   - Turn the faucet off with a paper towel. Do not touch the faucet or sink with your clean hands.
4. Inspect the medication label for the correct information:
   - Your name
   - Medication name
   - Correct dose
   - Expiration date not passed
   - If anything is wrong with the label, DO NOT USE THE MEDICATION. Contact your pharmacy company.
5. Inspect the fluid and its container for the following:
   - Cloudy fluid
   - Particles floating in the fluid

- Leaking or damage to the container
- If any of these problems are present, DO NOT USE THE FLUID OR CONTAINER. Contact your pharmacy company.

6. To administer the IV medication or fluid.

   a. Make sure the medication is at room temperature before administering.

   b. Remove the administration set or IV tubing from its sterile packing and close the roller clamp. Label the tubing with the date you opened the package.

   c. Pull the protective cover from the entry port of the medication bag. Do not touch the open port with your hands.

   d. Remove the cover from the tubing spike and push the spike firmly into medication port.

   e. Prime, or flush any air out of, the IV tubing. *If the infusion is to be by gravity,* make sure the IV pole is about 2½ feet above your IV insertion site. Hang the bag on the pole, squeeze the drip chamber until it is about ½ full, and open the roller clamp until fluid drips out. *If using a pump,* prime it as described for a gravity infusion, or use the pump to prime the tubing following the manufacturer's instructions. Loosen the end cap but *do not touch* the end of tubing.

   f. Program the pump as ordered or check the existing program for correct infusion rate and amount. Follow manufacturer's instructions.

   g. When all the air is expelled from the tubing, clean your IV device by scrubbing the cap or needleless valve with an alcohol pad.

   h. Open the clamps on the IV device, flush them with saline as ordered, and connect the IV tubing.

   i. For a pump infusion, make sure all clamps are open and start the pump, after checking the program again.

   j. For a gravity infusion, open the roller clamp and adjust the drip rate. While you watch the drip chamber, count the drops that fall in 1 minute and adjust the drip to the ordered rate using the roller clamp.

   k. Inspect the length of the IV tubing. You

should not be lying on the tubing. The tubing should not be kinked or twisted.

   l. Keep a record of when your medications are given.

   m. Take care while the infusion is in progress not to knock over the IV pole or pumps, as this could pull out or damage your IV access device.

7. After infusion is complete

   a. Close the clamp.

   b. Disconnect the tubing from the IV access. Make sure the cap or needleless valve remains tightly on the IV device.

   c. Flush the IV access as ordered.

   d. *If reusing the tubing,* leave the spike in the empty bag and place a sterile cap on the end of the tubing that was attached to the IV access device. If you accidentally touch the end, discard the tubing and bag. Place the used IV tubing into a clean plastic bag or leave it hanging on the IV pole for use with the next dose of medication.

   e. If the tubing is not going to be reused, discard the bag and tubing.

8. How to change bags when fluids are given continuously.

   a. Change the fluid bag while there is still fluid surrounding the tubing spike. This keeps air out of the tubing.

   b. Inspect the new bag for leaks or cloudy fluid.

   c. *For a gravity infusion,* clamp the tubing or *if using a pump* place the pump on hold.

   d. Remove the protective cover from the entry port of the new bag.

   e. Remove the near empty bag from the IV pole.

   f. Remove the tubing spike from the old bag, and push the spike into the entry port of the new bag.

   g. Hang the new bag on the IV pole.

   h. Readjust the drip rate with the roller clamp or reset the pump so that the fluid flows at the prescribed rate.

9. Dispose of used needles/syringes into a puncture-proof container with a lid. Dispose of full receptacle according to your town's requirements.

OTHER INSTRUCTIONS

How to Use Your Implanted Venous Port

Your implanted port is a special intravenous (IV) device that has been placed so you can receive IV medications and fluids. It is made up of a small chamber with a self-sealing silicon septum attached to a very flexible tube that goes to the large vein just outside your heart. The type of port you have is a _____ (brand). If properly cared for, the port should stay in place until your therapy is complete. For use, the port will be accessed with a special type of needle that will not damage the silicon septum. When not in use, your port will not be accessed with a needle and will need no daily care, only flushing with _____ milliliters (ml) of _____ every _____ days.

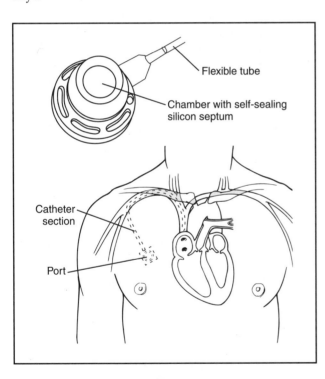

Flexible tube

Chamber with self-sealing silicon septum

Catheter section

Port

PREVENTING PROBLEMS

If your port is being used often for administration of medication or fluids, the needle may stay in place for up to 7 days. Because the port catheter is in your bloodstream, you must be careful that an infection does not develop around the port or enter your bloodstream while the port is accessed with a needle. A local anesthetic cream may be ordered before the needle puncture. A dressing must remain over the needle and port while it is accessed. The dressing over the needle site must be *occlusive*. This means the dressing sticks tightly to the skin and needle site, with no air pockets, moisture, or peeling edges. Gauze may be used to pad around or under the needle part that touches your skin. Tape may be used outside the dressing to secure the needle's extension tube for your comfort and help prevent the needle from being accidentally pulled out. Saline and heparin solutions are flushed through the port to keep it from becoming blocked.

This dressing should be changed

- Whenever it becomes wet, soiled, or starts to peel,
- Any time you note the needle pulling out of the port,
- Every _____ days.

GUIDELINES

Use the following guidelines to help you decrease your risk for infection and to keep the port needle in place and working properly.

1. Always wash your hands with antibacterial soap and running water before touching any part of the accessed port's tubing or extensions.
2. Keep the dressing dry. During bathing do not allow water to come in contact with the dressing or any tube outside the dressing.
3. Make sure the cap, needleless valve, or extensions stay tightly connected together and the clamp is closed between doses of medication.
4. Check to see that the needle is in place frequently before, during, and after use.
   a. Look for redness, swelling, or drainage.
   b. If you have a *fever* or the port is *tender, swollen, or draining, call the nurse immediately.*
   d. If the dressing starts to peel off, *call the nurse immediately* unless you have been trained to change the dressing.
5. Flushing your port will help keep it from becoming blocked.
   a. Flush with _____ milliliters (ml) of sodium chloride (saline solution) before administration of medications or fluids.
   b. Flush again with the same amount of saline after the medication or fluid is completed.
   c. Finally flush with _____ ml of heparinized solution (heparin lock flush).
   d. You may remember this as SASH: *Saline–Administration–Saline–Heparin.*
   e. Always use 10-ml syringes. Smaller syringes

make too much pressure and may damage your port.

6. Prepare the syringe for flushing as follows:
   a. Prepare a work surface by cleaning the selected area with soap/water or alcohol and allowing the area to air-dry.
   b. Wash your hands.
   c. Gather your equipment
      - 0.9% sodium chloride (saline),
      - Heparinized solution (heparin lock flush) _____ units/ml,
      - Sterile 10-ml syringes with needle attached,
      - Alcohol prep pads.
   d. Repeat steps e through j to prepare the saline and heparin syringes needed. Tag the heparin syringe with a label or piece of tape so you know the heparin is the last flush to be given.
   e. Pop the cap off the solution bottle, open an alcohol wipe, and use it to clean the rubber top of the bottle.
   f. Remove the cap from the needle and pull the plunger back to the _____ ml mark. *Do not touch the needle or the cleaned bottle top with your fingers. If you accidentally touch the needle, get a fresh one and start again.*

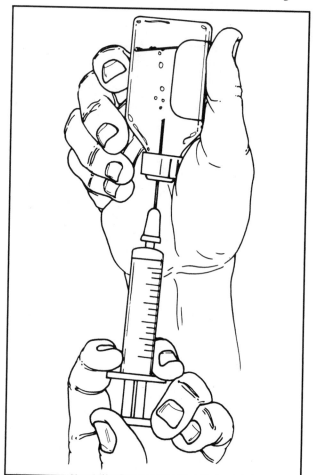

g. Insert the needle into the rubber top of the bottle.
h. Turn the bottle, needle, and syringe upside down. Inject the air and withdraw _____ ml of solution.
i. Remove the needle and syringe from the bottle. If air bubbles remain in the syringe, hold the syringe with the needle up. Draw the plunger back slightly and gently tap the barrel of the syringe until the bubbles rise to the top. Push the plunger slightly to get the air out.
j. Carefully re-cap the needle and lay the syringe down on the cleaned surface.

7. Flush your implanted port.
   a. Open any clamp present on the needle extension tube.
   b. Clean the cap or needleless valve with alcohol, scrubbing briskly.
   c. Allow it to air-dry.
   d. While leaving the needle on the syringe, puncture the cap or remove the needle from the syringe for direct connection of the syringe to the valve.
   e. Inject the fluid by pushing the plunger, until the full amount is used. If resistance is met, *do not* force the fluid in. Stop and call your home care nurse. If you have pain or swelling around the port, stop and call your home care nurse.
   f. After flushing, close the extension clamp.
   g. Remove the syringe.
   h. Discard all used needles/syringes in a puncture-proof container with a lid. Dispose of full receptacle according to your town's requirements.

8. Before changing a dressing on a port accessed with needle, patient or care giver must have training and specific doctor's order.
   - Change your port dressing whenever it is wet, loose, or soiled, and routinely as ordered by your doctor.
   - Have sterile supplies or dressing change kits available.
   - Store your supplies in a clean, dry place away from children and pets.
   - Find a clean, well-lit work area. A mirror may be helpful if you change your own dressing.

9. Change your dressing.
   a. Prepare a work surface by cleaning the selected area with soap/water or alcohol and allowing it to air-dry.
   b. Wash your hands.
      - Remove all jewelry,
      - Wash with warm running water and liquid antibacterial soap,
      - Scrub fingers, nails, knuckles, back of hands, and up to 3 inches above the wrist,

- Rinse well.
- Dry your hands with paper towels, and turn the faucet off with those towels. Do not touch the faucet or sink after your hands are clean.
- If caring for someone else's dressing, care givers should put on clean latex gloves after washing and drying their hands.

c. Gather your supplies
  - Prescribed antiseptic cleanser,
  - Sterile dry swabs (large) or prepackaged antiseptic swabs,
  - Sterile dressing material (gauze or clear occlusive dressing) or
  - Prepackaged "dressing change kit" with all the above included,
  - Paper tape,
  - Bag for waste.

d. Set up your sterile supplies within easy reach.

e. Remove the old dressing by gently loosening the edges. Then remove the dressing over the insertion site by holding the skin and needle access with one hand and stretching the clear dressing out along your skin. Do not stretch up and out.

f. As the dressing is stretched and the adhesive is loosened, gently pull it away from the needle. Take care not to pull out the needle.

g. If sutures are in place, be careful not to pull them loose.

h. Discard the old dressing in the waste bag.

i. Wash your hands again and change to clean gloves.

j. Moisten a dry swab with the antiseptic cleanser or use a premoistened swab to cleanse the insertion site. Clean in a circular motion, working out away from the site about 3 to 6 inches. Include the needle (if present), as well as the skin. Look for signs of *redness, swelling, or drainage*. If any of these signs are present, finish the procedure and call your nurse.

k. Discard the swab in the waste bag, without touching the dirty end with your hands. Repeat twice more with a new, clean wet swab.

l. Gently wipe the needle and insertion site with an alcohol wipe. Clean from the insertion site down the extension tube away from your body. DO NOT REMOVE THE NEEDLE.

m. Air-dry your skin and catheter completely before replacing the dressing.

n. If padding for the needle is needed, use a sterile gauze pad.

o. If using a clear or transparent dressing.
  - Remove the paper backing from the clear dressing and apply the sticky side over the needle.
  - Place a piece of tape over the extension tube, where it comes out of the dressing, to anchor it to skin.

p. If using gauze and tape.
  - Place a gauze pad over the needle and cover the gauze pad completely with strips of tape.
  - Make sure no gauze is exposed.

q. Label the dressing with the date of the dressing change.

r. Dispose of used supplies.

10. How to remove a needle access from an indwelling port. Before deaccessing port needle, the patient or care giver must have training and specific doctor's order.

  a. Before taking the needle out, be sure to flush the needle. Clamp the extension while you still have pressure on the barrel of the syringe. This keeps positive pressure in the port so that blood is not drawn back into the catheter.

  b. Remove the old dressing by gently loosening the edges. Remove the dressing over the insertion site by holding the skin and needle with one hand and stretching the clear dressing out along your skin. Do not stretch up and out.

  c. As the dressing is stretched and the adhesive is loosened, gently pull it away from the needle. Be careful not to pull the needle out.

  d. Discard the old dressing in a waste bag.

  e. Hold the edges of the port pressing in with your thumb and first finger to stabilize it.

  f. Grasp the needle with your other hand. Pull straight out and away. Be careful to not stick yourself or anyone else with a bloody needle.

11. How to access an implanted port with a needle. Before accessing the port with a needle, the patient or care giver must have training and specific doctor's orders.

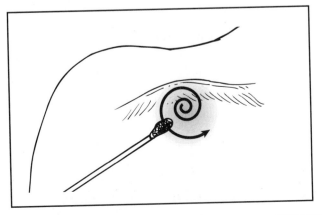

a. Prepare a work surface by cleaning with soap/water or alcohol and allowing it to air-dry.

b. Wash your hands.
  • Remove all jewelry.
  • Wash with warm running water and liquid antibacterial soap.
  • Scrub fingers, nails, knuckles, back of hands, and up to 3 inches of the wrist.
  • Rinse well.
  • Dry your hands with paper towels, and turn the faucet off with those towels. Do not touch the faucet or sink after your hands are clean.
  • If caring for someone else's dressing, care givers should put on clean latex gloves after washing and drying their hands.

c. Gather your supplies
  • Prescribed antiseptic cleanser
  • Sterile gloves
  • Noncoring needle size: _____ gauge _____ inches long (only non-coring needles should be used with an implanted port. The noncoring needle has a special point that protects the port.)

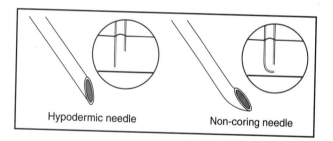

Hypodermic needle   Non-coring needle

  • 10-ml sterile syringe filled with saline
  • Sterile dry swabs (large) or prepackaged antiseptic swabs
  • Sterile dressing material (gauze or clear occlusive dressing) or prepackaged "dressing change kit" with all the above included.
  • Paper tape
  • Bag for waste

d. Set up your sterile supplies within easy reach.

e. Look at the skin over the port. Report any *redness, swelling,* or *broken skin* to your home care nurse.

f. Feel for the silicon septum.

g. Using sterile technique, put on the sterile gloves.

h. Clean the area over the port with an antiseptic swab, starting over the port and moving outward in a spiral motion to cover an area

about 5 inches in diameter. Allow the area to air-dry.

i. Connect the noncoring needle and extension set to the 10-ml saline syringe and push the saline through, removing all of the air.

j. Locate the port silicon septum with a sterile gloved finger.

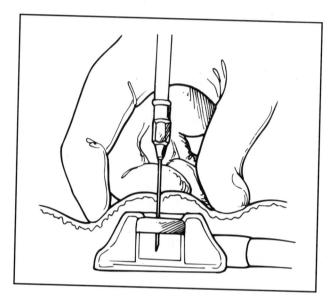

k. Insert the needle firmly through skin and straight into port septum to the bottom. Do not tilt or rock the needle once the septum is punctured.

l. Pull back the barrel of the syringe and check for blood return. If blood is pulled back, push the saline in and clamp the extension. If no blood is pulled back, remove the needle from the skin and start the procedure over with new sterile supplies.

m. When a blood return is noted and the port flushes without resistance, the needle is correctly placed in the port septum. Apply a dressing as instructed above in Guideline 8.

SPOTTING PROBLEMS

Call your home health nurse immediately if you experience any of the following:

Signs of Infection

• Swelling, pain, or drainage around the insertion site,
• Chills or fever over 101°F.

Signs of a Damaged or Blocked Port

- Inability to flush the port,
- Pain or swelling when you attempt to flush the port,
- Fluid leaking from the port during an infusion or while flushing the port.

Signs Your Dressing Is No Longer Occlusive

- Air pockets,
- Moisture,
- Loose or peeling edges.

Signs of Serious Complications That May Require Immediate Medical Treatment

If during infusion of medication or flushing of port you have any of these symptoms, activate the Emergency Medical System immediately (call 911).

- Sudden pain in your chest, shoulder, or lower back,
- Cough and shortness of breath,
- Pounding headache,
- Fast, irregular heartbeat,
- Dizziness or fainting.

OTHER INSTRUCTIONS

Therapeutic Agents

Angina Medications

WHAT THE MEDICATION DOES

1. Prevents angina
2. Relieves angina pain

HOW TO TAKE THE MEDICATION

1. Angina medications are made in different ways. Follow the directions for your type of medication.
2. Take as directed on the label.

Sublingual (Under the Tongue) Type

1. Take the tablet at the first sign of an angina attack.
2. Wet the tablet with saliva.
3. Place it under the tongue or between your cheek and gums.
4. Keep it under the tongue until it is completely dissolved.
5. Do not swallow or chew the tablet.
6. Sit down and rest.
7. If you have angina 5 minutes *after* taking the first tablet, take one more tablet.
8. If you still have angina 5 minutes *after* taking the second tablet, take one more tablet.
9. If you still have angina *after* taking the third tablet, call your doctor or the hospital. You may need medical care.
10. Store the tablets in a cool, dry, closed container away from light.
11. Carry at least six tablets with you at all times.
12. Remove cotton from the container. Cotton absorbs the medication.
13. New tablets are needed every 3 months. The tablets lose their strength quickly.

Tablets to Swallow

1. Take on an empty stomach. Take ½ hour before or 1 to 2 hours after meals.
2. Swallow the tablet whole. Do not break, crush, or chew it.

Tablets to Chew

Chew completely before swallowing.

Mouth Spray

1. Spray once or twice on top of or under the tongue.
   a. Do not inhale the spray.
   b. Count slowly to 10 before swallowing.
2. Take at the first sign of an angina attack.
3. Sit down and rest.
4. If you still have angina 3 to 5 minutes after the *first* spray, spray your tongue once or twice again.
5. If you still have angina 3 to 5 minutes after the *second* spray, spray your tongue once or twice again.
6. If you still have angina after the *third* spray, call your doctor or the hospital. You may need medical care.

Skin Ointment

1. Remove the old plastic film and wipe the skin clean.
2. Use the ruled paper (that comes with the medication) to place a thin, even layer of ointment on the skin. Do not get the ointment on your fingers.
3. Place the ointment on a hairless or shaved area of skin, such as the chest, upper arm, thigh, stomach, or back.
   a. Use a different area each time.
   b. Do not rub the ointment.
4. Cover the ointment with plastic film and secure it with tape if instructed to do so.

Skin Patches

1. Remove the old patch and wipe the skin clean.
2. Place the new patch on a clean, dry, hairless area. Use a different area each time.

SIGNS AND SYMPTOMS TO REPORT TO YOUR NURSE OR DOCTOR

1. Headache
2. Dizziness
3. Flushing of the face or neck
4. Redness and irritation of the skin (from ointment or patches)
5. Constipation
6. Nausea

SPECIAL POINTS

1. If you have headaches with the medication, your nurse or doctor may tell you to take aspirin.

2. Your nurse or doctor may instruct you to take an extra dose before certain angina-producing situations, such as stress or exercise.
3. To lessen dizziness, stand up slowly.
   a. Sit or lie down at the first signs of dizziness.
   b. Go up and down stairs slowly.
4. Do not drink alcohol.
5. Keep this and all medications out of the reach of children.

6. Obtain new tablets after 3 months, even if you have some left in the container.

MEDICATION INSTRUCTIONS

Medication Name: _____

Dose: _____

When to Take: _____

Special Notes: _____

OTHER INSTRUCTIONS

Antianxiety Medications

WHAT THE MEDICATION DOES

1. Decreases tension and anxiety
2. Produces a mild sedation

HOW TO TAKE THE MEDICATION

1. Take as directed on the label.
2. Do not overuse.
3. Consult with a doctor before stopping.

SIGNS AND SYMPTOMS TO REPORT TO YOUR NURSE OR DOCTOR

1. Drowsiness
2. Light-headedness
3. Diarrhea
4. Constipation
5. Dizziness
6. Dry mouth
7. Slurred speech
8. Overexcitement

SPECIAL POINTS

1. Avoid hazardous activities.
2. Avoid alcohol.
3. Do not stop the drug abruptly.
4. Chewing sugarless gum or eating hard candy may relieve dry mouth.
5. May be addictive with long-term use.

MEDICATION INSTRUCTIONS

Medication Name: _____

Dose: _____

When to Take: _____

Special Notes: _____

OTHER INSTRUCTIONS

Antibiotic Medications

WHAT THE MEDICATION DOES

1. Kills bacteria (germs)
2. Stops bacteria from growing

HOW TO TAKE THE MEDICATION

1. Take as directed on the label.
2. Some medications should be taken with food to lessen stomach irritation. Some medications should be taken ½ hour before or 1 to 2 hours after meals. Ask your nurse or doctor about your medication.
3. Finish taking the medication, even if you feel better.
4. If you forget to take the medication, take it as soon as you remember, *unless* it is almost time for your next regular dose, then take *only* the next dose as scheduled.

SIGNS AND SYMPTOMS TO REPORT TO YOUR NURSE OR DOCTOR

1. Nausea, vomiting
2. Diarrhea
3. Skin rash
4. Fever or chills
5. Dizziness
6. Headache
7. Vaginal itching or irritation
8. Mouth sores

SPECIAL POINTS

1. Tell your nurse or doctor if you have an allergy to medications. If you have an allergic reaction to an antibiotic, you should carry a medical identification card at all times.
2. Some medications may cause you to have false results on urine glucose tests.
3. Keep this and all medications out of the reach of children.

MEDICATION INSTRUCTIONS

Medication Name: _____

Dose: _____

When to Take: _____

Special Notes: _____

OTHER INSTRUCTIONS

Anticoagulant Medications

WHAT THE MEDICATION DOES

Prevents blood clots

HOW TO TAKE THE MEDICATION

1. Take as directed on the label.
2. Take at the same time daily.

SIGNS AND SYMPTOMS TO REPORT TO YOUR NURSE OR DOCTOR

1. Bleeding gums
2. Nose bleeds
3. Skin bruises easily
4. Blood in urine
5. Fever
6. Skin rash
7. Extra heavy menstrual flow
8. Black (tarry) stools
9. Vomiting blood

SPECIAL POINTS

1. Do not take aspirin or medication that contains aspirin unless your nurse or doctor tells you.

2. Take extra care to avoid bruising or cutting yourself.
   a. Brush your teeth with a soft toothbrush.
   b. Shave with an electric razor.
   c. Avoid contact sports.
3. Eating different amounts of foods that contain vitamin K can affect the way the medication works. Because green leafy vegetables have vitamin K, you should eat about the same amount each day.
4. Some medication my change the color of your urine.
5. Carry medical identification, with the medication name and dose, at all times.
6. Keep this and all medications out of the reach of children.

MEDICATION INSTRUCTIONS

Medication Name: _____

Dose: _____

When to Take: _____

Special Notes: _____

OTHER INSTRUCTIONS

Anticonvulsant Medications

WHAT THE MEDICATION DOES

Prevents seizures

HOW TO TAKE THE MEDICATION

1. Take as directed on the label.
2. Do not stop taking the medication unless your nurse or doctor tells you to.

SIGNS AND SYMPTOMS TO REPORT TO YOUR NURSE OR DOCTOR

1. Fever
2. Sore throat
3. Mouth sores
4. Skin bruises easily
5. Skin rash
6. Loss of appetite or nausea
7. Blurred vision
8. Trouble with coordinated movement

SPECIAL POINTS

1. The medication may make you sleepy or dizzy. Do not drive or perform any activities that require you to be alert.
2. Do not drink alcohol while taking this medication.
3. Keep this and all medications out of the reach out children.

MEDICATION INSTRUCTIONS

Medication Name: _____

Dose: _____

How to Take: _____

Special Notes: _____

OTHER INSTRUCTIONS

Antidepressive Medications

WHAT THE MEDICATION DOES

1. Decreases feelings of depression
2. Improves sense of well-being

HOW TO TAKE THE MEDICATION

Unless otherwise prescribed, take the full dose at bedtime.

SIGNS AND SYMPTOMS TO REPORT TO YOUR NURSE OR DOCTOR

1. Dizziness upon standing
2. Blurred vision
3. Dry mouth
4. Excessive sweating
5. Drowsiness
6. Palpitations
7. Confusion
8. Nausea and vomiting
9. Weight loss or weight gain
10. Constipation
11. Loss of appetite
12. Body rash
13. Inability to urinate
14. Retention of fluids in legs or ankles

SPECIAL POINTS

1. Avoid use of alcohol.
2. Avoid activities such as driving that need you to be alert.
3. Ask your doctor before taking any over-the-counter medications.
4. Avoid prolonged exposure to sunlight.
5. Don't stop taking the medication abruptly.
6. Avoid foods high in tryptophan (liver, kidney, fish, poultry, eggs, nuts, peanut butter, beans, wheat germ).
7. Avoid foods high in tyramine (aged cheese, wine, beer, avocados, chicken liver, soy sauce, bananas, meat tenderizers, salami, bologna, chocolate).
8. Avoid large amounts of caffeine.
9. May take 3 to 4 weeks for the drug to be effective.
10. Weigh yourself once a week at the same time of day, such as first thing in the morning. Report weight gains of more than 1 to 2 pounds a week to your nurse or doctor.

MEDICATION INSTRUCTIONS

Medication Name: _____

Dose: _____

When to Take: _____

Special Notes: _____

OTHER INSTRUCTIONS

Antipsychotic Medications

WHAT THE MEDICATION DOES

1. Improves ability to control behavior
2. Reduces excitability
3. Improves ability to separate fantasy from reality
4. Controls hallucinations

HOW TO TAKE THE MEDICATION

1. Take as directed on the label.
2. Keep taking the medication even if you feel better.

SIGNS AND SYMPTOMS TO REPORT TO YOUR NURSE OR DOCTOR

1. Involuntary body movements
2. Sedation
3. Dizziness upon standing
4. Dry mouth
5. Constipation
6. Headache
7. Sensitivity to sunlight
8. Excessive salivation
9. Blurred vision
10. Jitteriness
11. Inability to urinate
12. Increased heart rate

SPECIAL POINTS

1. Avoid prolonged exposure to sunlight. Use sunblock and wear long-sleeved shirts and pants when outdoors.
2. Avoid activities such as driving that require you to be alert.
3. Avoid the use of alcohol.
4. Check with your doctor before taking any over-the-counter medication.
5. Change position, especially sitting to standing, slowly.
6. The medication may take weeks to be effective.
7. The medication often needs to be taken on a long-term basis.

MEDICATION INSTRUCTIONS

Medication Name: _____

Dose: _____

When to Take: _____

Special Notes: _____

OTHER INSTRUCTIONS

Antitussive Medications

WHAT THE MEDICATION DOES

1. Reduces coughing
2. May help to loosen sputum

HOW TO TAKE THE MEDICATION

1. Take as directed on the label.
2. For liquid medication, wait at least 15 minutes after taking the medication before drinking fluids.

SIGNS AND SYMPTOMS TO REPORT TO YOUR NURSE OR DOCTOR

1. Loss of appetite
2. Nausea
3. Vomiting
4. Blurred vision

SPECIAL POINTS

1. The medication may make you sleepy or dizzy.
2. Drinking coffee or tea may help lessen drowsiness. Do not drink alcohol while taking this medication.
3. Drink about 6 to 8 8-ounce glasses of water daily.
4. If your mouth becomes dry, drinking cool drinks or eating hard candy may help.
5. Keep this and all medications out of the reach of children.

MEDICATION INSTRUCTIONS

Medication Name: _____

Dose: _____

When to Take: _____

Special Notes: _____

OTHER INSTRUCTIONS

Aspirin and Aspirin-Like Medications

WHAT THE MEDICATION DOES

1. Relieves pain
2. Lowers fever
3. Reduces swelling (inflammation)
4. Prevents blood clots

HOW TO TAKE THE MEDICATION

1. Take as directed on the label
2. Take with food, milk, or antacids to lessen stomach irritation, if allowed.

SIGNS AND SYMPTOMS TO REPORT TO YOUR NURSE OR DOCTOR

1. Ringing in the ears, hearing loss, or both
2. Nausea, stomach pain, vomiting
3. Bleeding gums
4. Skin bruises easily

SPECIAL POINTS

1. Do not give to children with chickenpox or flu (danger of Reye's syndrome).
2. May cause false urine glucose readings.
3. Do not take other medications that contain aspirin or prevent blood clotting, unless approved by your nurse or doctor.
4. Keep this and all medications out of the reach of children.

MEDICATION INSTRUCTIONS

Medication Name: _____

Dose: _____

When to Take: _____

Special Notes: _____

OTHER INSTRUCTIONS

Bronchodilators

WHAT THE MEDICATION DOES

Makes breathing easier.

HOW TO TAKE THE MEDICATION

1. Shake well before each use.
2. Clear throat and blow nose.
3. Breathe out (exhale), pushing out as much air from your lungs as you can.
4. Place the mouthpiece inside your mouth, close your lips around it.
5. Inhale deeply and slowly for about 10 seconds.
6. Hold your breath for several seconds.
7. Remove the mouthpiece and exhale slowly.
8. Use as directed by your doctor. The usual dose is two puffs four times a day.
9. If more than one kind of inhaler is ordered, wait 2 to 3 minutes before repeating the above steps.
10. If using a steroid inhaler: Use the bronchodilator first, wait 5 minutes, then use the steroid inhaler.

SIGNS AND SYMPTOMS TO REPORT TO YOUR NURSE AND DOCTOR

1. Dizziness
2. Nervousness
3. Tremors
4. Headache
5. Increase in heartbeat
6. Feeling that you need to move fast and do things quickly
7. Nausea and vomiting
8. Restlessness
9. Insomnia
10. Tightening of your chest
11. Bronchospasm after using the inhaler

OTHER INSTRUCTIONS

SPECIAL POINTS

1. Check with your doctor before taking any other drugs including over-the-counter medications.
2. Some inhalers turn sputum and saliva pink.
3. Use your inhaler(s) as directed. Overuse can lead to developing a tolerance to the drug so that it will not work for you.
4. If your breathing problems are not relieved by the inhaler, tell your nurse or doctor.
5. Rinse the plastic mouthpiece daily with warm tap water and then dry it.
6. Inhaled medications begin to take effect in about 3 to 6 minutes and usually last about 4 to 6 hours.
7. Keep the protective cap on the inhaler when not in use.
8. Refill your prescription when the canister is about one-fourth full. Place the canister in a bowl of water and use the picture as a guide to the amount of medication remaining in the container.

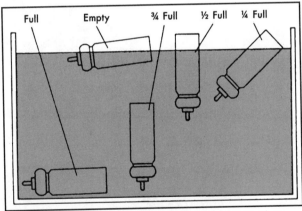

From Beare PG, Myers JL: Principles and Practice of Adult Health Care Nursing, 2nd ed. St. Louis, CV Mosby, 1994.

MEDICATION INSTRUCTIONS

Medication Name: _____
Dose: _____
When to Take: _____
Special Notes: _____

Diuretic Medications

WHAT THE MEDICATION DOES

Reduces the amount of water and salt in the body.

HOW TO TAKE THE MEDICATION

1. Take as directed on the label.
2. Take early in the day to avoid the need to pass urine during the night.

SIGNS AND SYMPTOMS TO REPORT TO THE NURSE OR DOCTOR

1. Weakness
2. Cramps
3. Sore throat
4. Fever
5. Ringing in the ears
6. Headache
7. Dizziness upon standing
8. Dry mouth
9. Fatigue

SPECIAL POINTS

1. With some medications, you may need to eat foods high in potassium, such as citrus fruits, bananas, tomatoes, dates, and apricots.
2. To lessen dizziness, stand up slowly.
   a. Sit or lie down at the first signs of dizziness.
   b. Go up and down stairs carefully.
3. Weigh yourself at least once a week at the same time of day, such as the first thing in the morning. Report weight changes of more than 1 to 2 pounds in 1 week.
4. Keep this and all medications out of the reach of children.

MEDICATION INSTRUCTIONS

Medication Name: _____

Dose: _____

When to Take: _____

Special Notes: _____

OTHER INSTRUCTIONS

Drug Safety

1. Keep each drug in its original, labeled container.
2. Make sure labels are legible. Your pharmacist will redo your labels if you cannot read them.
3. Discard outdated medications.
4. Always finish a prescribed drug unless otherwise instructed by your doctor or nurse. Never save a drug for future illness.
5. Dispose of drugs in a sink or toilet. Never place drugs in the trash within reach of children.
6. Never give a family member or friend a drug prescribed for another person.
7. Refrigerate drugs that require it.
8. Read labels carefully and follow all instructions.
9. Herbal and vitamin supplements and over-the-counter medications can affect certain medications. Always ask your doctor about supplements before taking them.

OTHER INSTRUCTIONS

Heart Medications

WHAT THE MEDICATION DOES

1. Slows the heart rate
2. Increases the strength of each pump of the heart

HOW TO TAKE THE MEDICATION

1. Take as directed on the label.
2. Take and record your heart rate (pulse) each day. If your pulse is less than 60 beats per minute, call your nurse or doctor.

SIGNS AND SYMPTOMS TO REPORT TO YOUR NURSE OR DOCTOR

1. Loss of appetite, nausea, or vomiting
2. Sudden increase or decrease in your pulse rate while resting
3. Change in the rhythm of your pulse while resting
4. Yellow-green "halos" around objects
5. Blurred vision
6. Constipation
7. Confusion
8. Dizziness
9. Difficulty passing urine
10. Fever
11. Skin rash
12. Headache
13. Ringing in the ears
14. Skin bruises easily
15. Diarrhea
16. Fatigue

SPECIAL POINTS

1. To lessen dizziness, stand up slowly.
   a. Sit or lie down at the first signs of dizziness.
   b. Go up and down stairs slowly.
2. If you have constipation, you may need a stool softener.
3. Do not drink alcohol while taking this medication.
4. Keep this and all medications out of the reach of children.
5. Weigh yourself at least once a week at the same time of day, such as first thing in the morning. Report weight changes of more than 1 to 2 pounds a week to your nurse or doctor.

MEDICATION INSTRUCTIONS

Medication Name: _____

Dose: _____

When to Take: _____

Special Notes: _____

OTHER INSTRUCTIONS

High Blood Pressure Medications

WHAT THE MEDICATION DOES

Lowers and controls blood pressure.

HOW TO TAKE THE MEDICATION

1. Take as directed on the label.
2. Keep taking the medication even if you feel better. High blood pressure cannot be cured, only controlled.
3. Take the medication at the same time each day.

SIGNS AND SYMPTOMS TO REPORT TO YOUR NURSE OR DOCTOR

1. Dizziness
2. Decreased mental acuity (sharpness)
3. Drowsiness
4. Difficulty sleeping, nightmares
5. Nausea, vomiting
6. Skin rash
7. Impotence
8. Nasal stuffiness
9. Dry mouth
10. Fever
11. Sore throat
12. Fatigue
13. Headache

SPECIAL POINTS

1. Do not drink alcohol while taking this medication.
2. To lessen dizziness, stand up slowly.
   a. Sit or lie down at the first sign of dizziness.
   b. Go up and down stairs slowly.
3. If you become pregnant, tell your doctor immediately.
4. Do not take any medications, even those you can buy without a prescription (like cold remedies), without checking with your nurse or doctor.
5. If you have side effects, your doctor may be able to change your medication.
6. If your mouth becomes dry, sipping cool beverages or eating hard candy may help.
7. Avoid hot showers; they can cause dizziness.
8. Weigh yourself at least once a week at the same time of day, such as the first thing in the morning. Report weight changes of more than 1 to 2 pounds in 1 week.
9. Keep this and all medications out of reach of children.

MEDICATION INSTRUCTIONS

Medication Name: _____

Dose: _____

When to Take: _____

Special Notes: _____

OTHER INSTRUCTIONS

Laxatives

WHAT THE MEDICATION DOES

Promotes regular and easy bowel movements.

HOW TO TAKE THE MEDICATION

Take as directed on the label.

SIGNS AND SYMPTOMS TO REPORT TO YOUR NURSE OR DOCTOR

1. Nausea or vomiting
2. Diarrhea
3. Abdominal cramps
4. Burning sensation in the rectum

SPECIAL POINTS

1. Increase fluid intake to 6 to 8 8-ounce glasses of water per day.
2. Increase intake of "bulky" foods and foods with fiber, such as bran and fresh fruits and vegetables.
3. Intended for short-term use only.
4. Excessive or long-term use may cause dependence on laxatives.

MEDICATION INSTRUCTIONS

Medication Name: _____

Dose: _____

When to Take: _____

Special Notes: _____

OTHER INSTRUCTIONS

Muscle Relaxants

WHAT THE MEDICATION DOES

1. Relaxes muscles
2. Relieves spasticity

HOW TO TAKE THE MEDICATION

1. Take as directed on the label.
2. Take with food or milk to lessen stomach irritation, if allowed.

SIGNS AND SYMPTOMS TO REPORT TO YOUR NURSE OR DOCTOR

1. Difficulty breathing
2. Skin rash
3. Fever
4. Constipation
5. Trouble passing urine

SPECIAL POINTS

1. The medication may make you sleepy or dizzy. Do not drive or perform any activities that require you to be alert.
2. Do not drink alcohol while taking this medication.
3. Some medications may change the color of your urine.
4. If your mouth becomes dry, sipping cool beverages or eating hard candy can help.
5. Follow your nurse or doctor's instructions for rest and activity.
6. Keep this and all medications out of the reach of children.

MEDICATION INSTRUCTIONS

Medication Name: _____

Dose: _____

When to Take: _____

Special Notes: _____

OTHER INSTRUCTIONS

Pain Medications

WHAT THE MEDICATION DOES

Relieves pain.

HOW TO TAKE THE MEDICATION

1. Take as directed on the label.
2. Take the medication when the pain begins. Do not wait until the pain becomes intense.

SIGNS AND SYMPTOMS TO REPORT TO YOUR NURSE OR DOCTOR

1. Difficulty breathing or slow breathing
2. Trouble passing urine
3. Nausea and vomiting
4. Constipation
5. Ringing in the ears
6. Skin rash
7. Excessive sleepiness

SPECIAL POINTS

1. Avoid activities that require alertness.
2. Medications may cause confusion or sleepiness.
3. Some medications may cause constipation. You may need to ask your nurse or doctor for a stool softener.
4. Do not drink alcohol while taking this medication.
5. Keep this and all medications out of the reach of children.

MEDICATION INSTRUCTIONS

Medication Name: _____

Dose: _____

When to Take: _____

Special Notes: _____

OTHER INSTRUCTIONS

Maternal Health

Breast Feeding

Breast feeding can be very satisfying for you and your baby. The following tips can help you.

GUIDELINES

Getting Started

1. Many babies need a few days before they nurse well. It may take 2 weeks for you and your baby to settle into a pattern. Do not worry if your baby does not want to nurse at every feeding.

2. Many nursing positions help breast emptying and reduce nipple tenderness. Make sure you are comfortable and that you support your baby. Support large, heavy breasts during feeding. Your baby can nurse while you are sitting, lying on your side, or holding the baby in a "football" hold.

   a. Hold your breast with your free hand in a C position (the hand on the opposite side you

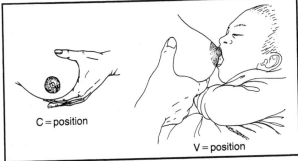

C = position

V = position

From Riordan J, Auerbach K: Breastfeeding and Human Lactation. © 1993 by Jones and Bartlett Publishers, Inc.

are breast feeding). Place your thumb above the areola (dark area surrounding the nipple) and your fingers underneath your breast (forming a "shelf"). Keep all fingers behind the areola.

   b. Turn your baby to you "tummy to tummy" with baby facing the breast directly. Tickle the baby's lower lip with your nipple. Wait

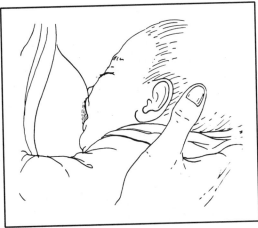

From Riordan J, Auerbach K: Breastfeeding and Human Lactation. © 1993 by Jones and Bartlett Publishers, Inc.

until baby opens his or her mouth very wide (like a yawn). When the baby's mouth is opened wide, bring the baby quickly to your breast. Be sure baby has about 1 inch of areola in his or her mouth.

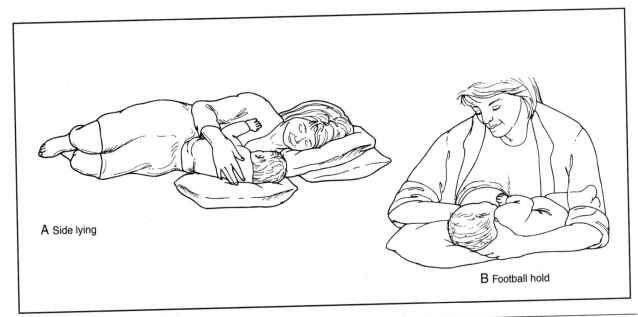

A Side lying

B Football hold

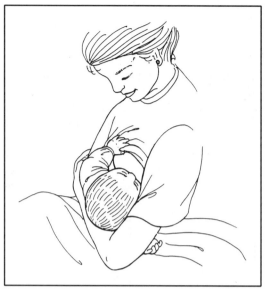

From Riordan J, Auerbach K: Breastfeeding and Human Lactation.
© 1993 by Jones and Bartlett Publishers, Inc.

c. Nursing should not hurt. If it hurts there usually is a problem with the baby's position or attachment on the breast.

d. If nursing hurts, break the seal quickly by inserting your finger gently into the baby's mouth between the gums (keep the finger in place while removing the breast) and start again. When the baby's nose is lightly touching the breast, the baby usually should clear the breast enough for breathing because babies have air channels on both sides of the nose.

Feedings

1. Let the baby finish nursing on the first breast. Baby can nurse as long as he or she wants. Burp baby before offering the second breast. Let baby nurse on the second breast as long as the baby wants.
2. If the baby does not want the second breast, start with that one at the next feeding. If the baby takes the second breast, offer it first at the next feeding. Baby usually takes more milk from the first breast offered. To help you remember, mark your bra strap with a safety pin on the breast side on which you have finished the feeding.
3. Burp the baby at the end of the feeding.
4. Breast-fed babies often want to eat every 1½ to 2½ hours because breast milk is easily digested. These frequent feedings will help to increase your supply of milk.
5. In the early days, the baby should not sleep more than about 4 hours between feedings. If the baby sleeps longer during the night, that is fine. Feedings should total at least 8 in 24 hours.

Basic Facts About Breast Feeding

1. Colostrum is the first food (milk) your baby receives from your breast. Colostrum is present in the breast only for the first few days. It is rich in disease-protective factors and acts as a laxative for the baby's stools.
2. Breast milk will "come in" around 2 to 6 days after delivery.
3. As long as you breast feed, the breasts will continue to produce milk. The quantity and quality of milk vary from woman to woman, day to day, and hour to hour. Breasts constantly produce milk, but do so more quickly during feedings.
4. Between feedings, your breasts make small amounts of a thin bluish milk (foremilk). This is what the baby drinks during the first few minutes at the breast.
5. "Hindmilk," which follows foremilk, is much creamier in color and helps the baby grow.
6. Sometimes, the pressure in the breast results in leaking and spraying of milk from the nipple ("letdown"). Letdown occurs a few times during a 30- to 40-minute feeding. You may feel only the first one. You may feel a slight fullness or tightness, "pins and needles," or a burning feeling from under the armpit to the nipple.

Nutrition and Diet

1. Your nurse and dietitian can teach you about good nutrition.
2. While breast feeding, you need to have a plan for nutrition.
   a. This may mean about 500 more calories every day.
   b. Plan to eat
      (1) 4 to 5 servings from the milk group,
      (2) 3 servings of protein,
      (3) 4 to 5 servings of fruits and vegetables,
      (4) 6 to 11 servings of whole-grain foods.
   c. Your baby can be affected by what you eat and drink, especially food and drink such as cauliflower, broccoli, and caffeine. If your baby seems fussy, try to avoid that type of food for a few days.

Rest

1. Try to nap when your baby does.
2. When possible, nurse in a chair (or bed), with your feet up.
3. During the first few weeks, give yourself permission to rest more, even if all of the housework is not done.

4. One of the hormones that helps you make milk is prolactin. Prolactin increases during feedings. Due to the increased prolactin, you may experience a very relaxed and tired feeling during nursing sessions. This feeling is a natural body response.

Helpful Hints

1. You can tell the baby is getting enough milk if
   a. He or she has five to eight really wet diapers a day, by 5 days of age.
   b. He or she continues to gain weight.
   c. He or she has daily stools (at least 2 to 3) for 4 weeks.
2. Your baby's stools
   a. Breast-fed babies have bowel movements that are usually looser and more frequent than those of bottle-fed babies.
   b. Constipation is rare. Even a couple of days between bowel movements may be normal for your older baby. Your nurse or doctor can answer questions you may have.
3. If your baby is fussy:
   a. Babies commonly have a regular time when they are fussy. It can be any time of the day or evening.
   b. Try burping and holding your baby. Check for wet diapers.
   c. If your baby is still fussy, try nursing.
   d. If you feel like you are losing patience with the baby and you do *not think* there is anything really wrong with him or her, put the baby in the crib. This may prevent your unintentionally hurting the baby. Call your nurse or the help line phone number you may have been given if you are having difficulty coping with the baby.
   e. If your baby cries, pick up and cuddle him or her. That way you help baby learn that all-important sense of trust in his or her world.

Expressing Breast Milk

1. Hand (manual) expression
   a. Wash your hands.
   b. Hold a clean cup under your breast.
   c. Hold your breast at the edge of the areola, with your thumb above and your fingers beneath.
   d. Push your thumb and fingers back toward the chest wall. Then compress the breast with your fingers.
   e. Do this at several different spots around the areola, moving your fingers clockwise.
2. Breast pumps
   a. There are many different types of breast pumps: electric, battery, and manual.

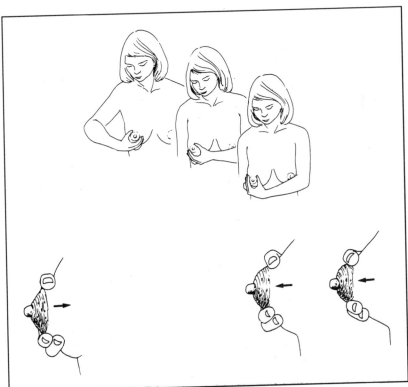

From Lawrence R: Breastfeeding: A Guide for the Medical Profession, 4th ed. St. Louis, Mosby–Year Book, 1994.

b. You may never need to pump your breasts.

c. If you are going back to work or wish to pump for other reasons, speak with your health care professional to receive information regarding pump purchase and use.

Storing Breast Milk

1. Milk may be stored in the refrigerator for 72 hours.

2. Use glass jars, plastic jars, or bottles. Special "freezer" type bags for breast milk only are also available.

QUESTIONS

1. Your nurse or health care professional can answer any questions you have.

2. Your local La Leche League may also have reading material.

OTHER INSTRUCTIONS

Breast Feeding: Special Conditions

Breast feeding can result in certain conditions. Your health care professional may give you special instructions for your condition.

CONDITIONS

Breast Engorgement

What It Is. A painful swelling of the breast.

What It Feels Like. The breasts feel hard, tender, and tight. The baby may have difficulty latching on.

When It Happens. Usually 2 to 3 days after delivery. The swelling usually decreases 2 to 5 days after it starts.

What to Do. Try to prevent it by changing breasts during feeding and nursing often.

1. Wear a well-fitted, 100% cotton supportive bra.
2. Nurse often and, if necessary, manually express or pump breasts.
3. Drink more fluids. Drink fluids each time you sit down to nurse.
4. If your breasts become engorged, you may be instructed to
   a. Place a towel soaked in hot water (not hot enough to burn the skin) or a small hot water bottle wrapped in a towel on the breasts for about 15 minutes before nursing or pumping.
   b. Take a warm or hot shower.
   c. Use cool wet compresses or ice packs covered with a cloth between nursing or pumping to reduce swelling.
   d. Take a pain reliever if your doctor permits.
   e. Use a breast pump before the feeding to soften the breast.

Sore Nipples

What It Is. Nipple irritation (red, chapped nipples).

What It Feels Like. Tender, sore nipples during and after nursing.

When It Happens. It can happen at any time.

What to Do. Treat sore nipples as soon as possible.

1. Do not use soap on nipples (soap causes drying and cracking).
2. Use *only* lanolins that do not need to be washed off the nipples before each feeding. Your nurse or doctor may suggest pure medical-grade lanolin.
3. Keep nipples dry. Change breast pads often.
4. Expose nipples to the air between feedings to help with healing.
5. Ice can be used on the nipple a few minutes before nursing to ease nipple pain. Crushed ice wrapped in a wet washcloth or a dampened washcloth that has been frozen works well. Numbing the nipples can slow down the "letdown" reflex.
6. Start nursing on the less sore breast. In about 10 minutes, switch your baby to the other breast. If both nipples are sore, try to hand express milk until you have a letdown. Nurse the baby after letdown occurs.

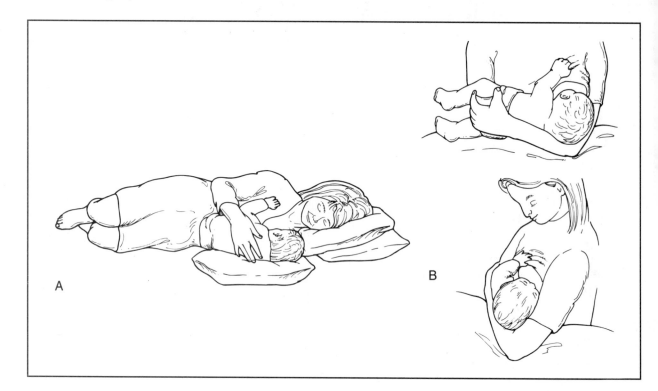

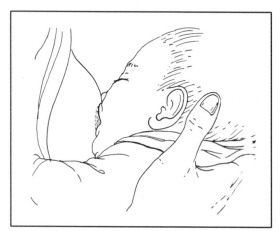

From Riordan J, Auerbach K: Breastfeeding and Human Lactation.
© 1993 by Jones and Bartlett Publishers, Inc.

7. Change your position at each feeding. Lie down or sit up. Hold the baby in different positions. This will change pressure to different parts of the breast.

8. Be sure the baby is taking as least 1 inch of the areola into his or her mouth. Do not let your baby take just the nipple or chew on the nipple.

9. You can still nurse with bleeding or cracked nipples. You may decide not to nurse for 48 hours to let the nipples heal. Pump your breasts and feed baby with an alternative feeding method as instructed by your health care professional.

Clogged Milk Duct

What It Is. Milk cannot pass through one of the milk ducts (passages).

What It Feels Like. Tender spot or sore lump on your breast.

When It Happens. It can happen at any time. A bra that is too tight can cause pressure on the ducts.

What to Do.

1. Check to see if your bra is too tight. If you wear an underwire bra, try one without a wire or remove the wire from the bra.
2. Allow the baby to breast feed more often on the involved side.
3. Change your position at each feeding. Lie down or sit up. Hold the baby in different positions. This will change the pressure to different parts of the breast. Gently massaging the affected area toward the nipple during nursing or pumping may help.
4. Pump the breast with the clogged duct after each feeding. Try to empty the breast as much as possible.
5. If you see a dried crust covering the nipple, wash off the nipple before and after feeding with warm water only.
6. You may apply heat to the breast by doing one of the following:
   a. Soak the breast in warm water as you lean over a basin.

b. Apply a hot water bottle wrapped in a towel to the breast.

c. Apply a towel soaked in hot water (not hot enough to burn the skin) to the breast. Try to nurse the baby or express some milk after soaking by hand or pump.

7. Do not stop nursing. If you stop suddenly, your breasts will get too full and you may increase chances of developing a breast infection.

Breast Infection

What It Is. An infection of some of the breast tissue, usually in the ducts.

What It Feels Like. You may have a headache, fever, flu-like feeling, painful engorgement (breast fullness), breasts that feel hot and tender to touch, and breast skin that looks red.

When It Happens. It can happen at any time.
What to Do.

1. Call your doctor immediately for treatment.
2. Get plenty of rest.
3. Keep the breast empty by frequent nursing. The baby will not be harmed.
4. Drink enough to urinate every hour during the daytime.
5. Take pain relief medication that your health care professional recommends.

QUESTIONS

Discuss any questions with your nurse or doctor. If you have had breast surgery, check with your doctor about your ability to produce enough milk.

OTHER INSTRUCTIONS

Guidelines for Pregnancy

GENERAL INFORMATION

Pregnancy is a time of great change in your body. Making healthy choices in receiving regular prenatal care and following a healthy diet and lifestyle will help you and your baby.

It is important to become more aware of your body and your environment while pregnant. Your nurse or doctor can provide you with much information about having a healthy pregnancy. The following instructions are some of the more important guidelines.

Guidelines

Making healthy choices means

1. Eat healthy foods and drink at least 8 to 10 8-ounce glasses of water every day.
2. Get regular exercise.
3. Ask for help if you are having trouble coping with pregnancy.
4. Plan rest periods daily. Lie on your side when resting.
   a. Do not eat uncooked meat or eggs because of harmful bacteria.
   b. Do not eat raw cookie dough or batters (uncooked eggs).
   c. Caffeine in coffee, tea, soda, and chocolate may need to be limited.
5. Stop cigarette smoking. Avoid being near others who are smoking.
6. Do not drink alcohol.
7. Do not use any drugs, medications, or herbal supplements unless approved by your doctor.
8. Avoid working with chemicals and inhaling aerosols (such as room deodorizers).
9. Avoid hot tubs/saunas, hot baths, and steam rooms because they can raise the body temperature to more than 102°F (39°C).
10. Avoid changing cat litter. Some cats carry the *Toxoplasmosis* virus in their feces.
11. Always tell any health care worker that you are pregnant before having any tests done. It is important to tell an x-ray technician this even if you only think you might be pregnant.

How to Feel and Time Contractions

When your uterus (womb) contracts, it will get tight or feel hard to the touch. It is normal for your uterus to contract at times during your pregnancy. You may have contractions after activity or after sex. Before 37 weeks of pregnancy, too many contractions can cause your baby to be born too soon.

Steps to follow:

1. Empty your bladder.
2. Lie down on your left side. Use pillows for support if needed.
3. Drink one to two full glasses of water, juice, or milk while lying down.
4. Put your fingertips on your upper abdomen.
   a. If you can easily press your fingertips in and it feels soft, this is not a contraction.
   b. If you cannot press your fingertips in and it feels hard, this is a contraction.
5. Write down the number of contractions in 1 hour. Write the time each contraction starts and how long it lasts.
6. If four or more contractions are counted, call your doctor or go to the emergency department.

How to do "kick counts" to check on your baby's activity

1. Plan to do kick counts during the baby's most active time of day.
2. Lie on your left side.
3. Count your baby's kicks, turns, or twists
   a. After you have walked for 5 minutes.
   b. One-half hour to 1 hour after you have finished a meal.
   c. After you eat or drink something cold.
4. Write down the time you start and put a checkmark each time the baby moves.
5. You should feel about four to five movements in an hour. If you do not feel the baby move, call your doctor or nurse.
6. Do kick counts every day or as directed.

Warning Signs in Pregnancy

Call your doctor or nurse for any of the following:

1. Bleeding from the vagina
2. Your water breaks (fluid leaking from the vagina)
3. You have constant severe pain or cramping that does not go away. Do not wait for a whole hour to check your contractions.
4. Absence of or decrease in baby movement for more than 4 to 6 hours
5. Chills or fever

6. Changes in your vision like flashing bright lights or spots, dim or blurred vision
7. Severe headaches that are not normal for you
8. Increased swelling or puffiness in your feet, hands, or face
9. Your abdomen gets hard and stays hard
10. Frequent vomiting for more than 1 day
11. Pain or burning on urination or a decrease in the amount you are urinating
12. Vaginal itching, irritation, or foul-smelling discharge
13. Fall or car accident

Signs of premature labor

1. Contractions are 12 to 15 minutes apart (may be painless)
   a. More than four to six contractions in 1 hour
2. Cramping just above the pubic bone. It may be constant or come and go
3. Dull low backache that may be constant or come and go

4. Feeling like the baby is pushing down
5. Increase in or change in vaginal discharge or a gush of fluid from your vagina
6. Stomach cramps like gas pains, with or without diarrhea
7. Feeling that something is not right
8. What to do
   a. Empty your bladder.
   b. Lie on your left side and check contractions.
   c. Drink three to four glasses of water while lying down.
   d. Write down your contractions.
      (1) If contractions are less than 10 minutes apart, call your doctor *right away.*
      (2) If contractions are 15 minutes apart or are becoming closer after 1 hour of rest and drinking fluids, call your doctor.
   e. If you cannot reach your doctor, go to the emergency department.
      (1) Do not drive yourself.
      (2) Call emergency services if you need help.

OTHER INSTRUCTIONS

How To Tell When Labor Begins

DUE DATE

Your due date is a "guestimate." It helps you and your doctor plan for the safest possible birth for your baby. Most women do not give birth on their due dates. Instead, they give birth as much as 2 weeks before or after the date. This is normal.

LABOR

In the last 3 to 4 weeks of pregnancy, your stomach might get hard and then get soft at irregular intervals. These irregular contractions are called false labor pains, or Braxton-Hicks contractions. They might become uncomfortable and you might think you are in labor. Since false labor usually occurs close to your due date, it is sometimes hard to tell if you are really in labor. One way to tell the difference is to keep a record of the contractions for an hour. Compare your record to the table in the right-hand column. Call your doctor if you think you are in true labor or if you are not sure.

Differences Between False Labor and True Labor

Differences	False Labor	True Labor
Timing	Contractions occur at irregular intervals and do not get close together.	Contractions occur at intervals and get closer and closer together.
Change	Contractions usually stop when you walk or change position.	Contractions continue and may get worse when you move around.
Location	Contractions are usually felt in the lower abdomen and groin.	Contractions are usually felt in the back coming around to front.

CALL YOUR DOCTOR

If any of the following happen, call your doctor immediately:

1. You have bright red bleeding from the vagina, any amount, or a large amount of dark, menstrual-type blood.
2. You have constant severe pain. Do not wait for a whole hour to check your contractions.
3. Your water breaks, even if you are not having any contractions.

OTHER INSTRUCTIONS

Nutrition Management During Lactation

DESCRIPTION

A healthy, well-balanced diet is also important during lactation to help the quality and quantity of breast milk, as well as maternal postpartum nutritional status. Use the pregnancy dietary guidelines (see page 421) and add an additional one to two servings of milk or milk products and 1 to 2 ounces of meat, poultry, fish, beans, eggs, and nuts. Calcium sources are important.

From Chilton Memorial Hospital, Pompton Plains, NJ.

ADEQUACY

This diet is adequate in all nutrients.

GUIDELINES

1. Getting enough fluids is important during lactation. It is important to drink to satisfy thirst; drink about 8 to 10 8-ounce glasses of fluid per day. This ensures adequate volume of breast milk.
2. Both alcohol and caffeine should be limited during lactation.
3. Talk with your nurse or doctor before dieting for weight loss while nursing.
4. Ask your doctor before taking vitamins and over-the-counter or herbal medications.

OTHER INSTRUCTIONS

Nutrition Management During Pregnancy

DESCRIPTION

A well-balanced diet during pregnancy is essential to meet the increased nutritional needs of the mother and to promote the normal growth and development of the fetus. Recommended Daily Allowances of practically all nutrients are increased during this period. *The Recommended Daily Allowance for most nutrients is increased during pregnancy; however, the recommended increase in calories is only 300 additional calories a day after the third month. Therefore, foods should be carefully chosen to provide adequate nutrients without providing excess calories. A weight gain of 25 to 35 pounds is appropriate for healthy women of normal weight before pregnancy. Women who may be overweight or underweight before pregnancy should have the optimal weight gain goal adjusted by their doctor.*

ADEQUACY

This diet is adequate in all nutrients recommended for the average pregnant or lactating woman.

Follow the plan for a regular diet with the following adjustments:

Breads, cereals, rice, and pasta	9 servings per day
Vegetables*	4 servings per day
Fruit*	3 servings per day
Milk, yogurt, cheese	3 (4 to 5 for teens) servings per day
Meat, poultry, fish, beans, eggs, and nuts	6 ounces
Fats, oils, and sweets	Use sparingly

*Be sure to include at least one serving of citrus fruits and dark green or yellow vegetables every day.

From Chilton Memorial Hospital, Pompton Plains, NJ.

GUIDELINES

1. *Caffeine and herbal teas should be limited during pregnancy.*
2. Certain foods that are high in calories and contribute little nutritional value (for example, potato chips, fried foods, sweets, candy, soft drinks) should be avoided when your weight gain is too much, indicating that calories should be limited.
3. Salt should be iodized.
4. Mild nausea and vomiting may occur early in pregnancy. This may be overcome by consuming high-carbohydrate foods such as crackers, dry toast, jelly, or hard candies before arising. Frequent small meals may be preferable to the three large ones. Fluids should be taken between meals rather than with meals. Fried foods, pastries, desserts, excessive seasoning, strong-flavored vegetables, and coffee in large quantities may be restricted or eliminated if nausea persists or if the patient complains of heart burn or gastric distress.
   a. Select low-fat protein foods such as lean meats, broiled fish, skinless poultry, and eggs.
   b. Select easily digested carbohydrates such as pasta, fruits, rice, potatoes, toast, and crackers. Foods that cause digestive disturbances should be avoided.
   c. Cold foods may be preferred due to reduction in food odor.
5. For constipation
   a. Increase the amounts of fluids and foods high in soluble fiber such as fruits and whole grain cereals.
   b. Exercise regularly as allowed by your doctor.
   c. Try drinking prune juice.
6. For heartburn
   a. Eat small meals every 2 to 3 hours.
   b. Avoid large meals before bedtime.
   c. Avoid lying flat for 1 to 2 hours after eating.
   d. You may need to elevate your head at bedtime by adding an extra pillow.
7. Alcohol, drugs, and smoking should be avoided during pregnancy because they can harm the baby.
8. Prenatal vitamins and/or medications, herbal medications or teas should be used only as prescribed by your doctor.

OTHER INSTRUCTIONS

Postpartum Care

The postpartum period, or time after birth, can be hard on a new mother. There are many demands on her time and energy. Life is different after the baby is born and, for most women, more difficult! You might find that you are spending most of your time on others and neglecting yourself. Or you feel that everyone is making a big fuss over the baby and totally ignoring you.

During this stressful time, make sure to take care of yourself, so that your feelings do not overwhelm you. Remember, if you are feeling good about yourself, you will feel good about all the new changes in your life.

GUIDELINES

1. Try to get regular physical exercise. Your prenatal book has exercises you can do.
2. Avoid being alone too much. Share your feelings—good and bad—with family members or friends.
3. Take a nap or lie quietly and rest when your baby is napping. You probably will not get 8 hours of sleep each night, so try to get rest periods during the day.
4. Arrange for someone to watch your baby and take a warm, relaxing shower. Wash yourself every day. Keep your genital area clean to avoid infection. Wipe this area gently from front to back.
5. Eat healthy foods. Ask your nurse for a copy of *Nutrition Management During Lactation and Nutrition Management During Pregnancy*.
6. Drink at least 8 to 10 8-ounce glasses of water every day.
7. Follow up with your doctor. Your next appointment is _____ .
8. Schedule special time alone with your husband or partner and share why you each think the other is special. Give a trusted relative or friend the opportunity to babysit so that you and your partner can really focus on each other.
9. Practice cleanliness around your home. Ask your nurse for a copy of *Infection Control for the Home*.
10. Wash your hands often.
11. If you have hemorrhoids: Wash your anal area after bowel movements. Use Tucks pads as directed. Ask your doctor for a stool softener. Increase your fluid intake. Increase your intake of dietary fiber (whole grain foods, bran, fruits, green leafy vegetables, prunes).
12. Do not have sex until your doctor tells you it is okay. Usually this is after your 6-week checkup.

CALL YOUR HOME CARE NURSE OR DOCTOR

If any of the following happens, call your home care nurse or doctor:

1. You have difficulty sleeping.
2. You do not have any energy.
3. You cry for no reason—and it happens a lot.
4. You feel like you cannot do a good job taking care of your baby.
5. You do not feel like eating.
6. You feel ugly and worthless—and these thoughts do not go away.
7. Everyone and everything they do irritate you.
8. Most of the time you feel hopeless and alone.

If any of the following happens, call your home care nurse or doctor IMMEDIATELY:

1. You do not want to take care of your baby.
2. You do not want to talk to or play with your baby.
3. You want to hurt yourself or your baby.
4. You think your baby wants to hurt or punish you.
5. Your genital/anal area is painful or very uncomfortable.
6. You have a fever and/or chills.
7. You have pain and/or burning when you urinate. You have to urinate often. When you have to urinate you have no time to waste.
8. You have a bad-smelling discharge from your vagina.
9. You have pain, swelling, or warmth in your legs.
10. Your heart rate or breathing rate suddenly gets very fast.
11. You have a persistent headache.
12. Your breasts are red and painful.

OTHER INSTRUCTIONS

Appendix

EQUIVALENT MEASURES OF FLUIDS

BLANK MONTHLY CALENDAR

ILLUSTRATIONS

Equivalent Measures of Fluids

Household Measures

Drops	Teaspoons (Tsp)	Tablespoons (Tbsp)	Cups	Pints	Quarts	Ounces (oz)	Milliliter (ml)/ Cubic Centimeters (cc)
60	1	⅓					5
	3	1				½	15
		2				1	30
		8	½			4	120
		12	¾			6	180
		16	1			8	240
			2	1		16	480
			4	2	1	32	960

IMPORTANT NOTE: Not all spoons and containers conform to a standard size. Test the size of the spoons and containers that you are using to make sure they meet the standard equivalents listed above.

MONTH _____

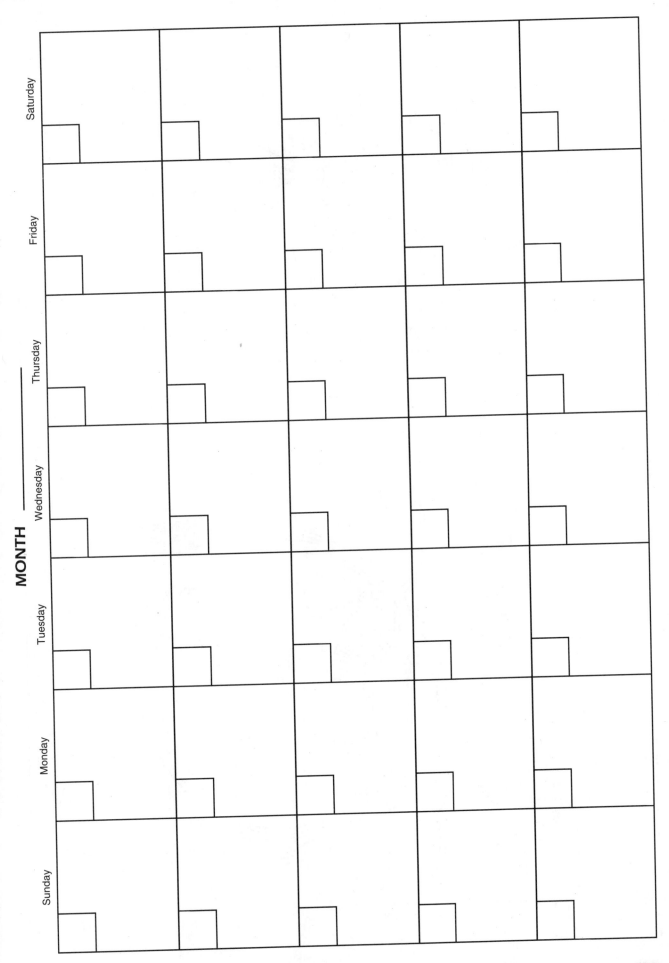

EYE

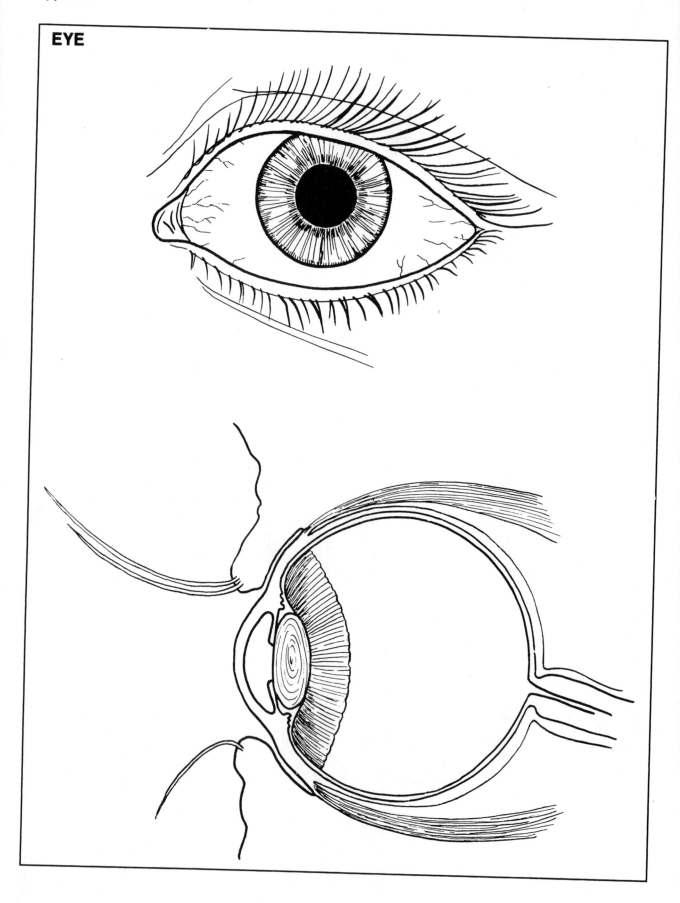

EAR

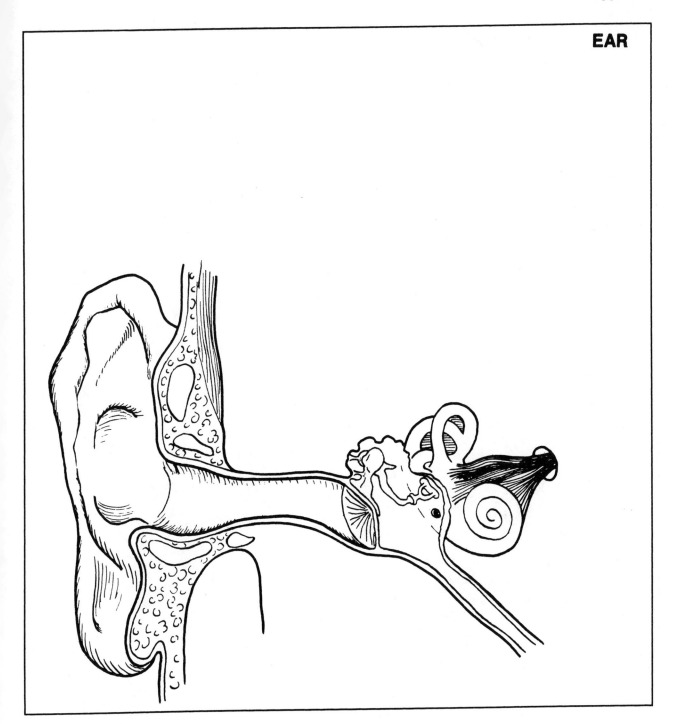

NOSE AND THROAT

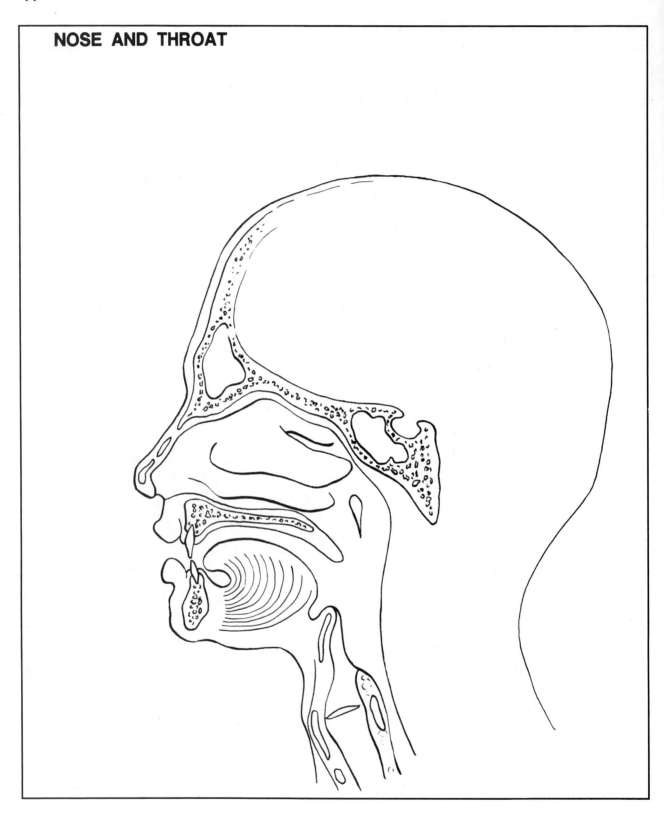

SINUS CAVITIES

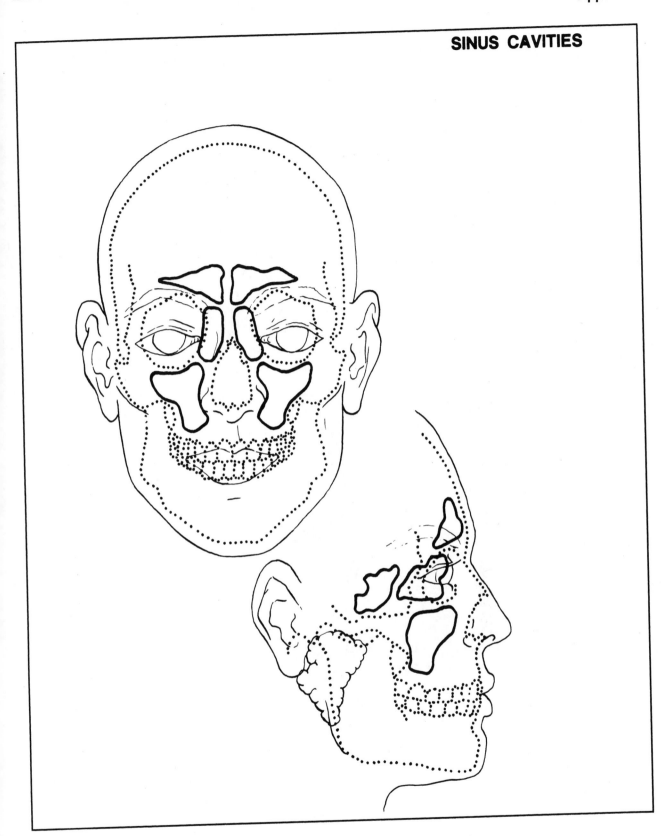

TRACHEA AND LARYNX

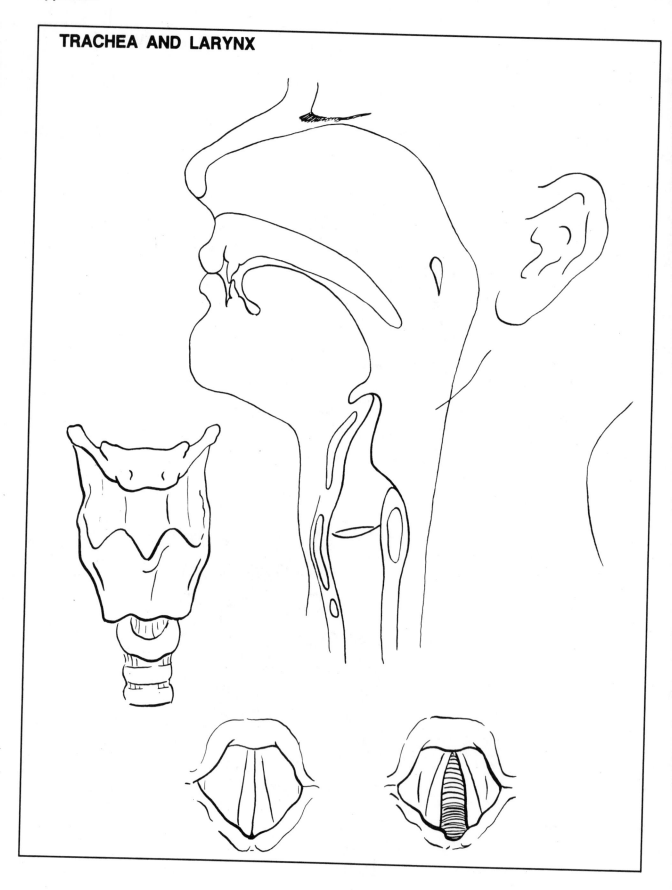

LARYNX AND THYROID GLAND

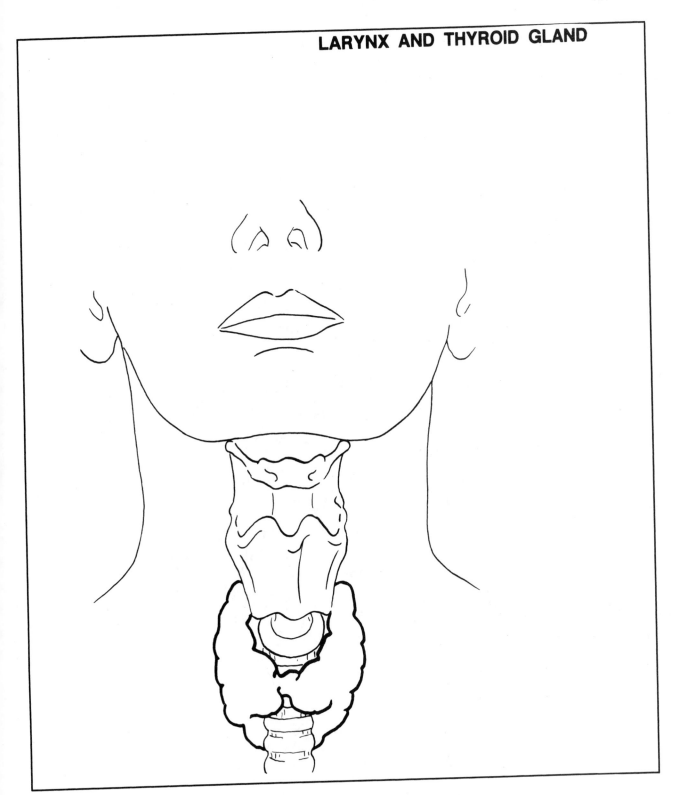

BRONCHIAL TREE AND LUNGS

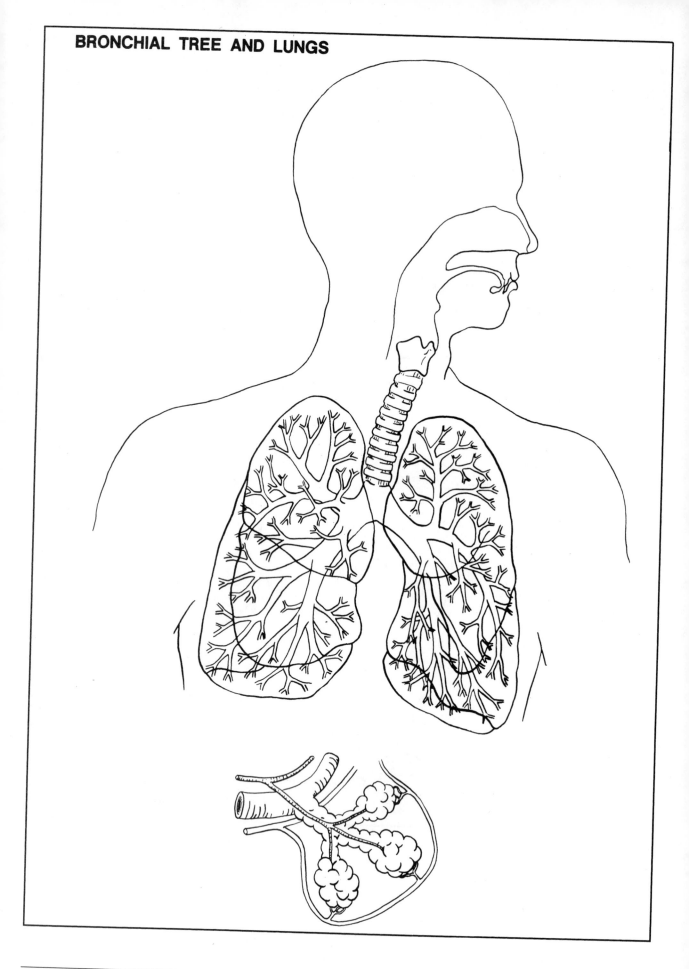

HEART, Showing Coronary Arteries

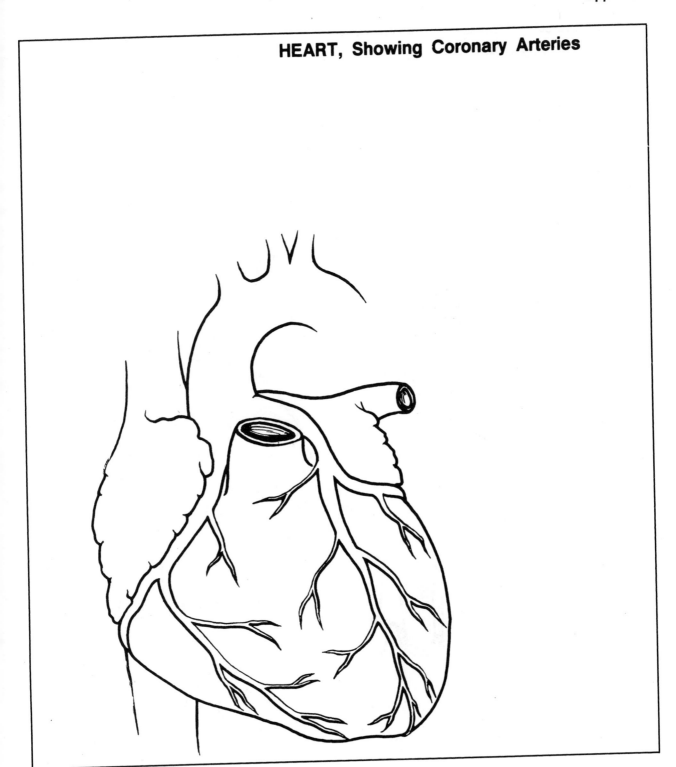

HEART, Schematic Cross-Section

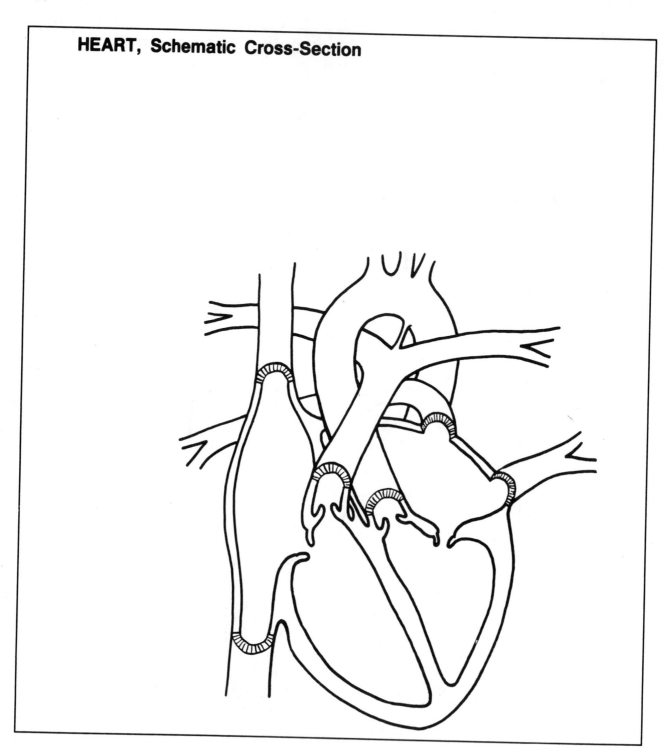

GASTROINTESTINAL TRACT

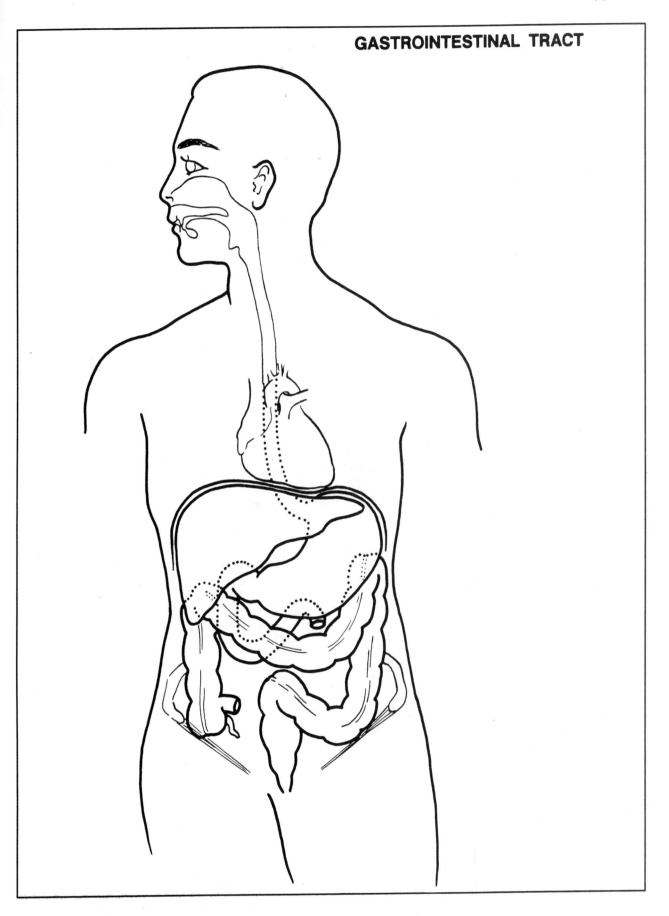

STOMACH, LIVER, GALLBLADDER, AND DUODENUM

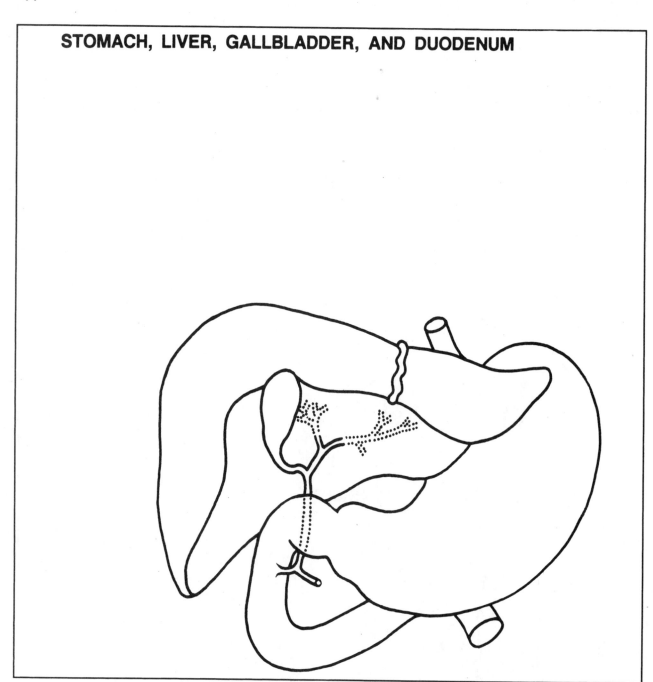

URINARY TRACT

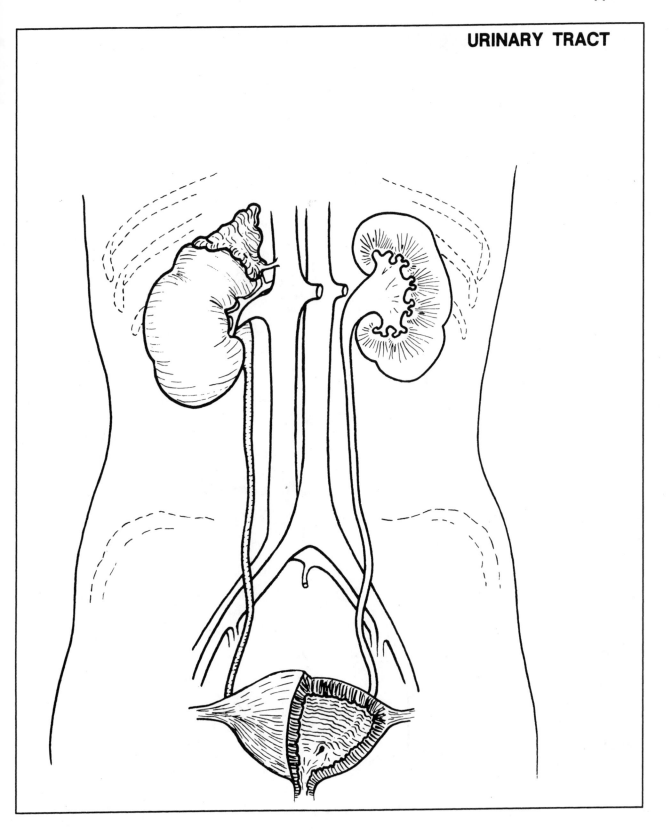

ENDOCRINE SYSTEM, Male and Female

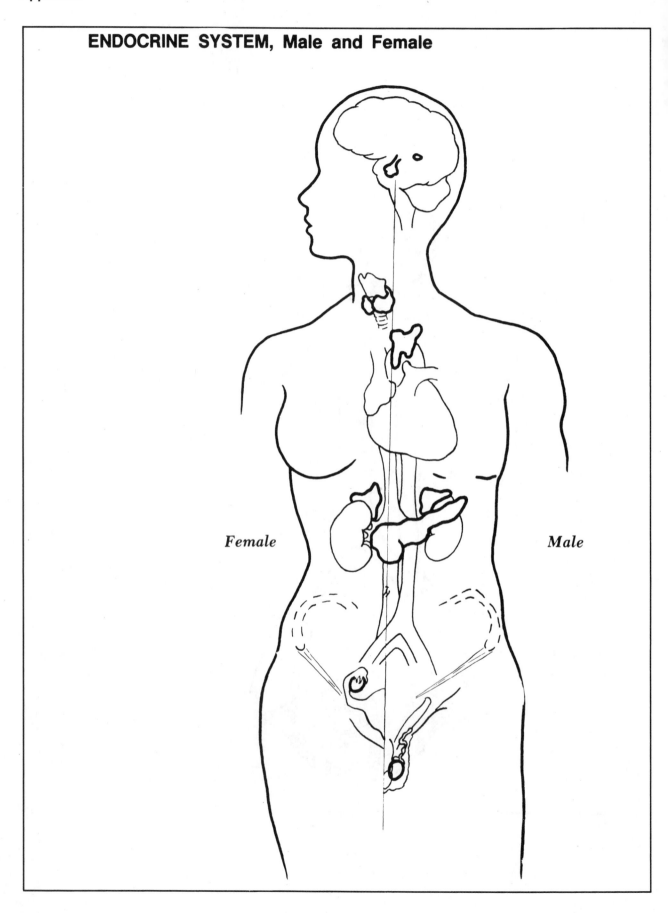

Female

Male

FEMALE GENITAL ORGANS

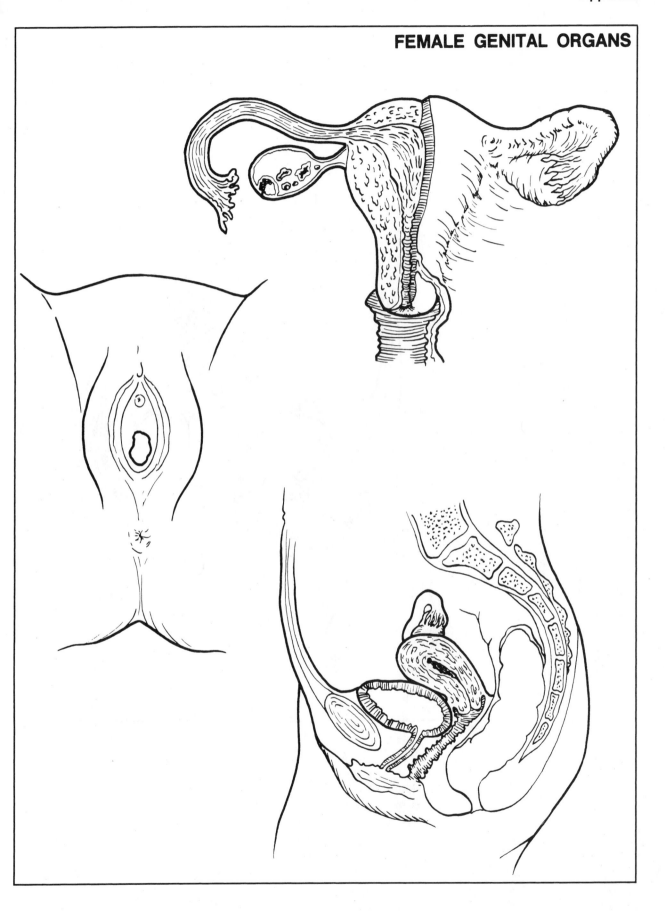

MALE GENITAL ORGANS

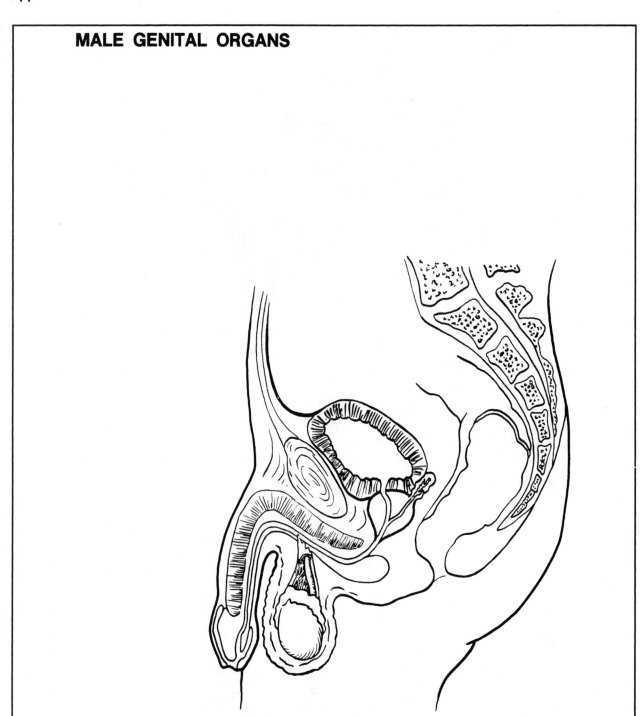

SKELETAL SYSTEM, Showing Major Bones and Joints

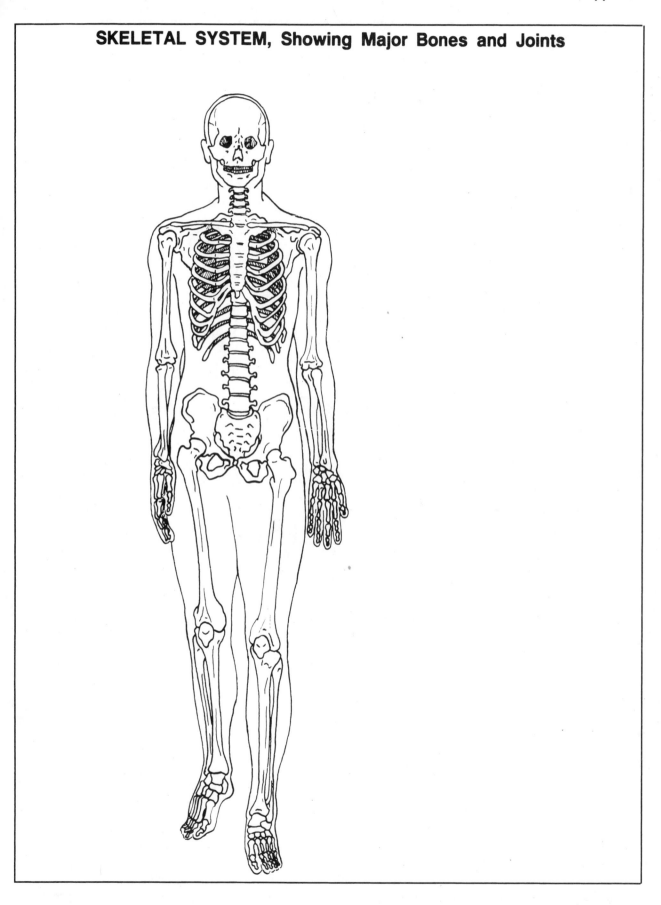

FRACTURES

Hip Fracture Through
Trochanter of Femur

Hip Fracture Through
Neck of Femur

Greenstick

Spiral

Comminuted

Transverse

Compound

Compression

Index

Note: Page numbers in *italics* refer to illustrations; page numbers followed by t refer to tables.